Veterinary Laboratory Medicine

CLINICAL BIOCHEMISTRY AND HAEMATOLOGY

To my mother:
in gratitude for the winter of the millennium

Veterinary Laboratory Medicine

CLINICAL BIOCHEMISTRY AND HAEMATOLOGY

Second Edition

Morag G. Kerr

BVMS, BSc, PhD, CBiol, FIBiol, MRCVS
(Formerly Lecturer in Clinical Pathology, Royal Veterinary College)
Vetlab Services
Unit 11
Station Rd
Southwater
Horsham
W. Sussex

Blackwell
Science

© 1989, 2002 by
Blackwell Science Ltd
Editorial Offices:
Osney Mead, Oxford OX2 0EL
25 John Street, London WC1N 2BS
23 Ainslie Place, Edinburgh EH3 6AJ
350 Main Street, Malden
  MA 02148 5018, USA
54 University Street, Carlton
  Victoria 3053, Australia
10, rue Casimir Delavigne
  75006 Paris, France

Other Editorial Offices:

Blackwell Wissenschafts-Verlag GmbH
Kurfürstendamm 57
10707 Berlin, Germany

Blackwell Science KK
MG Kodenmacho Building
7–10 Kodenmacho Nihombashi
Chuo-ku, Tokyo 104, Japan

Iowa State University Press
A Blackwell Science Company
2121 S. State Avenue
Ames, Iowa 50014-8300, USA

First edition published by Blackwell Scientific
Publications Ltd 1989
Second edition published by Blackwell Science Ltd 2002

Set in 10/12.5pt Gillsans Medium
by DP Photosetting, Aylesbury, Bucks
Printed and bound in Great Britain by
MPG Books Ltd, Bodmin, Cornwall

DISTRIBUTORS

Marston Book Services Ltd
PO Box 269
Abingdon
Oxon OX14 4YN
(Orders: Tel: 01235 465500
           Fax: 01235 465555)

USA and Canada
Iowa State University Press
A Blackwell Science Company
2121 S. State Avenue
Ames, Iowa 50014-8300
(Orders: Tel: 800-862-6657
           Fax: 515-292-3348
           Web www.isupress.com
           email: orders@isupress.com)

Australia
Blackwell Science Pty Ltd
54 University Street
Carlton, Victoria 3053
(Orders: Tel: 03 9347 0300
           Fax: 03 9347 5001)

A catalogue record for this title is available from the
British Library

ISBN 0-632-04023-8

Library of Congress
Cataloging-in-Publication Data
is available

For further information on
Blackwell Science, visit our website:
www.blackwell-science.com

Contents

Introduction

Laboratory medicine and the veterinary surgeon

Since the first edition of this book was published in 1989, there have been many changes in veterinary laboratory practice – some very much for the better, others less so.

The most striking change is the much greater volume of biochemistry and haematology investigation being carried out. To a large extent this is a good thing, though a note of caution has to be sounded against using blood tests as a substitute for thorough clinical examination and history-taking, and anyone who finds themselves paralysed to act in an emergency because blood results are unavailable really ought to be reconsidering their priorities. In general, however, the more relevant information which is available to the clinician the more likely it is that the correct diagnosis will be arrived at, and so long as the laboratory data is *in addition to* the clinical data then more widespread use of laboratory investigation is to be welcomed. Indeed, the much greater readiness of practitioners to embark on laboratory investigation of the more challenging cases and to seek laboratory confirmation of the presumptive diagnosis in the more straightforward ones has made laboratory medicine a very rewarding discipline.

Following on from that, a more recent development has been the emergence of more veterinary surgeons specializing in clinical pathology/laboratory medicine at postgraduate level. Twelve years ago only a minority of commercial veterinary laboratories were under professional veterinary direction, with the majority run by technicians (often trained only in analysis of human samples) providing a results-only service without any professional interpretation. Now only a few laboratories remain in the latter category, and practitioners have a good choice of professionally-run laboratories offering not simply a string of numbers but a full range of advice covering selection of tests, interpretation of results and recommendations regarding treatment. Practitioners now recognize the laboratory as a second-opinion referral service, made extremely convenient and accessible by the fact that only the blood (or other) samples have to be referred rather then the entire patient.

In parallel with this there has also been an enormous increase in the amount of laboratory work carried out within veterinary practices. This is a bit of a mixed blessing. A near-patient facility designed to complement the professional laboratory and enable quick (if sometimes approximate) results of appropriate tests to be obtained as an interim measure in emergencies and out-of-hours, and to allow simple monitoring of already-diagnosed patients on treatment is invaluable. Certain items (e.g. the pocket glucose meter, the refractometer, the microhaematocrit centrifuge and, of course, the microscope) are so easy for the non-technician to use, so cheap and so useful, that it really is a case of 'every home should have one'. On the other hand, what is sometimes not appreciated is the enormous gulf between this type of side-room facility and a professional laboratory. However conscientiously those concerned with teaching the subject at undergraduate level try to instil a few of the principles of analytical procedure into veterinary students, a veterinary course is far removed from the sort of training a laboratory technician receives, and although some laboratory component is included in the veterinary nursing syllabus, this again should be regarded as helping equip nurses to perform the near-patient type of testing competently rather than expecting them to run a full laboratory service in between setting up drips and monitoring anaesthetics.

The main driving force of the 'practice lab' has been, as expected, the dry-reagent biochemistry analyser. Twelve years ago these machines were just emerging, having been developed for near-patient testing of human samples. It was clear that there were substantial problems when non-human samples were analysed by these methods, apparently due to what is termed the 'plasma matrix effect', but the optimistic view was that these problems would be solved and that there was good cause to hope that a wide range of reliable biochemistry results might be available in the practice side-room. Unfortunately this hope proved to be unfounded. There have been very few published studies comparing results of dry-chemistry methods to standard wet-chemistry methods for animal samples (and most of those are, for some reason, in German), but it is quite clear that for most of the methods the correlation is far poorer than would be required for professional laboratory application. Thus, although some practices owning these machines still do rely on them for routine work-up of non-emergency cases, many now realize that their place, if they are used at all, is in the near-patient emergency testing category, confining their use to the tests which are less poor performers (such as urea), concentrating on gross deviations from normal and not trying to read subtleties into smaller abnormalities which the accuracy of the methods is not really good enough to support.

Thus the thrust of this edition, contrary to expectations of twelve years ago, is much more towards the practitioner in partnership with the professional laboratory, performing relevant side-room tests where appropriate, but relying on the referral laboratory for the bulk of the routine testing and non-emergency case work-up.

So, does that mean that the clinical student or the practitioner can put this book down, sit back, and wait for the clinical pathologist to tell him or her what is wrong with the patient and what to do about it? Well, no. Two heads are always better than one: the person who has actually seen the patient has an insight into the case which cannot be replicated simply by reading even the best-expressed clinical history, even the smartest clinical pathologist occasionally misses the blindingly obvious, and really successful use of the laboratory relies on an intelligent dialogue between the clinical pathologist and a well-informed and interested practitioner.

The format of the book remains based on the lecture notes approach. Some sections of comparatively basic science have been included, but the rule has been to cover only those areas which are genuinely relevant to clinical use. The information is initially organized on a test-by-test basis as this is still the essential way into the subject for the student, and it is important to have some way of assessing all the possible clinical implications of a single result. However, the systematic reassembly of the data has been expanded to give more emphasis to the pattern recognition approach to interpretation of laboratory reports. Detailed information regarding treatment and case management is given for a few specific conditions, but in general, information which is easily available in other basic texts has not been duplicated. Very unusual and rare conditions have also been omitted, as have tests which are not likely to be available to the general practitioner, and for information on these subjects the reader is referred to more advanced textbooks such as those listed on p. 355.

Laboratory medicine in case management

The most common use of laboratory work in veterinary practice is as an ancillary diagnostic aid. Other applications such as assessment of severity of the disease, prognosis and response to treatment tend to be secondary to this. It is therefore useful to consider where this type of procedure fits into the general management of a case.

The first rule of laboratory medicine is, *first catch your differential diagnosis*. This is something which must be arrived at, at least to a first approximation, on clinical grounds, for the very simple reason that only when you have at least some theory about what is going on can you begin to decide which tests to carry out to prove it.

At the most basic level, one first has to decide whether laboratory investigation (blood analysis or microbiological investigation), or radiography or other diagnostic imaging, or electrocardiography or whatever, is the most promising initial route to pursue.

The second step is to try to *ask the lab a specific question*. The clearer you are in your own mind just what question you want answered the easier it will be to decide which tests to ask for, to interpret the results when you get them back, and to realize when your question is, in fact, not one which a laboratory can really answer. For example, to consider a dog with severe acute vomiting, you may decide to ask 'Does this dog have acute pancreatitis or is it in renal failure?', which leads straightforwardly to one set of test requests (amylase, lipase and urea and creatinine), or you may want to know 'How dehydrated is this dog and which i/v fluid should I be giving?', which leads to a different set of requests (total protein, albumin and electrolytes). Both questions are quite valid, both questions can be answered by the laboratory, but only you can decide which one you want to ask or whether you want to ask both. Or to consider a different point, 'Is this cow hypocalcaemic?' is obviously a realistic question, but 'Does this cow have a fractured pelvis, or obdurator paralysis?' is not really something which a laboratory is going to be able to answer with any real certainty. Here the formulation of the question, as opposed to just writing 'downer cow', can help clarify both the extent and the limitations of the information which the laboratory can be expected to provide. It is important in this context to realize that while laboratory data can be highly revealing in a large number of areas, there are certain areas of medicine where general 'routine' blood tests are usually not particularly informative, at least in a diagnostic sense. These include respiratory disease, most orthopaedic conditions and the majority of neurological cases.

Next, translate your question into a *request for specific tests* to be done. In order to do this it is necessary to know what information can be gained from each of the available tests and what is its likely applicability to the situation under consideration. This aspect occupies the bulk of the scope of this book. However, in spite of this, it is probably the actual formulation of the question which requires the most clinical skill, and turning this into a specific request soon follows on naturally. A single result is seldom pathognomonic for a particular disease, however, and the judicious selection of the most appropriate range of tests for each case is very important. It is necessary to strike a balance between requesting dozens of tests (which can be very expensive and may even lead to the relevant information being overlooked in the deluge of results), and the often false economy of restricting requests to one or two tests per sample. As one becomes more familiar with the extent and limitations of the information available from each test this process of acquiring maximum information from a reasonably small number of tests becomes easier and easier (the approach to this is outlined in Chapter 15). In addition, many laboratories have now adopted the approach to profiling first outlined in the previous edition of this book, where profiles are designed around common major presenting signs rather than on an organ-by-organ basis. Profiles designed in this way provide a short-cut to the most rational selection of tests by ensuring that all the differential diagnoses are covered which should realistically be considered when that presenting sign is present – for example, the polydipsia profile for dogs will include calcium, as hypercalcaemia is an extremely important but uncommon cause of polydipsia which might otherwise be forgotten when selecting tests. Nevertheless, it is still good practice to 'engage brain before ticking boxes', as sometimes an extra test or two might be needed to cover particular circumstances, or you might be confident enough that certain conditions are *not* on the cards to allow a less extensive range of tests to be requested. Once you have decided on what information you require from the laboratory and which tests you need to acquire it, you are ready to collect and submit your sample.

The fourth step is to *consider the results in the context of the whole clinical picture*. The conscious act of formulating your original question will make this step much easier, in that when you ask a specific question you tend to have some idea in mind of the answers you are likely to receive, and of your probable response to these answers. However, this stage is definitely the time for some lateral thinking. Even in cases where the answer to the original question seems fairly straightforward, it is well worth asking 'Is there any *other* explanation which could fit all the facts of this case?', and in cases where unexpected or even apparently inconsistent results appear then it is essential to consider the situation in some depth. There is a sort of laboratory 'cringe' which says 'where the clinical picture and the lab results disagree then you should always believe the clinical picture', but this view is misleading. Results from a *reliable* laboratory should never be ignored just because they don't fit your cosy little theory – and if you can't rely on your laboratory, you shouldn't be using it. When arriving at a diagnosis it is essential to look every single fact straight in the eye and to come to a conclusion which can be reconciled with *all* of them. A laboratory result, normal or abnormal, is a fact just like any other piece of clinical information and should be given its *due consideration*. Obviously in each case some facts will weigh more heavily than others, and the decision as to just how much importance to give to each item involves a great deal of clinical skill which takes time and experience to acquire. Unfortunately there are no easy generalizations like 'clinical facts are always more important than lab facts' (or vice versa!) to help here, and there is really no substitute for a *thorough* knowledge of the significance and implications of *all* your findings.

The final maxim to bear in mind is *sample before treatment whenever possible*. The rather desperate approach to laboratory medicine which views lab investigations as a last resort when all attempts at 'diagnosis' by response to treatment have failed causes some veterinary surgeons to come unstuck at this point. It is true that antibiotic treatment is not often a direct cause of trouble with haematology or biochemistry tests (though it can play havoc with any bacteriology you may subsequently decide to do) but the ubiquitous corticosteroids have a wide range of haematological and biochemical effects which can mask vital information of diagnostic significance. Other culprits are fluid therapy (especially when the fluid contains glucose) and mineral preparations such as calcium borogluconate. Clearly, it is difficult to avoid the situation where a farmer has administered every nostrum in his cupboard before you arrive, but it is good practice, whenever treatment is about to be instituted, to consider 'Am I likely to want any laboratory work done on this case, and if so, am I going to regret not having a pre-treatment sample?' Even in circumstances where treatment must be started before any results will be received – a fairly frequent occurrence – a pre-treatment sample can be invaluable and can save a lot of time and trouble in the long run.

Basic principles of haematology and biochemistry

Haematology is the study of the cellular elements of the blood and the associated clotting factors, and can be extended to include cytology of non-blood fluids such as cerebro-spinal fluid (CSF). It is a subject which can provide a great deal of useful information, but, like all diagnostic tests, intelligent assessment of the results is vital. In some ways haematology can be easier to cope with than biochemistry, if only because the easy option of a 'full blood count' or 'general series' examination is available on all lab request forms. This means that it is actually quite easy to bypass the mental disciplines outlined above which lead up to the selection of individual tests. However, if you omit this prior consideration of *why* you are taking this sample and what conclusions you might expect to derive from the results, you must expect to compensate by a particularly thorough assessment of the findings once you receive the results. Remember also that haematology can only tell you what is happening, directly or indirectly, to a fairly small number of circulating cell types, and that the actual number of tests available is quite limited. For general metabolic investigations the wider range of tests and the more direct nature of the information offered by clinical biochemistry is at least as helpful, possibly more so, and normal practice should be to consider *both* disciplines side by side when deciding on the range of tests required for each case.

Clinical biochemistry is a very different subject from pure biochemistry and an antipathy to the latter acquired in early student days should not deter anyone from tackling the former. Basically, clinical biochemistry involves the analysis of samples of body fluids, principally plasma (though occasionally other samples are used such as urine, faeces, CSF and pleural and peritoneal fluids), and the use of the results to clarify the clinical picture. The nature of the subject and the much larger number of 'routine' tests on offer mean that, in general, a wider range of specific information is available from biochemistry than from haematology, but also that a single group of tests cannot be regarded as a basic 'profile' applicable to all (or nearly all) situations. Judicious selection of the appropriate tests for each individual case is therefore of particular importance in clinical biochemistry.

'Normal values'

Many publications quote apparently rigid 'normal values' for biochemical and haematological measurements, sometimes to an extraordinary number of significant figures. The fact that it is extremely rare to find two publications in absolute agreement on these numbers demonstrates clearly the artificiality of this situation.

The spread of values from 'normal' individuals for most constituents (excluding some enzymes) takes the form of a normal distribution curve (see Fig. A.1). If the limits of this curve are defined as the mean ± 2 standard deviations then very rigid values to any number of significant figures can be derived. However, these limits will of necessity exclude 2.5% of all *normal* individuals on each side of the curve – how can you know that your individual patient is not one of this 5%? In addition, it is important to realize that a value *within* these limits is not necessarily 'normal' for every individual animal – one which was towards the lower part of the range when healthy may have a genuinely pathologically evaluated value when ill, which is still within the statistically 'normal' limits. Thus on either side of every 'normal range' there is a grey area where a result may be normal or may be abnormal, and only statistical probabilities of its being one or the other can be quoted. In dealing with individual results in these grey areas it is particularly important to take other factors into consideration, both clinical signs and other laboratory results.

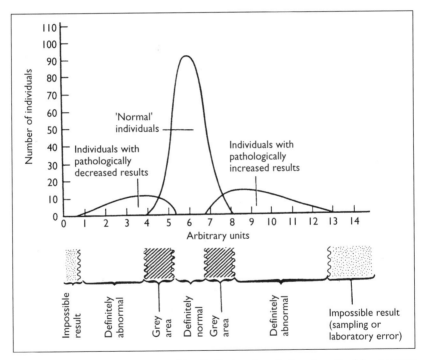

Fig. A.1   Schematic representation of the distribution of results for a figurative laboratory test showing overlaps of 'normal' and pathological ranges.

As a consequence of this, only approximate guideline values are given in this book for each constituent, and when interpreting actual results the modifying effects of species (only the very major species differences are highlighted), breed, sex, age, diet and management systems must be taken into account. It is this multiplicity of species, breeds and patient 'lifestyle' differences which make veterinary laboratory medicine a bit of an art as well as a science, and there is no doubt that the best way to become proficient in interpreting laboratory data is to examine numerical results for as many actual cases as possible. In particular, remember that it is much more important to know what degree of weight to attach to a particular *level* of deviation from normal (e.g. insignificant– ill–dying) than to be able to quote glibly memorized 'normals'.

There is also the question of methodological variation. Since the advent of external quality assessment in NHS laboratories in the 1960s, great attention has been paid to uniformity of reference ranges and results between laboratories. This 'inter-laboratory precision' ensures that patients with chronic illnesses who move from one part of the country to another do not run into serious problems when their new consultant is faced with results from an unfamiliar laboratory with unfamiliar reference ranges. University, state and commercial veterinary laboratories have also benefited from these schemes and participated in them, and nowadays any discrepancies between laboratories' reference ranges should be minor and insignificant (with perhaps a few specific exceptions such as alkaline phosphatase (ALP), where method differences can still have an appreciable effect). Thus it is possible to quote general guideline values which are fairly universally applicable, and it should not be necessary either to completely relearn the subject when changing laboratories, or to be constantly enquiring 'what is *your* reference range for this analyte?'.

Units

The changeover from the old 'conventional' (mostly gravimetric in biochemistry) units to the modern 'SI' (mostly molar in biochemistry) units has created some considerable confusion, particularly among clinical users who just want to know what is wrong with the patient and don't want to be bothered with technicalities. This was probably inevitable at the time, but now that it is at least 25 years since the actual changeover it is about time things settled down.

In haematology there has been comparatively little trouble, in that the adoption of the litre as the standard volume of measurement has usually involved either a simple change in the name of the units (or in the power of 10 included in it) while leaving the actual number unaffected, or at the most there has been a shift in the position of the decimal point. So, mean corpuscular volume (MCV) has moved from cubic microns (μ^3 or cu.μ) to femtolitres (fl) with no change in the number (as they are actually the same thing), while packed cell volume (PCV) has changed from a percentage to a decimal fraction, which in effect moves the decimal point two places to the left (the decimal fraction is sometimes labelled 'l/l', but this is a non-unit in which the top and bottom cancel out – gallons/gallon would be equally valid, as PCV is in fact a v/v ratio). One place where care is required is where a unit of '$\times 10^3$/mm^3' or 'thousands/cu.mm' has been replaced by '$\times 10^9$/l', as with white cell and platelet counts. The numerical result has not in fact changed, but as some people were in the habit of quoting the figure as so many *thousand*, it is possible to fall into the (sometimes potentially dangerous) trap of reporting a result as several thousand $\times 10^9/l$, which is of course out by three orders of magnitude.

Biochemistry unit changes have been more complex because the actual numbers involved have been affected. Historically, plasma constituents were measured by weight (usually mg/100 ml), but subsequently all branches of chemistry and pure biochemistry adopted molar concentration units as the only realistic way to describe reaction processes. In the early 1970s clinical biochemists also changed to molar (SI) units to describe concentrations of plasma constituents, as these are obviously much more meaningful in real terms. However, a few countries have lagged behind in this and the USA in particular has still failed to address the situation even at the beginning of the twenty-first century. This means that the old gravimetric units are still to be found not only in pre-1975 books and journals, but in modern American publications, and the table of conversion factors given below (Table A.1) should be used to convert these figures to the SI equivalents whenever they are

Table A.1 Conversion from old 'gravimetric' biochemistry units to SI units

Constituent	Gravimetric unit	SI unit	Conversion factor
Total protein, albumin, globulin	g/100 ml	g/l	10
Sodium	mg/100 ml*	mmol/l	0.435
	mEq/l		no change
Potassium	mg/100 ml*	mmol/l	0.26
	mEq/l		no change
Chloride	mg/100 ml*	mmol/l	0.28
	mEq/l		no change
Calcium	mg/100 ml	mmol/l	0.25
	mEq/l*		0.5
Magnesium	mg/100 ml	mmol/l	0.41
	mEq/l*		0.5
Phosphate	mg phosphorus/100 ml	mmol/l	0.32
Copper	µg/100 ml	µmol/l	0.16
Urea	mg nitrogen/100 ml (BUN)	mmol/l	0.36
	mg urea/100 ml		0.17
Creatinine	mg/100 ml	µmol/l	88.4
Ammonia	µg/100 ml	µmol/l	0.59
Glucose	mg/100 ml	mmol/l	0.056
Bilirubin	mg/100 ml	µmol/l	17.1
Cholesterol	mg/100 ml	mmol/l	0.026
Triglycerides	mg/100 ml	mmol/l	0.011
Tri-iodothyronine (T_3)	µg/100 ml	nmol/l	15.4
Thyroxine (T_4)	µg/100 ml	nmol/l	12.9
Cortisol	µg/100 ml	nmol/l	27.6
Urine protein/creatinine ratio	g/g	g/mmol	0.113

*Less commonly encountered units.

encountered. When doing this, take care to avoid acquiring extra, spurious, 'significant' figures which may be misleading. (This is another source of the unrealistic number of significant figures seen in some lists of normal values.) It is important to avoid trying to interpret results in gravimetric units as they stand. For one thing, it is quite enough work to become completely familiar with one set of units and probably impossible to become fluently 'bilingual'. If, on the other hand, you persist in converting everything back into old units you will find yourself regarded as somewhat out of touch by the clinical biochemistry establishment in the UK, where SI units have been solidly established for at least 25 years now!

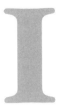

Haematology

Haematology is the study of the cellular elements of the blood, which can be divided into three categories:

(1) The erythrocytes or red blood cells.
(2) The thrombocytes or platelets.
(3) The leucocytes or white blood cells.

Occasionally other cells which are not normally present in circulation can also be detected in a blood sample, such as mast cells or plasma cells – usually because the cells are neoplastic.

The red cells are responsible for oxygen transport from the lungs to all the tissues of the body, the platelets are responsible for routine maintenance and repair of the blood vessels, and the white cells (at a wild generalization) are responsible in various ways for repelling foreign invaders. Haematological examination may in a sense be regarded as a 'biopsy' of these systems.

1 The Red Blood Cells (Erythrocytes)

The erythron

The 'erythron' is the name given to the organ of the body, technically classified as connective tissue, which comprises all the red cells plus all the red cell producing tissue – essentially the relevant fractions of the blood, the spleen and the bone marrow. In so far as the red cells are concerned, a blood sample can be thought of as a biopsy of this organ. The single function of the erythron is oxygen/carbon dioxide transport between the tissues and the lungs, with haemoglobin as the O_2/CO_2 carrier, and the main reason that the haemoglobin is contained within cells rather than being free in the plasma like all the other blood proteins is simply that the sheer amount of protein involved (100–150 g/l whole blood as opposed to only about 40 g/l whole blood of all other proteins) would cause massive disruption of the osmotic pressure. Functionally speaking, therefore, mature red cells are little more than very flexible bags of haemoglobin in the shape of a slightly biconcave disc.

Red cell production (erythropoiesis)

This takes place in the red (haemopoietic) bone marrow (not in the white fatty marrow). This haemopoietic bone marrow is much more extensive in young animals than in mature ones, where it retreats to the centres of the bones. This tends to make effective bone marrow biopsy rather more difficult in older animals. The stages of development of the red cells are shown in Fig. 1.1.

As the erythrocytes mature they become very readily deformable (necessary in order to pass through small capillaries) and when they are flexible enough they can slide into the circulation through openings in the sinusoidal walls. The total maturation time varies between species from about 4–5 days in cattle to about 1 week in the dog. Normally about 10–15% of developing red cells die before reaching maturity (ineffective erythropoiesis) and this percentage can increase in certain disease situations.

When there is an increased demand for red cells (e.g. haemorrhage, oxygen

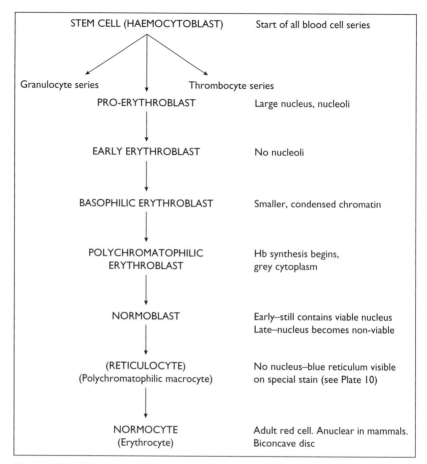

Fig. 1.1 Simplified representation of the stages of erythropoiesis.

starvation) production is increased firstly by allowing younger forms (reticulocytes, normoblasts) to enter the circulation, and secondly by allowing the
maturation stages to merge and skip so that erythropoiesis speeds up. The
former is not seen in all species – for example, dogs demonstrate reticulocy-
tosis very readily, cattle only on extreme provocation such as severe acute
haemorrhage, and horses never. The latter occurs in all species and sometimes
leads to the appearance of a few imperfect erythrocytes in circulation, such as
Howell–Jolly bodies, poikilocytes and leptocytes.

Erythrocyte lifespan

This varies between species from about 2 months in pigs to over 5 months in
cattle. Sheep are unique in having two populations of red cells, one short-lived
(70 days), the other long-lived (150 days). These differences mean that the rate
of progression of a hypoplastic anaemia varies between species. In certain

disease situations the survival time of the erythrocytes is shortened, particularly some nutritional deficiencies (iron, vitamin B_{12}, folic acid), congenital porphyria in cattle and congenital pyruvate kinase deficiency in basenji dogs.

Erythrocyte breakdown

This occurs in three ways. The cell may be fragmented into pieces small enough for the reticulo-endothelial system to take up, or when the enzymes present in the cell membrane are used up the much more fragile cell breaks up and is phagocytosed, or the whole cell may be phagocytosed directly.

The haemoglobin from a defunct red cell is also broken down. The (protein) globin fraction is lysed into its component amino acids which join the general body amino acid pool, either being restructured into new proteins as needed, or being deaminated with the amino residue excreted as urea and the carbohydrate residue entering the fuel metabolism pathways. The haem fraction loses its iron atom, which is *not* excreted but is recycled into a new haemoglobin molecule. The remaining part of the haem complex becomes bilirubin which, in its original form, is non-water-soluble and so must be transported in the plasma bound to albumin. On reaching the liver it is conjugated to glucuronic acid or a similar substance, which renders it soluble so that it can be excreted in the bile. After some recycling round the hepatic circulation and further metabolism most of this is excreted in the faeces as urobilin and stercobilin – these give the faeces their characteristic colour. Some is also excreted in the urine as urobilinogen. Investigation of these metabolites can be useful in the differential diagnosis of hepatobiliary disease in man, but only bilirubin seems to be of any real clinical use in veterinary species.

Control of erythropoiesis

Normally, production and destruction of red cells are kept in balance so that total erythrocyte numbers (i.e. erythron size) are constant – in a 15 kg dog about 800 000 red cells die and are replaced every second!

The hormone responsible for the regulation of the rate of erythropoiesis is a glycoprotein with a molecular weight of about 60 000–70 000 daltons, called *erythropoietin* (EP; it is sometimes referred to as EPO, but this invites confusion with evening primrose oil). It is not species specific, but bird and mammal hormones are not interchangeable. Fetal and maternal EP are quite separate because the hormone does not cross the placenta. The principal site of EP production is the kidney – in dogs this is the only site and thus the hormone is totally absent in nephrectomized animals, but there is an additional extra-renal site in some species (e.g. rats) which has not been identified. The fundamental stimulus to EP production is tissue hypoxia, and so the concentration in plasma is related to the ratio of oxygen supply to oxygen demand.

Erythropoietin affects red cell production in four ways:

(1) More stem cells differentiate to red cell precursors.
(2) Stages of red cell development are speeded up.
(3) Transit time out of bone marrow is reduced.
(4) Immature red cells are released (depending on species).

(1) is the normal method of obtaining fine control over the size of the erythron. (2), (3) and (4) only occur in response to large doses of EP, usually because of an acute requirement for more erythrocytes. The actual mechanisms involved are not fully understood but may be connected to the rate of haemoglobin synthesis.

Measurement of plasma EP concentration is becoming increasingly used in human medicine to aid differentiation of the causes of anaemia, and has recently become available in the veterinary field. EP is also available as a therapeutic drug in human medicine, most importantly in long-term renal failure patients being maintained on dialysis. It has also become a drug of abuse among endurance athletes. Its high cost and restricted availability have meant that only a few small-scale trials have been carried out in animals. It certainly does increase the packed cell volume (PCV) in chronic renal failure cases, but this is of little clinical benefit if the excretory capacity of the kidneys continues to deteriorate. Effects of changes in EP concentration can often be readily appreciated on examination of routine haematology results, and certain other hormones which affect EP synthesis can be used to stimulate its production. The endocrine organs involved in the modification of EP production are the pituitary, adrenals, thyroid and gonads. The hormones in question actually affect cell metabolism and hence tissue oxygen requirements, and so have a feedback on EP synthesis.

(1) *Hormones which increase EP production:* androgens, cortisol, thyroxine, adrenaline, noradrenaline, angiotensin, prolactin, growth hormone, thyroid-stimulating hormone (TSH) and adrenocorticotrophic hormone (ACTH).
(2) *Hormones which decrease EP production:* oestrogens.

Resultant clinical effects are quite wide ranging. By these mechanisms apparently unrelated occurrences can have a marked and unexpected effect on an animal's erythrocyte status.

(1) Males tend to have a higher PCV than females – this is a hormonal effect abolished by castration and spaying.
(2) Excess of a hormone in the first group will lead to an increase in PCV – the most common example is excess cortisol in Cushing's disease (hyperadrenocorticism).
(3) Deficiency of a hormone in the first group will lead to a decrease in PCV, i.e. slight anaemia. Examples are hypothyroidism, Addison's disease (hypoadrenocorticism) and anterior pituitary insufficiency. However, note that patients with untreated Addison's disease are nearly always dehydrated, which can cause the PCV to rise back into the normal range.

The anaemia will only be apparent as such when rehydration has been achieved.

(4)   Excess of oestrogens will lead to decreased erythropoiesis and in some cases to complete (and fatal) bone marrow aplasia. This has been recorded as a spontaneous occurrence in unmated ferrets in prolonged oestrus, but most cases are iatrogenic as a consequence of oestrogen treatment for misalliance incontinence or enlarged prostate (see true aplastic anaemia, p. 27).

Basic interpretation of red cell parameters

When investigating the red cells there are several different but related measurements which can be made, and these can be combined to produce several more figures which are descriptive of red cell status. It is important to be aware of the meaning of each of these different numbers and of their relationship to one another in order to make sense of a haematology report.

The primary red cell measurement which gives a basic assessment of the size of the (circulating) erythron is the *packed cell volume* (PCV) or haematocrit. This is simply a measurement of the fraction of the blood volume which is occupied by erythrocytes and is expressed either as a percentage or as a decimal fraction (35% = 0.35). Normal values vary slightly with species: about 0.30–0.40 in large animals, about 0.30–0.45 in cats and a wide-ranging 0.35–0.65 in dogs, with the greyhound/whippet/lurcher type breeds showing the highest values.

Next, information about the morphology of the red cells is provided by the *mean corpuscular volume* (MCV) and *mean corpuscular haemoglobin concentration* (MCHC) values, which are both calculated parameters in veterinary haematology.

The *MCV* is a measure of the size of the red cells and is obtained by simple arithmetic from the PCV and the total red cell count of the sample:

$$\text{MVC (fl)} = \frac{\text{PCV (\%)}}{\text{RBC } (\times 10^{12}/\text{l})} \times 10 \quad [1 \text{ femtolitre (fl)} = 10^{-15} \text{ l}]$$

The '$\times 10^{12}/\text{l}$' does not enter into the actual calculation, e.g. a sample with a PCV of 0.35 (35%) and RBC count of 4.89 $\times$ $10^{12}/\text{l}$ has an MCV of 71.6 fl. Normal values vary widely with species, and are completely independent of the size of the individual animal (Table 1.1).

Young animals tend to have rather smaller red cells than adults; in particular calves often have an MCV as low as 30 fl. Paradoxically, neonates actually have red cells at least as large as the adult.

The size of the red cells can also be assessed by looking at a well-made blood film. This is done partly by comparing the red cells with the white cells, which vary very little in size (see Plate 7), and partly by appreciating that where abnormal cells are present normal red cells are usually also present, and with practice the comparison is easy to make. In particular, abnormally large cells

Table 1.1 Erythrocyte size

Species	Approximate mean red cell volume (fl)
Man	90
Dog	70
Pig	60
Cow (adult)	50
Cat	45
Horse	45
Sheep	30
Goat	15

(macrocytes) are nearly always polychromatophilic (blue-mauve coloured) which makes them easy to spot (see Plate 8). Where a calculated MCV value disagrees with the appearance of the blood film, *believe what you see*, particularly if the red cell count was done manually. The manual method is not very accurate and often gives falsely high (or sometimes low) MCV values.

The *MCHC* is a measure of the haemoglobin concentration in the red cells and is obtained arithmetically from the PCV and the total haemoglobin concentration of the sample:

$$\text{MCHC (g/100 ml)} = \frac{\text{Whole blood haemoglobin concentration (g/100 ml)}}{\text{PCV (decimal fraction)}}$$

The normal value is about 35 g/100 ml irrespective of species or size of the red cells, i.e. for any given PCV the total amount of haemoglobin per unit volume of blood will be the same irrespective of species. In the sheep it is contained in a large number of small packets; in the dog it is contained in a smaller number of larger packets.

Corpuscular haemoglobin concentration can also be assessed by eye on a well-made blood film, with the hypochromic cells (low haemoglobin concentration) having noticeably pale centres (see Plate 9). Again, where a numerical value disagrees with the appearance of the blood film, believe what you see. Sometimes only a proportion of the cells are hypochromic, not enough to lower the MCHC value (which is, after all, a *mean*), but enough to be clinically significant.

An abnormally *high* MCHC is not possible as such; there is no such thing as a hyperchromic red cell. However, because of the way the figure is obtained, MCHC values of over 40 g/100 ml are sometimes obtained. There are three possible reasons:

(1) Haemolysed blood sample (either due to bad collection technique or, more rarely, genuine intravascular haemolysis). Since the calculation of MCHC assumes that all the haemoglobin is inside the cells, when in this case it is not, a falsely high value will be obtained.

(2) Other interfering substances in the plasma (e.g. lipaemic plasma) may cause an erroneously high haemoglobin reading and hence an erroneously high MCHC.

Table 1.2 Effects of sample artefacts on calculated RBC parameters.

	MCV	MCHC
Old sample	↑	↓
Lipaemia	—	↑
Haemolysis	—	↑
Underfilled tube	↓	↑
Autoagglutination	↑	—

(3) Excessive osmotic shrinkage of the red cells. This is rarely an *in vivo* phenomenon, but is common when an EDTA tube is underfilled leading to an excessive concentration of EDTA in the sample.

(4) Simple laboratory error in either haemoglobin or PCV measurements.

A third red cell parameter which can be calculated is the *mean cell haemoglobin* (MCH), measured in picograms (pg). This obviously varies with cell size and so with species, and is therefore not often used in veterinary medicine. It can be useful in assessing whether hypochromic macrocytic cells actually have the normal absolute amount of haemoglobin in them or not.

Total *red cell count* (RBC or RCC) and whole blood *haemoglobin concentration* (Hb) should *not* be interpreted clinically. Clearly, they vary almost exactly in parallel with the PCV and can tell you nothing more than the PCV result as they stand. Their function is to allow calculation of the MCV and MCHC, respec-

---

Case 1.1

A 6-year-old cairn terrier bitch was presented on a Friday afternoon with malaise and poor appetite. Rectal temperature was 39.2°C. By the time the results were received 4 days later, she had completely recovered. Can you explain the abnormalities?

PCV	0.61	raised
Hb	17.6 g/100 ml	
RBC count	$7.35 \times 10^{12}/l$	
MCV	83.0 fl	raised
MCHC	28.9 g/100 ml	low
Total WBC count	$12.4 \times 10^9/l$	

Film comment. RBCs: normal
WBCs: too degenerate to differentiate
Platelets: adequate

Comments

The haematology was in fact completely normal. The 'abnormalities' are artefacts caused by a 3-day delay in analysis due to weekend post. Erythrocytes swell, causing the MCV to increase and the PCV to rise, but as the haemoglobin content of the cells (MCH) remains unchanged the MCHC decreases. Leucocyte morphology degenerates, and unless a blood film made at the time of sample collection is sent with the specimen a differential WBC count will not be obtained.

tively, and these are the figures which should be interpreted. The only exceptions are where a sample is so badly haemolysed that the micro-haematocrit simply cannot be read (but the haemoglobin result may still be valid), or perhaps where a very approximate side-room haemoglobin estimation may be all that is available.

Erythrocyte sedimentation rate (ESR) involves measuring how fast red cells will settle out on standing, a measurement which depends to some extent on plasma viscosity, which alters when inflammatory proteins are present. It is an old-fashioned test, but still favoured by some general practitioners as a general indicator as to whether a patient is actually ill or not. However, results are extremely species specific, and the test has no place in veterinary medicine. In particular, the tendency of equine erythrocytes to form rouleaux means that the cells sediment extremely quickly, and the result is almost entirely a factor of the PCV. Feline cells often behave in a very similar manner. In contrast, bovine cells barely sediment at all. Some attempts have been made to produce tables of correction for PCV to allow the test to be used on canine samples, but the results appear to have little clinical relevance.

Abnormalities of the erythron: polycythaemia (abnormally high PCV)

Polycythaemia can be divided into two fundamentally different classes:

Relative polycythaemia

This is defined as an increase in PCV *without* any increase in the actual size of the erythron as a whole, and is by far the more common type of polycythaemia. In veterinary species there are two possible causes.

(1)   *Water deficiency (dehydration)*. In a dehydrated animal the plasma water content will be reduced, and as the red cells cannot escape from the circulation their concentration, and hence the PCV, will rise. Plasma proteins are also to a large extent (though not completely) trapped in the circulation and so in dehydrated patients the total plasma protein concentration will rise along with the PCV and by approximately the same percentage. However, as other smaller molecules are more or less freely diffusable into the interstitial fluid and tend to be under tighter homeostatic control, concentrations of these are of no use in assessing dehydration; attention should therefore be restricted to PCV, total plasma protein and albumin for this purpose.

(2)   *Splenic contraction*. Excitement, apprehension or fright will cause the smooth muscle in the spleen to contract, expelling the stored red cells into the circulation. This is part of the adrenergic 'fight or flight' reaction. Horses, particularly hot-blooded breeds, show this response very readily (it can be very difficult to get a baseline PCV result on a highly-strung

racehorse), but it can occur in all veterinary species. During this occurrence the total plasma protein concentration remains unchanged.

In human medicine the PCV is frequently used alone as a measure of state of hydration, as human subjects do not have a contractile spleen and so apprehension will not affect the results. Also, the normal range for PCV in man is quite narrow. In veterinary medicine it is generally good practice to use both PCV and total plasma protein concentration in conjunction, as the contractile spleen can seriously influence results, especially in horses. In dogs, splenic contraction is usually less of a problem, but the very wide normal range can make interpretation of a single PCV result impossible so far as assessing dehydration is concerned.

The absence of a contractile spleen in human athletes is the reason for the presumed efficacy of altitude training (where the natural effect of the hypoxia of high altitudes is used to induce an increase in PCV which persists advantageously for several weeks after the athlete has returned to sea level), erythropoietin administration and 'blood doping' (where a unit of blood removed from the athlete a few weeks earlier is auto-transfused just before competition to boost the PCV, which has recovered to normal by then). These stratagems produce an artificially increased PCV which improves the oxygen carrying capacity of the blood and so should improve athletic performance, but doubt has been expressed as to whether these procedures have any real effect and they can be dangerous. Altitude training is legal, blood doping and erythropoietin administration are not. In the horse the contractile spleen acts as a natural, endogenous 'blood doping' mechanism, with the PCV of a racehorse commonly increasing from 0.35 at rest to over 0.60 during a race. This means that 'blood doping' as practised by human athletes is a complete waste of time in horses. It also means that assessment of red cell status (PCV, Hb or RBC) is totally useless for predicting either stage of fitness or performance potential of racehorses. This does not prevent it from being widely used for these purposes!

Absolute polycythaemia

In this case the increase in PCV is a consequence of a genuine increase in the absolute size of the erythron. Absolute polycythaemia is much less common than relative polycythaemia. There are several possible causes.

(1) *Polycythaemia vera* is a rare type of myeloproliferative disorder characterized by a marked overproduction of normal-looking, adult red blood cells. It may be thought of as a type of bone marrow tumour. Its diagnosis depends on finding a PCV of around 0.70 or more in a normally hydrated, non-excited animal in the *absence* of any demonstrable respiratory, cardiovascular or endocrine disorder (see secondary polycythaemia, below). Erythropoietin levels, if measured, are normal.

In the past this was treated by repeated phlebotomy, but recently hydroxyurea has come into use as an effective medical treatment.

(2) *Erythropoietin-producing neoplasm of the kidney* is a very rare condition which can be distinguished from polycythaemia vera by a more regenerative RBC picture and higher circulating levels of erythropoietin.

(3) *Secondary polycythaemia* is the term used where the increase in erythron size is a secondary consequence of disease in another organ system. Secondary polycythaemia can itself be divided into two groups, depending on whether or not it accompanies low tissue oxygen tension. Where lowered tissue oxygen is a consequence of disease (as opposed to altitude), cyanosis is usually present and the organs involved are either the respiratory system (e.g. obstructive pulmonary disease) or the cardiovascular system (heart defects involving right-to-left shunting of blood, e.g. tetralogy of Fallot). Blood gas measurements can be helpful in these cases. The causes of secondary polycythaemia unassociated with decreased tissue oxygen tension are mainly endocrine problems where the primary hormone abnormality has a direct effect on erythropoietin production, for example excess cortisol in Cushing's disease. These cases are not cyanotic. In general the PCV values measured in secondary polycythaemia are less spectacularly abnormal than those seen in polycythaemia vera.

Summary, differentiation of the causes of polycythaemia

Relative, erythron size not increased

(1) Dehydration (total plasma protein also raised).
(2) Splenic contraction (total plasma protein unchanged).

Absolute, erythron size increased

(1) Polycythaemia vera (primary disease of the erythron, no evidence of cardiac, pulmonary or endocrine disease. No cyanosis). Erythropoietin-producing tumour may be a differential diagnosis here, but the condition is extremely rare.
(2) Secondary polycythaemia (due to disease of other organ). The only class to consider if many immature cells in circulation.
    (a) Result of low tissue oxygen tension, usually respiratory or cardiovascular disease (cyanosis may be present).
    (b) Tissue oxygen tension normal, usually endocrine disease with hormonal stimulation of EP production (cyanosis absent).

Abnormalities of the erythron: anaemia (strictly oligocythaemia, abnormally low PCV)

Anaemia is almost always absolute. Overenthusiastic administration of i/v fluids may occasionally push the PCV down to abnormally low levels, some cases of

Case 1.2

A 10-year-old black cat was presented as vaguely unwell. Much of the clinical examination was unremarkable, but the mucous membranes were observed to be dark blue in colour. There were no observable cardiac abnormalities. The following haematology results were received. What is the likely diagnosis, and how might it be further investigated?

PCV	0.72		
Hb	23.7 g/100 ml		high
RBC	$15.68 \times 10^{12}/l$		
MCV	45.9 fl		
MCHC	32.9 g/100 ml		
Total WBC count		$5.8 \times 10^9/l$	
Band neutrophils	0%	$0 \times 10^9/l$	
Adult neutrophils	76%	$4.4 \times 10^9/l$	
Eosinophils	2%	$0.1 \times 10^9/l$	
Basophils	0%	$0 \times 10^9/l$	
Lymphocytes	19%	$1.1 \times 10^9/l$	
Monocytes	3%	$0.2 \times 10^9/l$	

Film comment. RBCs: normal
WBCs: normal
Platelets: adequate

Comments

Such an extremely high PCV should always arouse suspicions of polycythaemia vera, particularly if it is consistent over more than one sample collected on different days. Other causes of polycythaemia (heart disease with right-to-left shunt, obstructive pulmonary disease, dehydration) would be expected to show clinical signs by the time the PCV reached this level. Mucous membrane colour in polycythaemia vera is usually intense red, and the blue appearance in this cat did initially give rise to suspicions of a heart condition, but none could be demonstrated. Erythropoietin concentration was normal, which confirmed the diagnosis, and clinical response to hydroxyurea was good.

congestive heart failure do become a bit waterlogged now and again, and it can be surprising how low the PCV of a depressed horse with no splenic tone can sometimes go, but in general an anaemia means that the size of the erythron is reduced.

Causes of anaemia can be divided into three basic aetiological classes: hae-morrhagic, haemolytic and aplastic (or hypoplastic). The primary aim when attempting to diagnose a case of anaemia is to ascertain which of these three basic causes is involved – only then can a more precise diagnosis be investigated. The very first step, however, is to decide whether the onset of the anaemia is acute or chronic.

Acute onset anaemia

Severe anaemia cases often appear to present as acute onset even when the progress of the disease is actually chronic. This is because in a sedentary animal a gradual insidious decline in PCV, causing a very gradual onset of lethargy and exercise intolerance, often goes unnoticed by the owner until the condition is severe enough to cause obvious distress and/or fainting fits. However, the genuine acute onset anaemia cases are quite easy to distinguish on clinical grounds.

Acute haemorrhagic anaemia

The usual clinical signs are pallor, tachycardia, hyperpnoea and possibly collapse. Diagnosis is nearly always very easy as most cases have clear external evidence of extensive haemorrhage. Only where the haemorrhage is into the abdominal cavity is diagnosis difficult, as the clinical signs can be difficult to distinguish from simple shock, for example, post road traffic accident (RTA). In these cases the presence of blood in the abdomen may be suspected on palpation and confirmed by paracentesis. If there is doubt as to whether the fluid obtained is frank blood or a bloodstained transudate, measure the PCV of the fluid. Frank blood will have a PCV at least as high as the circulating blood, probably higher, as the water is reabsorbed into the circulation before the cells. (Cases of acute haemorrhage into pleural or pericardial cavities do not present as anaemia unless there is concurrent haemorrhage elsewhere, as signs of pulmonary collapse or cardiac tamponade will develop first.) In the very early stages of acute haemorrhage haematological investigation is of little use: because when whole blood is being lost the haematology of what remains will be quite normal (even to a normal PCV) although the animal may be in acute hypovolaemic shock. Over the next few hours as plasma volume is restored the PCV will fall, but haematological evidence of regeneration (immature cells in circulation) will not appear for a day or two. Two aetiologies should be considered.

(1)   *Trauma.* Usually due to a road accident; also severe cuts, gunshot wounds, etc. Evidence of haemorrhage is accompanied by signs of trauma – torn claws on cats, road dirt in coat, obvious wounds. Blood clotting is normal. Most of these cases are straightforward, but it is important to check for unseen intra-abdominal bleeding as described above (e.g. ruptured spleen). The first treatment priority is restoration of circulating volume. Plasma expanders (e.g. polygeline 3.5% with electrolytes (Haemaccel: Intervet)) are usually sufficient, as an animal can survive losing up to two-thirds of its blood volume without requiring blood transfusion so long as hypovolaemic shock is prevented. Anaemia due to surgical haemorrhage should be treated in the same way as that due to accidental trauma. However, if severe intractable haemorrhage occurs as a result of minor or routine surgery, particularly in young animals, a clotting defect should be suspected (see Chapter 2).

(2) *Ruptured neoplasm.* Certain neoplasms, especially haemangiomas and haemangiosarcomas, consist largely of blood-filled 'cysts'. When they grow large enough they are prone to rupture with little or no provocation, and it is possible for an animal to bleed out into the abdominal cavity when such a lesion on the spleen or liver suddenly breaks open. However, the first rupture is not often fatal, and the more usual clinical presentation is of intermittent collapse (see p. 20).

(3) *Warfarin poisoning.* Warfarin is an anticoagulant of the coumarin type which acts as an antagonist to vitamin K. Vitamin K is an essential co-factor for the synthesis of prothrombin and several other clotting factors in the liver, and warfarin essentially halts production of these factors, causing a severe clotting deficiency. It is used as a rodenticide and therapeutically to treat navicular disease in horses. Poisoning occurs in small animals due to the consumption either of the rat bait itself or of rodents poisoned by warfarin – the manufacturers claim that it is safe for pets because the irritant bait is supposed to induce emesis in non-target species, but poisoning cases are common. Horses become affected due to overdosage of the therapeutic drug.

Warfarin poisoning in *small animals* is characterized by widespread haemorrhage without any real signs of trauma, obvious wounds, etc. Petechiation of gums, subcutaneous bruising/haematoma formation and blood in faeces and urine are often seen. Bleeding points are usually numerous, and serious intra-abdominal haemorrhage without external evidence of bleeding is unusual. These cases can be distinguished from RTA victims by lack of evidence of trauma and marked clotting abnormalities. Observation of whole blood collected into a test-tube is a very poor guide, but a properly performed clotting time (see p. 296) will show an increase from a normal of under 5 minutes to 10 minutes or more. More specifically, plasma prothrombin time will be prolonged from about 8–10 seconds to several minutes. In *horses* the condition is often less severe, presenting as marked haematoma formation after minor bumps, but occasionally substantial intra-abdominal bleeding can occur without other signs of haemorrhage – these cases can present as colic. To prevent this, all horses on warfarin therapy should have their prothrombin times checked regularly and the dosage reduced if this goes above 16–20 seconds (normally 10–12 seconds in horses).

Treatment is by administration of vitamin K_1 (phytomenadione– Konakion: Roche), a synthetic vitamin which is as biologically active as the natural vitamin (K_2). Note: vitamin K_3 (menadiol, formerly marketed as Synkavit) a water-soluble form of the vitamin intended for oral administration in patients suffering from fat malabsorption, is *not* an effective treatment for warfarin poisoning. Dose rate of Konakion (contrary to the human information on the package insert) is at least 2 mg/kg, and the route of administration should be chosen according to the severity of the case. Intravenous administration will begin to reverse the hypoprothrombinaemia in about 4 hours while with i/m administration 12 hours are required. (It has been suggested that s/c administration may be at least as effective as i/m, which seems reasonable, as vitamin K is a fat-soluble vitamin.) If ongoing haemorrhage is severe enough to endanger life in less than 4 hours, whole blood transfusion is necessary. The dose is 10–20 ml/kg depending on need, from a donor of the same species. The primary reason for transfusion is to give the patient active clotting factors, so the blood must be *fresh*. (Stored blood, or even blood removed from the patient's own pleural cavity and auto-transfused via a filtered giving set, will provide emergency oxygen transport but will not aid haemostasis.) Chest drainage may be necessary to prevent respiratory failure, but blood in the abdomen should not normally be removed as it will eventually be reabsorbed into the circulation. Konakion treatment should be repeated at 12-hour intervals for several weeks as the poison tends to persist – once the prothrombin time has returned to normal oral administration is usually sufficient. The use of 'second-generation' coumarins such as bromodiolone is becoming more widespread. These are extremely persistent and dogs have been known to suffer sudden haemorrhage even months after the initial episode. When these agents are involved it is prudent to continue oral Konakion for two or three months – this can be expensive, but so is emergency drainage of a chest full of blood! It is best to check the prothrombin time 4–6 days after the last tablet and restart treatment if an abnormality is found.

Acute haemolytic anaemia

As with haemorrhage, these cases present as collapsing, hyperpnoeic animals with marked tachycardia and a haemic murmur. However, pallor may not be evident – instead, jaundice is often present. In these cases PCV is reduced even from the earliest stages of the condition as no plasma is being lost concurrently. Initially free haemoglobin is seen in the plasma (but great care must be taken to avoid causing haemolysis of the sample by poor blood collection and handling, or diagnosis may be misleading), and as the disease progresses this is replaced by bilirubin (unconjugated), which gives rise to icterus or jaundice. However, note that the degree of clinical jaundice is seldom so marked as that seen in liver disease. Both haemoglobin (red) and bilirubin (orange-yellow) can be seen in the plasma layer of a micro-haematocrit PCV tube. Where there is free haemoglobin in the plasma the calculated MCHC will appear higher than normal, as the calculation assumes that this haemoglobin is inside the cells. In addition, haemoglobinuria is often present and may be demonstrated in a urine sample by a dipstick test (free haemoglobin in urine can be differentiated from red cells on the strip if only small amounts are present, or by centrifugation where large amounts are present, see p. 304). While unconjugated bilirubin should not, theoretically, appear in the urine (as it is albumin-bound), animals which are jaundiced as a result of haemolysis usually do show a positive urine bilirubin test. However, beware of false positives in this test (see p. 171).

In any one species the specific diagnoses associated with acute haemolytic anaemia are limited. Causes can be:

(1) *Infectious*, for example *Haemobartonella felis* (acute cases), *Leptospira icterohaemorrhagiae*, *Babesia* spp., bacillary haemoglobinuria (*Clostridium haemolyticum*), and others. In the UK, babesiosis does occur in cattle in tick-infested areas. Canine babesiosis has been reported in dogs entering the country under the Pet Passport scheme, and equine babesiosis is occasionally seen in imported horses. Ehrlichiosis and leishmaniasis have been rare in the UK but increased vigilance is wise following the relaxation of the quarantine laws. Feline infectious anaemia (FIA, caused by *Haemobartonella felis*) is occasionally seen in its own right. However, the other conditions are rare, and even FIA usually manifests secondarily to immunosuppression caused by such things as feline leukaemia virus (FeLV) and feline immunodeficiency virus (FIV).

(2) *Toxic*, for example copper poisoning (sheep) – due to chronic excess of dietary copper stored in the liver suddenly being released to cause massive acute haemolysis (see p. 98). Acute brassica poisoning (see p. 22) may also be included here.

(3) *Ag/Ab reactions*, for example haemolytic anaemia of the newborn. This is a condition of horses similar to the 'Rhesus baby' syndrome, in which the mare forms antibodies to the 'foreign' red cells of her foal. Like the Rhesus baby problem it does not affect the first pregnancy, but second and subsequent foals with maternally incompatible red cell antigens will be affected. Unlike the Rhesus babies, which are affected *in utero*, these foals are healthy until they are born and begin to drink the colostrum, due to the different mare placental structure which does not allow antibodies to cross. Affected foals must not be allowed to suck but should be fostered or hand-fed. A similar condition has been described in cats, usually associated with cross-suckling in households where more than one queen is nursing a litter at the same time. Transfusion reactions, due to a second transfusion of incompatible blood, are also included in this category.

Autoimmune haemolytic anaemia (AIHA), which is common in dogs and occurs occasionally in cats, can present as acute haemolysis. However, a more chronic presentation is more usual and so the condition is discussed under that heading (see p. 22).

Treatment is specific to the cause of the condition, plus blood transfusion (transfusion of packed red cells is even better) if the PCV falls dangerously low (below about 0.15 in acute cases). The safest transfusion for a foal with haemolytic anaemia is *washed* red cells from the mare (*not* whole blood, which contains the offending antibodies). Failing this, whole blood from a horse (preferably a gelding) which is not related to the foal's father can be used. As hypovolaemia does not occur, i/v administration of non-blood fluids is merely supportive and may aid renal function where this is impaired by excessive free haemoglobin in circulation.

Gradual onset anaemia

In gradual onset anaemia the PCV falls gradually over a period of days or weeks, plasma volume expands concurrently to compensate, and patients are not presented in acute hypovolaemia. Before considering the differential diagnoses it is important to consider the severity of the condition as this will affect the presenting signs and the interpretation of the haematological findings.

Mild/moderate anaemia (PCV below normal but still above 0.20–0.25) is often found when a full haematological examination is performed on an animal presented with a history apparently related to something quite different. In these cases the low PCV should be considered together with all other clinical and laboratory findings when arriving at a diagnosis, and can often be very helpful in this. However, as most animals will not be particularly inconvenienced by a PCV which is over 0.25, the anaemia is unlikely to be the main presenting sign, and so its investigation will not necessarily be the first priority in assessment of the case.

Severe/very severe anaemia (PCV below 0.20–0.25 down to about 0.05–0.06 which is more or less fatal) often presents as sudden onset illness because the insidious deterioration of the animal as the anaemia progresses has not been noticed by the owners. However, once the PCV falls to about 0.12–0.15, collapse and fainting will occur. These cases are weak, have poor exercise tolerance, show marked tachycardia with a pronounced haemic murmur (perhaps also tachypnoea/hyperpnoea) and have a history of collapse. If the extreme pallor of the mucous membranes is overlooked these may be mistaken for signs of cardiac disease. When an animal presents with these signs and a PCV below 0.20 the investigation of the anaemia is usually the first priority.

In any investigation of anaemia the major aim is to discover which of the three possible aetiologies is involved – haemorrhage, haemolysis or bone marrow failure. This is done by a combination of the examination of the *morphology* of the red cells, which is different in each case, and the piecing together of a number of other haematological and biochemical tests. Once the aetiology has been discovered, the basic cause of the problem can be investigated.

Chronic haemorrhagic anaemia

In cases of chronic haemorrhage the loss of blood is not always easy to appreciate and it is often necessary to establish the fact of haemorrhage first by other methods, then look for the source.

Red cell morphology

In small animals, there will be evidence of regeneration: many polychromatophilic cells are present together with some nucleated red cells. In the early stages the polychromatophilic cells will be macrocytes (large, i.e. MCV will be increased) and the adult cells will be normocytic and normochromic (see Plate 8). However, in long-standing cases the continuing loss of red cell constituents (iron, protein, etc.) leads to a secondary bone marrow exhaustion. This results in the cells becoming gradually more and more hypochromic (i.e. MCHC is reduced, due to iron deficiency) and smaller, and in very long-standing cases even the young cells, although still polychromatophilic, become hypochromic and microcytic (see Plate 9). Misshapen cells – poikilocytes, folded cells, cup/bowl cells and sometimes target cells – may appear. With the exception of extremes of starvation and some rather obscure malabsorption conditions, chronic haemorrhage is the only cause of iron deficiency anaemia seen in adult animals.

In large animals morphological evidence of red cell regeneration (i.e. young cells in circulation) is often absent, particularly in horses, but again as the condition progresses signs of bone marrow exhaustion will appear. This means that in these species diagnosis may have to be made on grounds other than erythrocyte morphology, and particular care must be taken to differentiate long-standing haemorrhage cases from primary bone marrow problems.

Other haematology

In cases where the haemorrhage is not caused by thrombocytopenia, the platelet count will often be raised (i.e. over 400×10^9/l); this is known as reactive thrombocytosis and is due to the consumption of platelets at the site of the lesion feeding back to step up production. Other coagulation tests (e.g. clotting time and prothrombin time) may be *slightly* abnormal due to excessive consumption of clotting factors. If the site of haemorrhage is infected, neutrophilia and/or monocytosis may also be present. In cases with a primary clotting defect the platelet count and/or coagulation tests should provide the diagnosis; see Chapter 2.

Biochemistry

As plasma is being lost along with the red cells, a progressive hypoproteinaemia, particularly hypoalbuminaemia, will develop. Plasma bilirubin will usually not be elevated unless liver disease is also present, but mild jaundice is occasionally seen when a large haematoma or intra-abdominal haemorrhage is being reabsorbed.

Site of haemorrhage

Possible sites of chronic haemorrhage where the bleeding can go unnoticed by the owners are gut, urinary tract and skin (bloodsucking ectoparasites).

Intestinal bleeding is the most common. There may be altered blood in the vomit ('coffee-grounds' appearance), and blood will always be detectable in the faeces. If the lesion is low down in the large intestine this may be seen as obvious fresh blood, but more usually the lesion is higher up (stomach/small intestine) and so the blood is digested and appears in altered form as a black colour in the faeces, called melaena. This 'occult blood' can be specifically demonstrated by the guaiac acid paper test (see p. 173). Carnivorous animals can show false positives due to haemoglobin in the diet, and so ideally these should be put on a meat-free diet for 3 days before testing (although as the patient is often anorectic this is not always necessary). Licking of a superficial bleeding wound and swallowing coughed-up blood will also produce positive results. Lesions to look for are ulcers (single or multiple), bloodsucking endoparasites (e.g. hookworm), bleeding ulcerated tumours, etc. In addition, liver failure patients are frequently hypoprothrombinaemic, and this, combined with increased portal venous pressure, can produce diffuse intestinal bleeding.

Urinary tract bleeding is easy to demonstrate, as a urine sample will give a positive blood result on dipstix test. Where only small amounts are present it is possible to distinguish whether this is due to blood cells (i.e. haemorrhage) or free haemoglobin (as a result of *haemolytic* disease) simply by examining the reagent patch for a stippled appearance (blood cells). However, where large amounts are present it will be necessary to centrifuge the sample and examine the sediment microscopically (see p. 304). Clinical conditions involved include severe chronic cystitis with bladder ulceration, and chronic bracken poisoning in cattle (a carcinogen in bracken leads to numerous small haemorrhagic, neoplastic lesions in the bladder). It is, however, quite unusual for enough blood to be lost from the urinary tract to cause anaemia in small animals.

A heavy infestation of bloodsucking ectoparasites (particularly lice and ticks, but fleas may also be to blame) should not be difficult to detect, but the owner may have treated the animal before presenting it, and so this should be suspected if the coat is poor and suggestive lesions are visible. It is surprising how severe an anaemia can result from a heavy flea infestation in cats, especially young kittens.

Intermittent intra-abdominal haemorrhage

This is a type of haemorrhagic anaemia which often presents differently from those discussed above. The animal (usually a dog, often a German shepherd dog) is presented with a typical history of anaemia (pallor, weakness, etc.), but even if no treatment is given it may recover almost miraculously by the following day. Several episodes of this nature may occur before one is severe enough to be acutely fatal. A blood sample taken when clinical signs are evident will show the typical low PCV and low plasma protein concentration of haemorrhage cases, but the red cell picture is often not particularly regenerative. A blood sample taken the following day may be absolutely normal, again often without signs of excessive regeneration. This is because blood lost into the abdomen will be reabsorbed (cells, protein and all) back into circulation within a day or so of the haemorrhage; therefore the bone marrow does not need to put in any special effort and the animal improves almost as if it had been given a blood transfusion. This is diagnosed by demonstrating frank blood (high PCV) on paracentesis. In addition, it is sometimes possible to recognize two distinct populations of red cells on a blood smear – one of very normal cells which have never left the circulation and one of misshapen and crenated cells which have been traumatized by their passage through the peritoneal cavity. The usual lesion involved is a haemangioma or haemangiosarcoma of an abdominal organ (often liver or spleen). More chronic cases often strongly resemble autoimmune haemolytic anaemia (AIHA), haematologically (see p. 22) – the red cell picture becomes regenerative but not especially hypochromic, as red cell components are not being lost from the body, while lysis of the more fragile reabsorbed cells can produce slight jaundice. Again the presence or absence of demonstrable blood on paracentesis is often the most important diagnostic criterion.

Treatment is by surgical removal of the tumour; this is comparatively easy when the spleen is the site, but difficult to impossible for hepatic lesions. It is unwise to assume that a tumour is a haemangiosarcoma simply on macroscopic appearance, as other lesions can look very similar. As the prognosis varies so much (very poor for haemangiosarcoma, often very good with benign lesions) it is important to identify the precise nature of the tumour histologically.

Chronic haemolytic anaemia

In many conditions the distinction between acute and chronic haemolytic anaemia is not at all clear-cut, the former being simply a more severe manifestation of the same basic problem; for example, severe *Haemobartonella felis* infection may present as acute haemolytic anaemia while a milder case may present as chronic haemolytic anaemia.

Red cell morphology

With the single exception of some cases of autoimmune haemolytic anaemia (AIHA) in dogs, small animals with haemolytic anaemia will also show a regenerative cell picture (see Plate 8). This can to some extent be distinguished from haemorrhagic anaemia by the fact that quite markedly misshapen cells may be seen even from the early stages of the condition, in particular crenated cells are typical (but remember that an old or mishandled blood sample will also contain crenated cells). As the condition progresses there is no loss of blood constituents from the body and so signs of bone marrow exhaustion do not appear.

Other haematology

In haemolytic anaemia, particularly in infectious cases, neutrophilia and/or monocytosis may occur. Other than this (and the red cell abnormalities) the haematology findings will be normal.

Biochemistry

As there is no loss of plasma from the body, plasma protein concentrations will not be reduced; in fact globulin concentrations are often increased. In chronic haemolytic cases free haemoglobin does not appear in the plasma and even jaundice is mild or absent. This is because in these less severe cases the release of haemoglobin is slower and can be coped with by the reticulo-endothelial system without large accumulations of bilirubin developing. Again, all the excess bilirubin will be unconjugated (i.e. albumin-bound), but in spite of this some bilirubin usually appears in the urine.

Causes of chronic haemolytic anaemia

These can be divided into four groups.

(1) *Infectious*. Consider less severe cases of the conditions listed on p. 17, also equine infectious anaemia, a viral disease of horses not present in the UK but fairly common in North and South America – imported horses are tested for this (by the Coggins' immunodiffusion test) but it should be suspected in horses recently imported or in contact with a recent import.

(2) *Toxic*. Toxins which may be involved include lead (which competes with iron and leads to the formation of fragile cells), and the brassicas (particularly kale and rape, which contain a compound which is converted in the rumen to dimethyl disulphide, which precipitates haemoglobin leading to a Heinz body anaemia). Post-parturient haemoglobinuria in cattle may also be related to brassica poisoning.

(3) *Ag/Ab reactions*. The only chronic disease of this type is *auto-immune haemolytic anaemia* which is virtually unheard of in species other than dogs, man and (less commonly) cats, but which seems to be becoming increasingly common in the canine population. There is some breed predisposition, particularly spaniels (especially springers) and Old English sheepdogs, and a degree of sex predisposition – more females than males seem to be affected. Most cases are around 2–8 years old on first presentation. Speculation that the apparently increasing incidence of the condition might be linked to increasing vaccine challenge of dogs with more and more antigens appears to be unfounded.

  AIHA can occasionally be very acute in onset, but is more commonly progressive over several days or weeks. The slower the onset the less likely the patient is to be jaundiced – gradual onset cases usually show no jaundice at all, but even acute cases are often only slightly yellow, certainly much less icteric than cases of liver disease. The anaemia can be very severe, as bone marrow regeneration is often insufficient to prevent continued deterioration. Other important presenting signs are persistent pyrexia and splenomegaly.

  Red cell morphology can vary considerably in this condition. Some cases show very marked regeneration, similar to that seen in a haemorrhagic condition but without signs of hypochromasia. However, many cases demonstrate only moderate regeneration, less marked than would be expected considering the severity of the anaemia, and a subset of dogs are presented with apparently non-regenerative anaemia which is often very severe. Abnormal erythrocyte forms are often visible – spherocytes in particular, also folded cells, cup/bowl cells, target cells, and occasional microcytes and poikilocytes. There may be cells with 'punched-out' centres which look hypochromic although the MCHC is not reduced. There is often a concurrent neutrophilia, and platelet count may be reduced or occasionally low – AIHA and auto-immune thrombocytopenia are closely related conditions and most cases are, in fact, attacking both erythrocytes and platelets, though to different degrees.

Plasma biochemistry usually reveals normal or only slightly depressed albumin concentration, and globulins may be slightly elevated. Slightly increased bilirubin concentration may be seen in the more acute-onset cases, but if haemolysis is gradual (as is often the case) then bilirubin will be normal. A Coombs' test should be performed on a blood sample collected *before* steroid treatment is initiated, as corticosteroids will cause a negative result. A positive result in suspicious circumstances may be taken as confirming the diagnosis, but some genuine AIHA cases are in fact Coombs' negative. The anti-nuclear antibody (ANA or SLE) test can sometimes be helpful in this situation, and is less affected by prior steroid treatment.

When a dog presents with severe regenerative anaemia, particularly if it is of the right age group, the first step is to search carefully for clinical evidence of haemorrhage (internal as well as external). If none can be found, AIHA is at the top of the list of differential diagnoses, and a presumptive diagnosis may be justifiable in many cases. There are, however, a few alternatives to bear in mind. Congenital conditions (inborn errors of metabolism) should be considered in breeds where these are known to occur – phosphofructokinase (PFK) deficiency in the English springer spaniel is the most obvious one (see p. 24). Thanks to the relaxation of the UK quarantine restrictions, parasitic diseases such as ehrlichiosis, babesiosis and leishmaniasis also have to be excluded.

A related condition which is comparatively unusual is *cold agglutinin disease*. In this condition autoagglutination and haemolysis only occur at temperatures below 37°C. The consequence is that anaemia is only mild, but dogs (and very occasionally cats) present in cold weather with necrosis and sometimes sloughing of the ear tips and the end of the tail. The paws may sometimes be affected also. Confirmation of diagnosis is by the 'cold agglutinin test' which is simply two Coombs' tests, one performed at 37°C and the other at 4°C – affected animals give a negative result at the higher temperature and a positive result at the lower.

The treatment is oral prednisolone at a dose rate of 2 mg/kg/day in two divided doses. The dog may take 4–14 days to respond but the response, when it comes, is often dramatic. The reticulocyte count goes up to around 30% and the PCV subsequently increases very quickly. In severe cases which take a little while to respond, a blood transfusion (packed red cells are even better than whole blood) is usually necessary to buy time to allow the prednisolone to take effect. Transfusion should be considered when the PCV falls below 0.10–0.12, depending on the clinical condition and the rate of PCV decrease. It is safer to begin treatment before transfusion so that the recipient is immunosuppressed before donor cells are encountered. While on prednisolone treatment, plasma ALT and ALP should be monitored to check for liver damage, as this dose rate is high enough to lead to steroid hepatopathy in a proportion of cases. This is reversible when prednisolone is withdrawn. Once PCV has increased and stabilized at a normal level, reduce prednisolone dosage *very* gradually over about a month (a faster reduction may be necessary if hepatic problems are encountered) and withdraw entirely. Some patients may never relapse. However, a sizeable proportion suffer repeated relapses and owners should be warned to be alert for early signs. These dogs usually respond to a repeat of prednisolone treatment, but it is probably wise to maintain such animals on a low dose permanently as this reduces the risk of relapse. Other therapeutic measures which have been advocated are azathioprine (for cases which do not respond to prednisolone) and splenectomy, as the site of haemolysis is said to be in the spleen. Anabolic steroids may also be of some help. Recently it has been suggested that there may be advantages to treating all cases with a combination of prednisolone and azathioprine (also at 2 mg/kg/day) from the outset, but this practice is not yet widespread due to the difficulty of handling azathioprine and the frequently good clinical response to prednisolone alone.

(4) *Congenital.* Certain inborn errors of metabolism, especially those involving enzymes relating to glycolysis and the Krebs' cycle, may present as episodes of haemolysis which are often associated with strenuous exercise. DNA testing for many conditions under this heading is available in the USA.

Phosphofructokinase (PFK) deficiency is seen mainly in the English springer spaniel, though there are reports involving American cocker spaniels and mongrels. Affected dogs may present as young adults (i.e. at approximately the same age as AIHA cases) and the springer spaniel features prominently in both conditions. However, PFK deficiency is usually a milder illness and animals will recover spontaneously without immunosuppressive treatment. Episodes of haemolysis are related to exercise; there is pyrexia, haemoglobinuria, pallor and sometimes jaundice. Exercise intolerance and muscle cramps (leading to high plasma CK activity) may also be noted, and the owner may report episodes of discoloured urine in the past. The condition is self-limiting with rest, and seldom life-threatening.

Pyruvate kinase (PK) deficiency is traditionally thought of as a condition of the Basenji dog, but it has also been reported in the West Highland White terrier, the Beagle and some breeds of cats (Abyssinian, Somali and domestic short hair). Once again the defect in energy metabolism leads to erythrocyte fragility, and a chronic, extremely regenerative anaemia. Dogs also develop skeletal lesions (osteosclerosis and myelofibrosis) and liver failure, and most die before the age of 4 years. Cats do not seem to develop these complications and may have a normal life expectancy.

Congenital porphyria is an uncommon condition encountered in several breeds of cattle which has also been reported in pigs and cats. This condition involves a block in haemoglobin synthesis giving rise to a deficiency of protoporphyrin III. As a result, abnormal quantities of uroporphyrin and coproporphyrin accumulate in the body, leading to pink pigmentation of the teeth, bones and urine. Clinical signs are photosensitization, poor growth, spontaneous fractures and a very regenerative anaemia with a markedly reduced red cell lifespan.

Hypoplastic/aplastic anaemia

By its very nature, this condition is always gradual in onset. Appreciation of the degree of severity is particularly important, as there is a great deal of difference between a mild bone marrow suppression which is secondary to some other disease, and primary bone marrow aplasia.

Red cell morphology

This varies to some extent with the particular condition involved, but is usually characterized by a complete absence of juvenile cells, with the adult cells sometimes showing marked abnormalities. Microcytes and hypochromic cells are often a feature, as are poikilocytes (misshapen cells) and leptocytes (cells where the area of cell membrane is too big for the amount of haemoglobin inside, leading to the adoption of odd shapes – folded cells, cup bowl cells and target cells). This can be distinguished from the secondary bone marrow exhaustion of chronic haemorrhage by the absence of polychromatophilic cells or reticulocytes.

Other haematology and biochemistry

These are specific to the various conditions involved.

Causes of hypoplastic anaemia

These may be divided into three main groups:
(1) Nutritional deficiencies:
    (a) Protein deficiency. Underfed animals are usually slightly anaemic (and

hypoalbuminaemic) – remember, haemoglobin is mostly protein. However, the malnutrition has to be quite prolonged for this effect to be apparent.

(b) *Mineral deficiencies* may also be involved, particularly iron, also copper and cobalt. Iron deficiency is, however, blamed for far more anaemia cases than it actually causes. In reality the only animals likely to be iron deficient are young animals on a milk-only diet (milk is very poor in iron) and which are prevented by husbandry conditions from access to their natural iron source, the soil. Specifically, this refers to intensively housed piglets (and veal calves) and these should be treated with i/m injection of iron dextran. Adults may develop iron deficiency as a result of chronic haemorrhage, but otherwise this will only occur in animals subjected to extreme starvation or in patients with severe malabsorption of iron, as dietary levels of iron in both carnivores and herbivores are more than adequate. The anaemia of protein and mineral deficiency is usually microcytic and hypochromic.

(c) *Vitamin deficiencies* are another possibility: B_{12}, folic acid, niacin, pyridoxine, thiamine or riboflavin may all be involved. B_{12}/folic acid deficiency also involves malabsorption; this can occur in dogs, and has been postulated in stabled horses (which seem to absorb these vitamins much less efficiently than grazing horses). However, it is unlikely that this equine peculiarity is severe enough to cause any appreciable anaemia. B_{12}/folic acid deficiency causes a red cell maturation arrest at the basophil erythroblast stage and so, unusually for a hypoplastic condition, the MCV is often increased (known as 'true macrocytic anaemia', as opposed to the macrocytosis of regenerating conditions, which is 'transitory').

Nutritional deficiency anaemia is usually mild and very seldom severe, and is not usually seen in animals on a good quality diet. However, animals whose athletic performance is disappointing are often treated with 'haematinics', nutritional supplements designed to correct a supposed slight anaemia which is blamed for the poor performance. The usefulness of these treatments is doubtful – most slow horses and greyhounds are not anaemic, just slow! A very 'laid-back' horse may appear to have a lower resting PCV than an excitable one, and this may have some correlation with performance – nevertheless, the placid horse is not anaemic, simply not undergoing splenic contraction so readily.

(2) *EP depression secondary to disease.* A variety of conditions can be involved.

(a) *Chronic renal disease* produces a primary EP deficiency as EP is produced by the kidney. The anaemia is initially normocytic, normochromic, but becomes microcytic as the condition progresses. In older animals the anaemia is often only mild, but young growing animals with chronic renal failure (often congenital) may present with severe anaemia before signs of the renal problem become obvious. Treatment with EP can have a dramatic effect on the PCV in these cases, but it is of no benefit to the underlying renal condition.

(b) *Hormonal disorders* where there is a deficiency of a hormone which usually stimulates EP production produce a fairly mild, normocytic, normochromic anaemia. The most common examples are hypothyroidism and Addison's disease; however, it should be borne in mind that the dehydration present in untreated Addison's disease will usually mask the underlying anaemia when the case is first presented.

(c) *Chronic debilitating disease* will also lead to a fairly mild, normocytic, normochromic anaemia. Examples are chronic infections, neoplasia, and some parasitic infections even when not bloodsucking (e.g. trichostrongylosis). Cats are particularly prone to developing anaemia secondarily to other disease conditions. A slightly different situation is seen in cases of neoplasia where there is tumour infiltration of the bone marrow (usually leukaemia/lymphosarcoma) when the anaemia may be very severe and can occasionally be slightly regenerative if there is some relatively healthy marrow which is trying to compensate.

Note that while nutritional supplements will be effective in cases of nutritional deficiency anaemia they will be quite ineffective in cases of secondary EP deficiency (or indeed of true aplasia) as they will simply not be utilized.

(3) *True aplastic anaemia* is a serious condition in which the entire bone marrow simply shuts down. Due to the different lifespans of the different cell types, the granulocytes (neutrophils, eosinophils and basophils) and platelets are affected first. Patients which present at this stage show severe pyrexia (due to lack of neutrophils) and haemostatic problems (due to lack of platelets). Total white cell and platelet counts will be very low, and most of the white cells which are present will be lymphocytes. PCV may simply be in the lower part of the normal range, but even if there has been substantial haemorrhage there will be no evidence of red cell regeneration. Some animals die at this stage, or are so severely ill that euthanasia is the only course open, but patients which survive this stage (and some in fact go through it without showing any symptoms, usually the ones in which the granulocyte and thrombocyte lines are less severely affected than the erythrocyte line) present as severe, progressive non-regenerative anaemia. Again granulocyte and platelet counts will be very low, and this is the best way of differentiating bone marrow aplasia (in dogs) from non-regenerative cases of AIHA, as in AIHA cases, even if there is no erythrocyte regeneration and a concurrent thrombocytopenia, the white cell count will be normal or even raised.

Factors which have been implicated in bone marrow aplasia are irradiation, acute bracken poisoning (in addition to the carcinogen mentioned above bracken contains a radiomimetic factor – these may actually be the same substance) and certain drugs. Oestrogen preparations are the most frequently implicated (used therapeutically for misalliance, urinary incontinence and prostatic hyperplasia) but the toxic effect is almost entirely confined to dogs and ferrets, also phenylbutazone (non-steroidal anti-inflammatory) and chloramphenicol (antibiotic). In the case of oestrogens the effect is individual and not particularly dose-related, so that a dose which has been used in many patients with no untoward effect may result in complete aplasia in one case. Introduction of lower-dose oestradiol regimes for misalliance and, more recently, the use of oestriol as an alternative have addressed this to some extent, but a degree of concern may still be justified. It is therefore wise to warn bitch owners that misalliance injections are in no way a safe substitute for contraception, and where long-term oestrogen treatment is instituted the dose should be as low as possible and the patient's haematology regularly checked for any sign of toxicity. The susceptibility of human bone marrow to phenylbutazone is such that the drug has been banned in human medicine, but animals usually seem less susceptible. Horses in particular do not appear to develop aplastic anaemia as a result of phenylbutazone; the toxic effect in this species is ulceration of the small intestine leading to protein-losing enteropathy and hypoalbuminaemia (see p. 77). Occasionally cases of bone marrow aplasia develop in the absence of any of these causative factors or any drug administration – unidentified 'toxins' have been suggested, but such cases are usually labelled idiopathic.

Blood transfusion will help bone marrow aplasia patients temporarily, and blood from a donor which has donated twice in fairly quick succession is said to be preferable (because it is high in EP). Testosterone and anabolic steroids may also be helpful, but as adverse drug reaction is often involved in the aetiology it may be best to avoid drug treatment as much as possible. There is, however, no reliable way to kick aplastic bone marrow back into action and severe cases are usually eventually fatal.

Summary, differentiation of the causes of anaemia

Acute

(1) Haemorrhagic (blood loss usually obvious).
   (a) Traumatic (obvious signs of trauma, clotting normal).
   (b) Ruptured neoplasms (blood on paracentesis).
   (c) Warfarin poisoning (no evidence of trauma, clotting and prothrombin times increased).
(2) Haemolytic (low PCV with free haemoglobin and/or unconjugated bilirubin in plasma, patient becomes jaundiced, haemoglobinuria).
   (a) Infectious.
   (b) Toxic.
   (c) Ag/Ab reactions.

Chronic (gradual onset)

(1) Haemorrhagic (regenerative red cell picture, signs of bone marrow exhaustion – platelet count often abnormal, usually high, occasionally very low – hypoproteinaemia, hypoalbuminaemia, usually no jaundice).
  (a) Intestinal (occult blood in faeces).
  (b) Urinary tract (haematuria, erythrocytes in urine sediment).
  (c) Bloodsucking ectoparasites.
(2) Haemolytic (regenerative red cell picture except in some cases of AIHA, crenated cells, not usually hypochromic – platelets usually normal – plasma proteins normal or high, bilirubin may be elevated).
  (a) Infectious.
  (b) Toxic.
  (c) AIHA (dogs, erythrocyte picture may be non-regenerative, bilirubin usually normal, thrombocytopenia may also be present – positive Coombs' test, often positive ANA test).
  (d) Congenital (PFK, PK deficiency, congenital porphyria, etc.).
(3) Hypoplastic/aplastic (non-regenerative red cell picture, often microcytic, hypochromic, leptocytes present).
  (a) Nutritional deficiencies – protein, minerals, vitamins. Mild to moderate anaemia.
  (b) EP depression secondary to other disease – renal failure, hormone deficiency, chronic debilitating disease. Also mild to moderate anaemia, usually normocytic, normochromic.
  (c) Neoplastic infiltration of bone marrow.
  (d) True aplastic anaemia (granulocytes and platelets also very much reduced) – irradiation, bracken poisoning, oestrogens/other drugs. Severe to very severe anaemia.

Terms used to describe erythrocyte morphology

Size

(1) *Macrocyte*: unusually large cell. Usually a juvenile cell, also polychromatophilic.
(2) *Microcyte*: unusually small cell. Usually a sign of bone marrow problem.
(3) *Anisocytosis*: variation in size of cells is unusually great.

Colour

(1) *Hypochromic*: very pale coloured cell, particularly in the centre. Due to low intracellular haemoglobin concentration.
(2) *Annulocyte*: extreme form of hypochromic cell. Reduced to a narrow ring of haemoglobin with nothing in the middle.
(3) *Polychromatophilic*: cell takes up blue stain as well as red, giving a mauve/purple appearance. Juvenile cells.

Shape

(1) *Crenated*: cells appear 'crinkle-edged'. Seen in old samples, also normally in pig blood even when fresh. Extensive crenation typical of some acute haemolytic conditions.

(2) *'Star' or 'burr' cell*: these appear to have spikes protruding from the circumference. Also typical of old samples.

(3) *Poikilocyte*: irregular pear-shaped cell, often microcytic, seen in a number of chronic anaemia conditions, e.g. 'tear-drop' cell.

(4) *Spherocyte*: cell lacking the normal biconcave disc shape. Typical of AIHA.

(5) *Leptocyte*: cell with too much membrane area for its size, resulting in folds and clumping of haemoglobin, e.g. folded cell, target cell, cup/bowl cells. Typical of bone marrow problems and AIHA.

Inclusion bodies

Take care not to confuse stain debris on the slide (very common) with inclusion bodies or red cell parasites.

(1) *Nucleated cell*: even younger than polychromatophilic macrocyte. Looks a bit like a lymphocyte but nucleus is smaller and denser, cytoplasm is more abundant and pink-tinged.

(2) *Howell–Jolly body*: blue dot in cell, a nuclear remnant (chromatin), occasional error in cell maturation. Commoner in very regenerative samples.

(3) *Heinz body*: another blue dot, this time precipitated haemoglobin. Common in cats (feline haemoglobin is naturally unstable) and in splenectomized animals (Heinz bodies are usually extruded from the cell in the spleen). Otherwise excessive numbers indicate an unstable haemoglobin.

(4) *Basophilic stippling*: multiple blue dots. Especially typical of the abnormal haemoglobin formed during chronic lead poisoning, also seen in red cell regeneration in ruminants.

Red cell parasites

(1) *Haemobartonella (a.k.a. Eperythrozoon)*: small cocco-bacillus, lives on the cell membrane, not in the cell. Acridine orange stain demonstrates it best; Giemsa is also used. This parasite is easily misdiagnosed from stain debris, and so care is required. *H. felis* and *E. ovis* are the most common.

(2) *Anaplasma*: also small round bodies, this time inside the cell. Tropical disease, very uncommon in Britain.

(3) *Babesia*: several forms, *B. divergens* the most common; seen in cattle in tick-infested areas. Stage of parasitaemia is very early in clinical disease so may be missed if patient sampled too late.

Blood transfusion

Indications

(1)   To provide oxygen transport.
  (a)   In acute haemorrhage where more than two-thirds of blood volume
        is being lost. In less severe cases plasma expanders will be sufficient
        and even in very severe cases correction of hypovolaemia is usually
        more urgent than providing red cells.
  (b)   In acute haemolysis where PCV shows signs of falling below about
        0.15.
  (c)   In any chronic anaemia where PCV has fallen below about 0.10–0.12
        depending on the clinical condition.
  In (b) and (c) packed red cells are better than whole blood if facilities for
  separating transfusion packs are available. When giving whole blood to an
  animal which is not hypovolaemic, particularly if under anaesthetic, take
  care not to overload circulation as blood pressure may become dangerously high.
(2)   To provide clotting factors.
  (a)   In acute warfarin poisoning, fresh whole blood transfusion (con-
        taining prothrombin) will stop the haemorrhage faster than phyto-
        menadione (Konakion) can act, even by the i/v route.
  (b)   In severe thrombocytopenia cases, the platelets in the donor blood
        have the same effect.

Fresh plasma (platelet-rich plasma for (b)) will have the same effect, but, as
these cases are usually also anaemic due to haemorrhage, whole blood is
usually used.

Immunological considerations

In man, the AB red cell antigens are identical to antigens found on the surface of
commensal gut bacteria. Hence all individuals who do not have either or both
of these antigens on their red cells are already sensitized to them as 'foreign'.
Thus even the first transfusion of ABO-incompatible blood will be attacked and
a haemolytic transfusion reaction will occur. Fortunately this situation does not
occur in animals (except sometimes in cats), and the *first* transfusion an individual receives is relatively safe (so long as the donor is the right species, of
course). It is also worth remembering that the antibodies take some time to
establish, and that a second unmatched transfusion within 7 days of the first is
usually safe.

After this time, second and subsequent transfusions carry a risk which is
minimized by either cross-matching between donor and recipient (a simple but
time-consuming procedure) or blood typing both animals and only transfusing

from a donor with the same blood type as the recipient. Simple blood typing kits have recently become available for dogs and cats (Rapid-vet H).

Choice of donor (dogs)

Preferably a large dog, 40 kg or over, if a full unit (450 ml) of blood is required. Young adult/middle-aged animal, tractable and patient enough to sit still with his head at a slightly uncomfortable angle for about 15 minutes with only gentle restraint. Avoid wrigglers – the donor *cannot* be sedated as most sedatives lower the blood pressure. Also avoid animals with fussy or over-anxious owners – nobody can avoid haematomas *every* time. Greyhounds are particularly good as they usually have a PCV of 0.50–0.65. If there is no suitable dog in the practice, (a) persuade your wife/husband/nurse to adopt one, (b) compile a register of clients with suitable dogs who are willing to volunteer their pet (a poster in the waiting room will often do the trick). When a privately-owned animal is used as a blood donor it is essential that the procedure be clearly explained to the owner, who should sign an appropriate consent form – this applies equally to animals owned by employees of the practice. The use of dogs presented for euthanasia is ethically somewhat dubious unless express permission has been given, and has the additional disadvantage of encouraging the use of stored, even outdated blood, when this is often not in the best interests of the patient.

Collection procedure (dogs)

Requirements are: three people (two at a pinch), a dog gently restrained in sitting position on non-slip table, about 1 ml of local anaesthetic with a 25G needle to inject it, commercial blood pack with suitable anticoagulant (citrate/phosphate/dextrose (CPD) is slightly better than acid/citrate/dextrose (ACD)) and 16G needle attached; special blood collection scales are optional but useful. Collect from the *jugular* vein. This is easier to visualize if some hair can be clipped off. Wipe the skin with spirit and allow it to dry. Inject a small amount of local anaesthetic s/c just over the vein (take care not to inject *into* the vein) and wait for a minute or two. The handler should hold the dog with its head raised and turned slightly away from the side of the venepuncture (see Fig. 16.3). The operator performs the venepuncture neatly (this may have to be done in two stages, i.e. skin first, then vein, as the needle is large) and holds the needle in the vein. The helper should hold the blood bag as low as possible, always mixing gently to avoid coagulation, and checking constantly that the blood is still flowing well. (If the blood flow stops for longer than a few seconds the blood in the tube will clot as there is no anticoagulant there.) If there is no helper, the operator must raise the vein and hold the needle in place with one hand (or grow a third arm!) and be able to look in two directions at once. Keep going until the bag is full. When the needle is withdrawn the handler should immediately apply pressure to the site of the venepuncture and keep it there for 5 minutes. Tie a knot in the collection tube near the bag, cut off the needle distal to the knot and dispose of it safely. The donor must *not* be allowed to pull against a collar for several hours (haematomas are harmless unless infected, and disappear quickly, but they are unsightly). Make sure the donor has water available afterwards as the fluid loss will cause thirst, and avoid strenuous exercise for the rest of the day.

Note: if a small donor must be used to collect a small volume, aspirate 2 ml anticoagulant from a blood pack (discard this afterwards) into one (or each of several) 20 ml syringe and proceed as for collecting a 20 ml blood sample.

Storage of blood

Stored blood is adequate for use in cases of acute traumatic haemorrhage (i.e. surgery cases or accident victims) where there is no clotting defect involved. However, for all other cases, fresh blood is immeasurably preferable. This is because fresh blood cells have a much longer lifespan and so are capable of buying very much more time for a patient with a continuing disease condition. This extra time can make all the difference to the outcome in conditions such as AIHA where instant correction of the cause of the anaemia is not possible. The other main reason is that stored blood does not possess an active clotting mechanism and so, in any condition where clotting factors are required (such as warfarin poisoning), this will prove unsatisfactory. It is therefore best to arrange for blood to be collected as required, as collection only takes about 15 minutes if the donor is on the premises. This avoids any waste of volunteer donor blood and removes the temptation to use blood in store for cases where fresh blood is really required. However, if you really must store blood, the *maximum* storage time at +4°C is 21 days. Whole blood should *never* be frozen.

Administration

The technique is exactly the same as for giving i/v fluids except that a giving set with a filter included is necessary to intercept small clots. Aim to give up to 20 ml/kg. The maximum safe rate depends on the size of the recipient, but unless the patient is hypovolaemic slow administration is essential to avoid overloading the circulation. Make sure the cannula is firmly taped to the leg along with a loop of the distal end of the giving set (an extension tube is useful here); the patient should be restrained by a lead shorter than the free length of the giving set tube.

Non-canine species

Large animals present few problems as jugular veins are easily accessible, but larger quantities of blood are obviously needed. Cats are a different matter. Collection from the donor is the first problem due to the small size. A 50 ml syringe containing 5 ml CPD (aspirated from a blood pack) may be used to collect 40–45 ml blood from a donor under short-acting anaesthesia. Jugular venepuncture is not especially satisfactory as there is a limit to the size of needle which can be used (20G is the practical minimum), though a butterfly or other flexible cannula can help considerably. Cardiac puncture (left ventricle) is favoured by some, but carries a very significant risk of haemopericardium. Neither procedure is without risk to the donor and it is probably unreasonable to expect volunteers. This is perhaps one situation where it might be justifiable to use an animal presented for euthanasia provided you have the owner's permission and you are happy that the blood collected will be suitable for transfusion (normal haematology, negative for FeLV, FIV and *H. felis* and no evidence of other infectious condition), or alternatively a large practice may choose to keep a donor cat or two on the payroll. Again, such cats should test negative for FeLV, FIV and *H. felis*. The second problem is immunological, as transfusion reactions are not uncommon in cats even to the first transfusion, and it is therefore necessary to check blood types or cross-match before administration in all cases. This should normally be done before collecting the blood for transfusion. Obviously blood transfusion in cats is not a procedure to be taken lightly, and it is necessary to weigh up both the risks and the benefits before proceeding. There is a significant danger of simply ending up with two dead cats instead of one. However, the temptation to give dog blood to a cat should always be resisted, as the danger far outweighs any short-term benefit.

The Platelets (Thrombocytes) and the Coagulation Factors

For a mechanically strong, haemostatic blood clot to form it is necessary to have both a sufficient number of functional platelets and a complete set of coagulation factors. However, for the purposes of investigating bleeding disorders it is less complicated to consider these two aspects separately.

Platelets

Platelet appearance

Mammalian platelets appear on stained blood films as pale blue granular fragments which are usually considerably smaller than the red cells. They are anuclear. Because of their size they are often overlooked, but it is good practice to assess platelet numbers and morphology routinely on blood smears. Platelets may be seen on several of the colour plates. Avian and reptilian platelets are much larger than mammalian platelets, though still smaller than the red cells, and they are true cells with nuclei (see Plate 12).

Platelet production (megakaryocytopoiesis)

Like erythropoiesis, this occurs in the bone marrow, and the stages of development are shown in Fig. 2.1. From stem cell differentiation to platelet production takes about 3 days. It appears that the megakaryocytes remain in the bone marrow to shed platelets and do not normally enter the circulation.

Circulating platelets

The numbers in circulation vary slightly with species, but are generally around $200-400 \times 10^9/l$. The main exceptions are the horse, where the lower limit of normal is about $90 \times 10^9/l$, and the goat where numbers as low as $50 \times 10^9/l$ are often found. About half as many again (one-third of the total platelet mass) are stored in the spleen, with constant dynamic exchange between circulating and stored platelets. In splenectomized animals the circulating platelet numbers

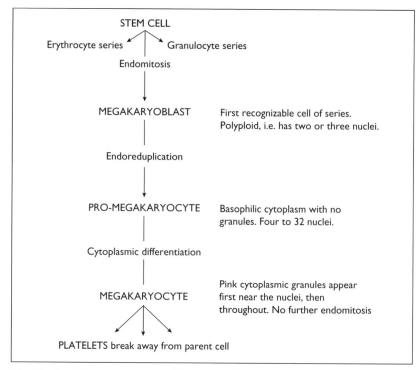

Fig. 2.1 Simplified representation of the stages of megakaryocytopoiesis.

increase by 50% because the total body stock of platelets remains the same and they are then all in circulation. Platelets survive for about 10 days.

Platelet function

(1) Normal running maintenance of the endothelium. Platelets are essential to maintain capillary endothelial integrity, and it appears that they are constantly being incorporated into the endothelium itself to perform this function. In cases of severe thrombocytopenia (platelet count under $20 \times 10^9/l$) the endothelium becomes weak and red cells may actually escape through the walls of intact uninjured capillaries. Petechiation, ecchymoses and even spontaneous haemorrhage then result.

(2) Repair of damaged endothelium. It is in this situation that the platelets function as an integral part of the clotting process.

    (a) An injury to the endothelium exposes underlying collagen and a single layer of platelets sticks to this (platelets do not normally stick to intact blood vessels).

    (b) Upon exposure of platelets to the collagen fibres of the vessel wall, serotonin, histamines and ADP are released into the ambient fluid ('platelet release'). The ADP causes adherence of the second platelet layer to the first and aggregation of a platelet plug.

(c) The plug retracts ('viscous metamorphosis') to form a mechanically strong patch which seals the hole. In time this is replaced by normal endothelium.

Platelet abnormalities

Thrombocytosis

(Increase in platelet numbers, i.e. platelet count greater than 500×10^9/l)

(1) Reactive. In haemorrhagic cases the consumption of platelets soon leads to an increase in circulating numbers via a feedback effect. Young platelets which are often very large are usually seen on a blood smear.
(2) Splenectomy. In splenectomized patients there is a redistribution into the circulation of the platelet mass normally stored in the spleen.
(3) Autonomous. Megakaryocytic leukaemia.
(4) Drug induced. Vincristine increases platelet shedding from the mega-karyocytes and may be used therapeutically for this purpose.

Thrombocytopenia

(Decrease in platelet numbers, i.e. platelet count less than about 200×10^9/l in most species)

(1) Functional. In the early stages of a haemorrhagic condition when demand is great but bone marrow production has not yet responded, a low platelet count will be seen.

Note: Spontaneous haemorrhage will not occur as a *result* of thrombocytopenia until the platelet count is less than 20×10^9/l. Therefore when a platelet count of $20-200 \times 10^9$/l is found in a haemorrhaging patient this is probably a functional thrombocytopenia and another cause for the bleeding should be sought. Normally these cases progress to a reactive thrombocytosis within 3 days.

(2) Thrombotic/thrombocytopenic purpura, disseminated intravascular coagulation (DIC) or consumption coagulopathy. This is a serious condition which is frequently fatal, and affected animals are invariably obviously systemically ill. The platelets are all used up in massive abnormal intravascular clotting so that few are left in peripheral blood – paradoxically, this may result in secondary haemorrhage. The intravascular coagulation is due to the release of tissue thromboplastin into the circulation and can be brought on by a number of triggering factors. The condition is fortunately quite rare in animals, but it may be associated with such things as persistent septicaemia, incompatible blood transfusion,

Case 2.1

A breeder presented a 6-year-old miniature pinscher dog, having noticed bleeding from the prepuce the day after the dog had mated a bitch. Examination revealed a 1 cm tear on the dorsum of the glans penis, but also widespread bruising of the mucous membrane of the glans. Oral mucous membranes were pale, and petechial haemorrhages were observed in the mouth. What is the most significant feature of the haematology report?

PCV		0.23	low
Hb		7.1 g/100 ml	
RBC count		2.64 × 10^{12}/l	
MCV		87.1 fl	high
MCHC		30.9 g/100 ml	
Total WBC count		13.6 × 10^9/l	
Band neutrophils	4%	0.5 × 10^9/l	
Adult neutrophils	81%	11.0 × 10^9/l	
Eosinophils	1%	0.1 × 10^9/l	
Lymphocytes	12%	1.6 × 10^9/l	
Monocytes	2%	0.3 × 10^9/l	

Film comment. RBC: moderately regenerative, slightly hypochromic
            WBCs: normal
            Platelets: none seen

Comments

The absence of platelets on the blood film is the most significant finding. The dog may well have been injured during the mating, but that is unlikely to explain the extent of the bruising, the petechiation in the mouth, or the severity of the anaemia. The probable diagnosis is autoimmune thrombocytopenia. It is possible that a degree of autoimmune haemolysis is also present, but it is also possible that the anaemia is a consequence of haemorrhage secondary to the haemostatic problem.

certain viral infections such as infectious canine hepatitis (ICH), neoplasia, obstetric complications and heat stroke. Treatment is by i/v administration of heparin, in addition to vigorous therapy directed at the underlying disease condition.

(3) Autoimmune, may or may not be accompanied by AIHA.

(4) Primary bone marrow suppression, e.g. bracken poisoning, drug sensitivity (e.g. oestrogens), see p. 27.

(5) Lymphosarcoma, in cases where the bone marrow is so severely infiltrated by neoplastic cells that everything else is crowded out.

(6) Equine infectious anaemia.

(7) Idiopathic, which is really an acceptable way of saying you have ruled out all the others and you don't know. Detailed specialist investigation may reveal more, e.g. congenital abnormality of the megakaryocytes.

Having said all this, in the dog, by far the commonest cause of thrombocytopenia is autoimmune disease, and this should always be the first suspicion. Treatment is as for AIHA (see p. 23).

Functional abnormalities (platelet count – and usually morphology – are normal, but some aspect of function is defective)

(1)   Hereditary conditions, the thrombasthenias and thrombopathias, are defects of platelet aggregation/clot retraction and platelet release, respectively. Several such conditions (e.g. Glanzmann's disease and Bernard–Soulier syndrome) are recognized in man, but they are rare in veterinary species. However, a condition of this type has been seen in basset hounds in the USA and the UK. This usually presents as intractable bleeding following surgery, including routine neutering operations. Von Willebrand's disease, which is also a hereditary problem of defective platelet function, does not strictly fall into this category as it is not caused by a defect in the platelets themselves; instead platelet function is impaired due to the absence of an essential plasma factor (see p. 42).

(2)   Acquired conditions are much more common in animals.

    (a)   Secondary to other disease situations, e.g. uraemia, liver disease, systemic lupus erythematosus (SLE), anaemias, leukaemias, myeloproliferative disorders.

    (b)   Drug induced, e.g. aspirin, phenylbutazone, other anti-inflammatories, promazine tranquillizers, oestrogens, plasma expanders, nitrofurans, sulphonamides, local anaesthetics, phenothiazines, live vaccines (also certain foods recognized in man). Most of these inhibit adhesive of platelets to sub-endothelium and/or platelet release, and are not usually serious.

Blood coagulation

Coagulation mechanism

The coagulation mechanism is a series of sequential activating steps where the substrate for each enzyme (or enzyme complex) is a pro-enzyme which becomes the active enzyme for the next stage of the reaction (Fig. 2.2). This functions as an 'enzymatic amplifier' so that a small stimulus at the beginning of the system can result in the production of large amounts of fibrin at the end. The system can be modified by negative or positive feedback. The sequence of reactions is usually referred to as a 'waterfall' or 'cascade', but it may be more helpful to consider it as a chain (or rather two converging chains) of dominoes set up to fall in sequence at the slightest touch. Thus the effect of amplification of the initial stimulus and the consequence of a missing domino can be appreciated.

The coagulation reaction can be initiated in two different ways – the

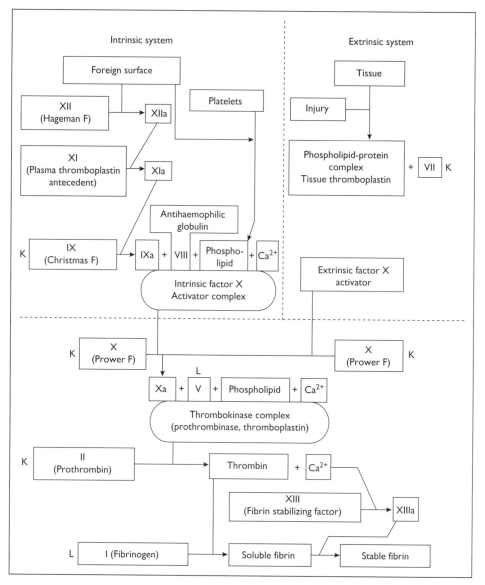

Fig. 2.2   Scheme of the coagulation system. An 'a' after the number of a factor indicates the activated form of that factor; for example, IXa is activated factor IX. K = factors requiring vitamin K for their synthesis; L = factors synthesized in the liver, not needing vitamin K.

exposure of the plasma to a foreign surface (intrinsic system) and the release of 'tissue thromboplastin' from injured tissue (extrinsic system). Fibrin produced by this system forms at the periphery of the initial platelet plug, and the platelet–fibrin mass subsequently grows, becomes covered by a cap of fibrin, and then contracts to produce a permanent seal. Thrombin itself is important in inducing aggregation of platelets and viscous metamorphosis.

Anticoagulants

The prevention of blood clotting is important when collecting blood for hae-matology, plasma harvesting, or for transfusion, and occasionally for the treatment of patients suffering from excessive coagulation, e.g. thrombosis or disseminated intravascular coagulation. Many of these anticoagulants involve the removal of calcium from the sample, e.g. *oxalate* (precipitates calcium as an insoluble salt), *EDTA* and *citrate* (chelate calcium). Citrate and its derivatives are useful where reversible action is required, e.g. for clotting tests (the plasma will clot when excess calcium is added) and for transfusion (citrate is metabolized by the liver). *Heparin* is a naturally occurring acid mucopolysaccharide found in liver, lung and intestinal mucosa, which interferes with thrombokinase for-mation and with the thrombin–fibrinogen reaction. It is used *in vitro* to prepare plasma for routine biochemistry and *in vivo* to treat DIC, and hyperlipidaemia in horses. It is also useful in eliminating lipaemia in dogs and cats where this is preventing biochemical analysis. (see p. 256). *Coumarin*-type anticoagulants are effective only *in vivo* by antagonizing vitamin K, so preventing the synthesis of prothombin (and also, to a lesser extent, of factors VII, IX and X). They are used as rat poison (e.g. warfarin) and therapeutically to treat navicular disease in horses and various types of thrombosis in man.

When collecting blood samples (or blood for transfusion) into anticoagulant, many people express surprise at the fact that blood which is clearly still liquid when it is mixed with the anticoagulant may be found clotted 10 minutes later. This is explained by the fact that while it may take 4 or 5 minutes for the whole row of dominoes to fall (and the clot to form), many anticoagulants act on a 'domino' which is very early in the chain, and if the cascade has passed this point before the blood encounters the anticoagulant then the reaction will go to completion regardless. Heparin, which acts very late in the chain, causes fewest problems in this respect, but in general the aim should be transfer of blood to the anticoagulant tube within a very few seconds of collection, ensuring that it is mixed immediately.

Clotting defects

One of the results of having so many factors involved in the clotting mechanism is that there are many opportunities for things to go wrong, either genetically (where a particular factor is either deficient, completely absent or present in a defective, inactive form) or as a result of disease.

Hereditary disorders

Many of the hereditary clotting deficiencies were first recognized in human patients, and animals with similar deficiencies have been used as experimental models for the study of the conditions more for their relevance to human haematology than for purely veterinary purposes. Some conditions are not yet recognized in animals at all (deficiencies of factors V, XIII, prekallikrein and high molecular weight kininogen). Animals known to have a heritable clotting defect are not normally allowed to breed unless for investigative purposes under laboratory conditions, and so some of these conditions are found only in laboratory-maintained lines and surface infrequently in the general population. However, the milder types of condition can go unnoticed for several genera-tions, and conditions associated with recessive genes (which is the case with nearly all such problems) are difficult to root out entirely. X-linked recessives are a particular problem as the progeny of an affected male will not themselves be affected. Thus hereditary clotting defects, while not common in animals, must always be considered where there is a history of a persistent haemostatic problem in a young animal. Clinical signs vary between conditions from the very severe (stillbirth, severe umbilical haemorrhage, recurrent haemarthrosis, early death) to mild (bruising tendency, haemostasis problems post surgery) or asymptomatic.

(1) Fibrinogen deficiency. Recorded in goats and dogs. This is generally severe, and homozygotes tend to die very young due to acute haemor-rhage.

(2) Prothrombin deficiency. Recorded (but very rare) in dogs. A milder syndrome with less severe bleeding in adults.

(3) Factor VII deficiency. Comparatively common in dogs, especially beagles. This is a mild disease with only some bruising tendency, and may be discovered during thorough 'routine' testing.

(4) Classic haemophilia (factor VIII deficiency). Occurs in dogs, horses and cats. Usually a severe disease which occurs only in males as the defective gene is an X-linked recessive. Most prevalent in the German shepherd dog due to a mildly affected male having been used extensively for breeding some years ago.

(5) Christmas disease (factor IX deficiency, also known as haemophilia B). Occurs in dogs and British shorthair cats. This is much rarer than classic haemophilia, and presents as a milder clinical disease.

(6) Factor X deficiency. Occurs in American cocker spaniels. Severely affected individuals appear to be 'fading puppies', while the milder disease shows as bruising tendency in adults.

(7) Factor XI deficiency. Occurs in cattle and dogs. This is usually mild but is associated with very severe bleeding after surgery – lethal haemorrhage can result from a minor surgical procedure.

(8) Hageman trait (factor XII deficiency). Asymptomatic, recognized in cats.

(9) Von Willebrand's disease. Occurs in pigs, dogs and rabbits. This is a multifactorial syndrome in which platelet function is impaired due to the absence of a necessary plasma factor. The clinical presentation varies from mild to lethal. This is the commonest inherited bleeding disorder in man and is not uncommon in certain breeds of dog including Dobermann pinschers and German shepherd dogs. It is not sex-linked.

Acquired disorders

Acquired coagulation disorders may occur at any age and usually do not present a great diagnostic problem as the possibilities are fairly limited. With the exception of warfarin poisoning, these disorders are secondary to quite severe systemic disease whose presence should be fairly obvious as such, quite apart from the clotting defect.

(1)   Warfarin poisoning or overdose. Deficiency of the vitamin K dependent factors, i.e. prothrombin and factors VII, IX and X, due to vitamin K antagonism, see p. 15.

(2)   Vitamin K deficiency. Vitamin K is a fat-soluble vitamin, and so patients with malabsorption or with a bile salt deficiency secondary to obstructive biliary disease may present with a clotting defect which is, in fact, identical to warfarin poisoning. Treatment is as for warfarin poisoning, but oral vitamin K will continue to be required so long as the primary clinical problem exists. This is what menadiol (vitamin K_3) is for; this formulation is more readily absorbed from the gut than phytomenadione (Konakion) in this type of patient.

(3)   Liver disease. The factors which require vitamin K for their synthesis (prothrombin and factors VII, IX and X), also fibrinogen and factor V, are all synthesized in the liver. Acute or chronic liver disease often results in a bleeding tendency, and coagulation tests which are relevant to these factors (e.g. prothrombin time) can be valuable in the diagnosis of liver failure. Vitamin K treatment tends to be much less effective. It is important that this aspect of liver failure be properly appreciated, as an exploratory laparotomy or a liver biopsy can have serious consequences if a clotting defect exists which has not been suspected prior to surgery.

Diagnosis of bleeding disorders

History and clinical presentation

It is usually possible to distinguish between hereditary and acquired problems on the basis of the history. A severe hereditary problem is nearly always evident early in life, and even milder cases usually have some history of previous episodes of bruising tendency or prolonged bleeding from minor wounds. The other common presentation is when a young, otherwise healthy animal develops intractable haemorrhage following routine surgery or an accident such as a deep cut.

Acquired problems can usually be divided into platelet-related conditions and coagulation factor disorders on the basis of clinical presentation. Platelet problems, of which autoimmune thrombocytopenia is by far the most common, usually present with marked petechiation and ecchymoses, with comparatively little actual haemorrhage. In contrast, coagulation factor deficiencies (warfarin poisoning in particular) generally show multiple haematomas and frank haemorrhage. The distinction is not absolute however – thrombocyto-penias sometimes show little more than a nosebleed, or can in severe cases look very much like warfarin poisoning on first examination.

Laboratory investigation

The first and simplest investigation in the practice is to check a blood film for the presence of platelets (see p. 294 and Plate 7b). Absence or virtual absence of platelets is a very strong pointer to a diagnosis of thrombocytopenia, though one should beware the very early case of something else (e.g. warfarin poisoning) where platelet numbers may be temporarily reduced due to sudden demand. The finding of adequate platelets on a blood film excludes thrombo-cytopenia for all practical purposes. By far the commonest cause of thrombocytopenia in the dog is autoimmune disease, and unless the pre-sentation is particularly unusual for this condition it may be reasonable to assume that this is what is going on and treat accordingly, rather than pursue specific autoimmune tests which are not particularly reliable in this condition and which often muddy the water more than they clarify the situation.

A clotting time should be performed at the same time as the blood film, preferably by the method detailed on p. 296. Simply observing the clotting of blood in a glass vial can be misleading, as sometimes this takes an inordinate time to clot even in a normal animal; however, if a sample like this clots in less than 5 minutes it is reasonable to assume that clotting time is normal. A normal clotting time rules out most of the cascade factor problems.

Clot retraction is another useful side-room test (see p. 297). Abnormal clot retraction will be seen in any type of platelet problem, including both thrombocytopenia and defective platelet function (including von Willebrand's disease). Bleeding time (see p. 299) gives similar information, and an abnormality points particularly to a platelet problem of some sort. It may be advisable to restrict the use of this test to cases which are not easily cate-gorized by other methods, as a severely affected animal may take quite some time to stop bleeding; nevertheless, in (for example) milder cases of von Willebrand's disease, this may be the only test which is abnormal. Clotting time, bleeding time and clot retraction obviously cannot be carried out on samples transported to a laboratory, so it is advisable to have the capability to perform these in the practice side-room.

In the majority of simple cases such as warfarin poisoning and autoimmune thrombocytopenia the above investigations can be quite adequate for initial case management. However, further investigation by the professional labora-tory is important for confirmation of diagnosis and monitoring progress. The minimum request should be for full haematology and prothrombin time, and note that it is *essential* to collect the sample for the latter (in a citrate tube) *before* administering any vitamin K to the patient. (Actual measurement of warfarin in a blood sample takes a long time and is usually reserved for post-mortem investigations, where of course measurement of prothrombin time is impossible.) Basic biochemistry tests are also useful to assess liver function etc. A suggested scheme for the rationalization of bleeding disorder diagnosis is shown in Fig. 2.3.

Precise diagnosis of hereditary bleeding problems, particularly the more obscure conditions, can be very difficult, and usually necessitates referring the patient to a specialist centre. However, an assay for von Willebrand's factor is available – but check sample requirements with your laboratory before sending in any material.

Treatment of bleeding disorders

Treatment specific to particular disease conditions

Certain of these have been discussed in more detail in earlier sections.

(1) *Warfarin poisoning and vitamin K deficiencies*: vitamin K (K_1 initially by injection in all cases, continuing oral treatment should be with K_1 for warfarin cases and K_3 for hepatic, biliary and malabsorption conditions).

(2) *Disseminated intravascular coagulation*: heparin. This is an anomalous case where an anticoagulant is used to treat as a condition which presents as a bleeding disorder. Vigorous treatment of the primary illness is also very important.

(3) *Autoimmune thrombocytopenia*: treatment is the same as for AIHA, i.e. immunosuppressive doses of prednisolone.

(4) *Hereditary deficiencies of clotting factors*: in man these conditions are treated by administration of the deficient factor purified from blood donations. This is impractical in animals because large, organized banks of non-human blood do not exist, and even if there were a surplus of the human factors these substances are antigenic across the species barriers. Treatment of severe disorders is usually pointless, but animals can live with the milder forms provided symptomatic treatment is given for bleeding episodes. There is one type of replacement therapy which might be attempted in cases of classic haemophilia or von Willebrand's disease, however. When fresh frozen plasma (separated from a blood donation) is thawed at $+4°C$ a 'cryoprecipitate' forms which contains concentrated factor VIII and fibrinogen. This precipitate can be separated and frozen, and is useful in the management of occasional acute bleeding episodes in patients with these two conditions.

Symptomatic and supportive treatment

(1) *Acute haemorrhage* should be treated in the usual way with plasma expanders, or whole blood if required to maintain the oxygen-carrying capacity of the blood. Haemorrhage arising during surgery may be controlled by diathermy, etc. Blood transfusion as a means of haemostasis (to

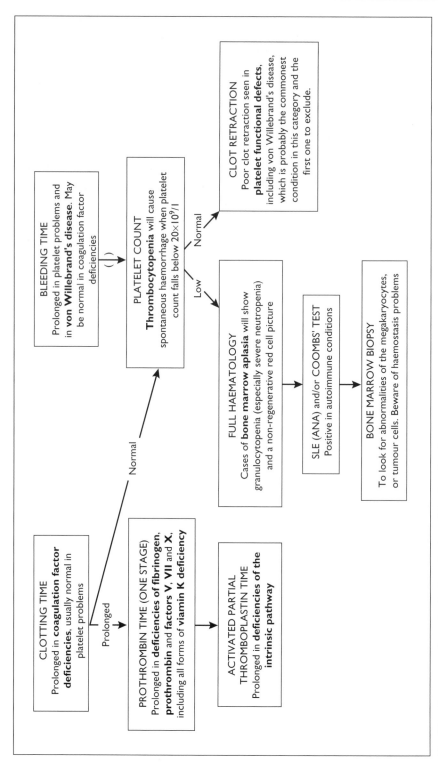

Fig. 2.3 Elementary scheme for the investigation of bleeding disorders.

provide clotting factors rather than red cells) is useful where platelets, prothrombin or fibrinogen are required; however, the very small amount of most of the other factors present in the donor blood means that no real benefit of this nature will accrue to, for example, haemophiliacs.

(2) *Chronic haemorrhage* often occurs in patients with clotting defects from lesions which would be very minor in normal animals. This can often be stopped by one dose of acetylpromazine, which lowers the blood pressure enough to stop the constant trickle of blood and allow some repair to take place. However, note that the promazine tranquillizers are among the drugs which interfere with platelet function, and so this strategy should be used with extreme caution, and no more frequently than once every 2 weeks. *Never* give ACP to a shocked or hypovolaemic patient, as the fall in blood pressure may be fatal.

Generally, patients known to have a coagulation abnormality should be, to some extent, 'wrapped in cotton wool'. Situations where bruising or injury may occur should be avoided, and very abrasive food should not be given. Avoid all non-essential surgery and in particular do not extract teeth unless these are already very loose. Avoid all drugs known to have an adverse effect on the clotting mechanisms.

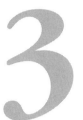

The White Blood Cells (Leucocytes)

General

The term leucocyte includes all white blood cells and their precursors. These cells use the bloodstream as a means of transport from their site of origin to the site in the tissues where they are required. The circulating numbers therefore reflect the balance between supply and demand, and usually range between about $5 \times 10^9/l$ and $14 \times 10^9/l$, depending to some extent on species. (Cats are often near the top of, or just above this range, while in pigs a white cell count of $20 \times 10^9/l$ or more is not unusual.) This range makes some allowance for what is known as 'physiological leucocytosis' which occurs during even moderate exercise, as white cells which have been sequestered in collapsed capillary beds during a period of rest are returned to the circulation.

The white cells can be divided into two basic categories – the *granulocytes* (or myelocytes) which include the neutrophils, eosinophils and basophils, and the *agranulocytes* which include the lymphocytes and monocytes.

White cell counting

The total white cell count is the primary measurement, and in some cases it may be sufficient to have this result alone. However, it is also absolutely essential to have a total white cell count before any attempt is made to make sense of a differential white cell count.

The differential white cell count is performed by examining a set number (usually 200) of white cells on a stained blood film and identifying them as neutrophils, lymphocytes, etc. The *initial* result is therefore expressed as a percentage. However, it is of no use whatsoever to declare that, for example, 90% of the white cells are neutrophils, unless the total white cell count is known. This is because the white cells tend to react independently to disease situations and the important figure for interpretation is not the percentage of a certain type of cell, which depends on how many of the other cell types are present, but the absolute number of that cell type in circulation. This is easily calculated from the total white cell count.

For example, to consider a bitch with pyrexia and polydipsia with a percentage differential white cell count of:

neutrophils   90%
eosinophils   3%
lymphocytes   5%
monocytes   2%

If the total white cell count is high, e.g. $28.6 \times 10^9/l$, the absolute numbers of the individual cell types are:

neutrophils $25.7 \times 10^9/l$
eosinophils $0.9 \times 10^9/l$
lymphocytes $1.4 \times 10^9/l$
monocytes $0.6 \times 10^9/l$

In this situation the eosinophils, lymphocytes and monocytes are more or less normal but the neutrophil count is extremely high.

However, if the total white cell count is low, e.g. $4.8 \times 10^9/l$, the same percentage differential count gives absolute values of:

neutrophils $4.3 \times 10^9/l$
eosinophils $0.1 \times 10^9/l$
lymphocytes $0.2 \times 10^9/l$
monocytes $0.1 \times 10^9/l$

In this situation the neutrophils, eosinophils and monocytes are more or less normal but the lymphocyte count is extremely low.

The clinical interpretation of these two situations is quite different. In the former case pyometra is an extremely probable diagnosis, while in the latter case the bitch does not have a pyometra and appears to be immunosuppressed for some reason.

Note that due to the uneven distribution of white cells on a manually-made blood film it is difficult to estimate the total white cell count from a blood film at anything better than a very rough guess. However, to an experienced eye this level of rough guess can be useful in an emergency.

Development of granulocytes

The granulocytes and monocytes develop almost exclusively in the bone marrow, and the stages of development are shown in Fig. 3.1. The lymphocytes develop mainly in the lymph nodes and spleen (and thymus in immature animals) and so are much less affected by a bone marrow aplasia, but under normal circumstances the bone marrow is also involved to a significant extent.

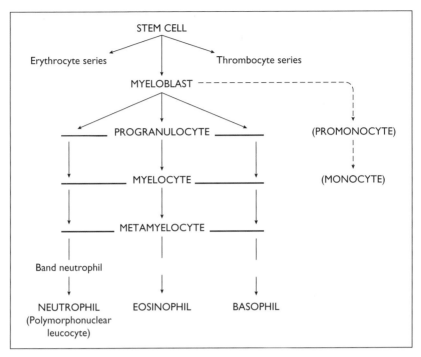

Fig. 3.1 Simplified representation of the stages of development of granulocytes and monocytes.

Neutrophils

Morphology

This has been studied in great detail including histochemistry and electron microscopy of the granules, but only a limited amount of this work has relevance to routine haematological examination.

Immature neutrophils (band cells) do not have a lobulated nucleus (see Plate 6a). The appearance of one indentation in the nucleus is enough to classify the cell as an adult, but the nucleus continues to become more and more pinched off into lobes as the cell ages and highly lobulated nuclei are characteristic of very mature cells, e.g. as a result of steroid influence reducing the removal of cells from the circulation. Failure of maturation of the nucleus is a rare hereditary condition in man called the Pelger–Hüet anomaly, where all the neutrophils appear as band forms. A few cases have been recorded in the dog. In the females of some species (including cats and dogs) a small proportion of neutrophils are seen to have a characteristic 'drumstick' lobe attached to the nucleus. This finding is not affected by spaying and is also seen in male tortoiseshell cats.

The cytoplasm of normal neutrophils is bluish in colour on a Leishman-type stain, with numerous dust-like pinkish granules (see Plates 2–5a). In generalized toxaemic conditions 'toxic neutrophils' can be seen in circulation with foamy, vacuolated cytoplasm and sometimes a scattering of blue granules (Döhle bodies). These appearances vary to some extent between species, and so a degree of experience is required when interpreting blood films.

Function and kinetics

Neutrophils function primarily as phagocytes and are particularly important in infectious conditions and in inflammation. Mature neutrophils are present in the body in three pools – the circulating pool, the marginal pool (comprising those neutrophils sequestered in inactive capillary beds) and the bone marrow pool. When there is a sudden demand for neutrophils this is initially met by mobilization of the bone marrow pool which can correct a neutropenia in a few hours, while for more long-term use more precursor cells differentiate to neutrophils. These cells take 4 – 6 days to mature and this cannot be speeded up.

Neutrophilia

This term refers to an increased number of neutrophils in circulation, over about $10 \times 10^9/l$ in monogastric animals or about $4 \times 10^9/l$ in ruminants. This can occur in a number of ways.

(1) A shift of cells from the marginal to the circulating pool – sometimes known as pseudo-neutrophilia as the total blood neutrophil pool actually remains unchanged. This occurs due to acute stress or exercise, and can be produced by injection of adrenaline.

(2) Steroid effects. In an acute steroid response there is an increase in circulating neutrophils due to a combination of decreased migration out of the blood vessels and increased mobilization of the bone marrow pool. In a chronic steroid response (e.g. prolonged therapy, intensive long-term athletic training, Cushing's disease) there is also increased neutrophil production.

(3) Response to infection. Initially the demand for neutrophils is met from the bone marrow pool, which in monogastrics is capable of releasing enough adult (and band) cells to produce a blood neutrophil count of up to twice the normal value within 1–2 days of the start of the infection. Increased neutrophil production is also stimulated, but these cells take about 4 days to reach the circulation. In chronic neutrophilia the half-life of the neutrophils is also prolonged, possibly because immature cells are released from the bone marrow and these cannot easily leave the circulation.

(4) 'Masked granulocytosis' refers to the situation which occurs during mild infections where, although the circulating neutrophil numbers are not increased, the size of the marginal pool is greater than normal. This is advantageous in that more neutrophils are available to enter the tissues in an early inflammatory response.

(5) Neoplasia. Myeloid/granulocytic leukaemia can be difficult to differentiate from a marked neutrophilia – sometimes the cells are all normal mature forms, or else the picture may be similar to a marked left shift. If a leukaemia is suspected, a bone marrow biopsy is essential.

Neutropenia

This term refers to a decreased number of neutrophils in circulation, under about $4 \times 10^9/l$ in monogastric animals or about $1 \times 10^9/l$ in ruminants. This can also occur in a number of ways and has in general been less well studied than the neutrophilias.

(1) Viral infection. This is the usual assumption where a neutropenia is demonstrated in a sick animal. It is often a correct assumption, as many viruses do cause this effect and some, such as feline parvovirus (feline infections enteritis, panleucopenia) and canine parvovirus, do so to a very marked degree. Cats with FIV often demonstrate a moderate to marked neutropenia. Horses with respiratory virus infections frequently show a moderate neutropenia, and this sometimes progresses to a post-viral malaise syndrome frequently characterized by neutropenia and hypo-globulinaemia (see p. 78). However, bear in mind that vague diagnoses of 'a virus infection' such as GPs hand out to human patients with upper respiratory symptoms are not necessarily justified in small animals. Dogs in particular suffer from a comparatively short list of viral ailments, most of which are well characterized, and if you can't put a name to the virus in question it is wise to consider other causes of neutropenia, in particular toxic insult (see point 3 below).

(2) Increased destruction of neutrophils in circulation. This may be the situation in cases of autoimmune neutropenia, an uncommon condition which is similar to AIHA but in which it is the neutrophils that are attacked by the autoantibodies.

(3) Increased movement of neutrophils into the marginal pool. This occurs shortly after endotoxin ingestion. This is the reason for the frequent finding of neutropenia in cases of food toxicosis in dogs and cats. The source of the toxin is generally the spores of bacteria (especially Clostridium perfringens) or fungi (e.g. Aspergillus nigrans or Mucor spp.) in contaminated food. Note that while (unsporulated) Clostridium perfringens is a normal (indeed necessary) component of normal bowel flora, the formation of the spore coat after passage of the organism in the faeces can produce a lethal toxin.

(4) Increased demand for neutrophils without compensatory inflow from the bone marrow. This can be the case during the first few hours of acute infection before the bone marrow has had time to respond, or in a chronic condition where the bone marrow is becoming totally exhausted. A neutropenia during infection is not uncommon in cattle as they appear to

have a smaller pool of neutrophil *precursors* in the bone marrow than, for example, dogs. Thus there can be a period of neutropenia occurring after the bone marrow pool of mature cells has been used up, before the increased production of neutrophils takes effect. This may explain the number of bovine (and ovine) cases where a neutropenia, usually regarded as a poor prognostic sign, is followed shortly by clinical recovery.

(5)   Decreased bone marrow production. A very marked neutropenia is a prominent feature of bone marrow aplasia (see p. 27), along with anaemia and thrombocytopenia. Radiation poisoning, radiotherapy and treatment with cytotoxic anticancer drugs produce a similar pattern. Protocols for cancer treatment allow periods of grace for the bone marrow to recover, and the dynamics of the situation are such that the effect on the neutrophil count tends to be the most dramatic feature. Bone marrow depression, principally presenting as neutropenia, is a recognised side-effect of carbimazole (Neo-Mercazole: Roche), used in the medical management of hyperthyroidism in the cat, but in practice the problem occurs relatively infrequently. Situations where the bone marrow is being taken over by tumour cells, e.g. some types of lymphosarcoma, will also lead to neutropenia, thrombocytopenia and anaemia. A 'cyclic neutropenia' has also been reported in silver-grey collies; this is a hereditary defect associated with the silver coat colour gene which results in cycles of neutrophil maturation arrest at the level of differentiation from the stem cell.

'Left shift'

This term refers to the appearance of immature neutrophils in circulation and refers to the 'Schilling index', a stylized table of blood morphology in which the immature cells appear on the left. During the early stages of a neutrophilia this is confined to the appearance of band cells, as no cells younger than that are stored in the bone marrow pool, but in more prolonged neutrophilias metamyelocytes or even younger may be released into the circulation. When a left shift accompanies a neutrophilia in this way it is known as a 'regenerative left shift' and is part of the normal response to acute infection. However, a left shift when neutrophil numbers are normal or decreased is a 'degenerative left shift'. This is most commonly a poor prognostic sign as it indicates that the bone marrow is unable to meet the demands being placed on it. However, in cattle a period of neutropenia with a left shift is common about 2–4 days into the course of an infection as described above and is not necessarily a poor prognostic sign.

Eosinophils

Morphology

Eosinophils appear very similar to neutrophils with the addition of very striking bright red cytoplasmic granules which appear to fill the whole cell (see Plates 2–5b). These are particularly prominent in equine eosinophils (see Plate 3b).

Function and kinetics

The major function of the eosinophils is detoxification by inactivation of histamine or histamine-like toxic materials. They also inhibit oedema production (stimulated by serotonin and bradykinin) and so are important in the allergic response, and they are capable of phagocytosis.

The bone marrow is again the major site of production of eosinophils although some production at other sites has been observed. The number of eosinophils in the blood is only a small fraction of the total number in the body. There are about 300 times as many in the bone marrow storage compartment, mostly mature, and about 100–300 times as many in the tissues, particularly skin, intestinal tract and lungs. The normal progression is that eosinophils randomly leave the bone marrow, spend some time in the bloodstream, and when they eventually enter the tissues they do not normally re-enter the circulation. Their lifespan from bone marrow to blood to tissues is around 8–15 days. Disturbances in circulating eosinophil numbers may be caused by various redistributions between these compartments as well as by alterations in production and destruction.

Eosinophilia

This refers to an increase in the circulating numbers of eosinophils. There is a diurnal variation in eosinophil numbers, and higher counts may be expected in samples taken at night. Normally there are about 0.5×10^9/l in circulation; an increase to over 1.0×10^9/l may be considered an eosinophilia. Contrary to popular opinion there are a number of causes of eosinophilia of which parasitism is only one – *eosinophilia is not synonymous with parasitism*.

(1) Allergy/hypersensitivity reactions. It is believed that the allergic response is, in fact, an antiparasite response becoming active in inappropriate circumstances or to gross excess; nevertheless, the allergic reaction is probably the most common cause of eosinophilia seen in routine small animal practice. Flea allergy is extremely common, and food allergies of various types probably the next most common. Food allergies in particular can manifest in a variety of ways such as dermatitis reactions (often around the eyes in cats) or eosinophilic enteritis. Contact dermatitis is another consideration, while atopic dermatitis (due to inhaled allergens) may not be as common as is sometimes supposed. Interestingly, there appears to be a relationship between eosinophilic enteritis and hyperthyroidism in the elderly cat.

'Hypereosinophilic syndrome' is the term given to extremely marked eosinophilias seen in the cat, often with juvenile (band) form eosinophils present. This is probably caused by a hypersensitivity reaction going completely over the top, and sometimes accompanies cutaneous eosinophilic plaques or rodent ulcers. Eosinophil counts can be very high, well over $10 \times 10^9/l$, and when figures of $50 \times 10^9/l$ are seen it can be difficult to say where hypereosinophilic syndrome ends and eosinophilic leukaemia begins. Some authors question whether the latter actually exists at all as a clinical entity, but where eosinophil counts of 90–100 $\times 10^9/l$ occur it is difficult to know what other conclusion to reach. Bone marrow biopsy may be helpful in resolving this question.

(2) Uncomplicated parasitism (without allergy). Eosinophilia occurs due to a sensitivity to the foreign protein of a parasite, which may be part of an immune phenomenon. Thus eosinophilia is likely to be seen when parasites are *migrating* through the tissues but need not be expected where they are, for example, free-living in the gut. Thus in addition to there being many causes of eosinophilia other than parasitism, not all parasitized animals will demonstrate an eosinophilia. While parasitism may be the first diagnosis to consider when encountering an eosinophilia in a large animal or a *young* (less than a year old) small animal, it is an uncommon cause in the adult dog or cat, and other causes should be considered in these animals.

(3) Tissue injury. Chronic eosinophilia is common in diseases of tissues which contain large numbers of mast cells, such as skin, lungs, gastrointestinal tract and uterus. Tissue injury leads to degranulation of mast cells and histamine release, and since histamine is chemotactic for eosinophils these are attracted from the bone marrow into circulation. Thus eosinophilia is not diagnostic of any single disease entity but is seen in a variety of conditions where chronic mast cell degranulation occurs. One study has demonstrated that pulmonary eosinophilic infiltrate is possibly the commonest cause of an initially unexplained eosinophilia in the dog.

(4) Mast cell tumours. Patients with a mast cell tumour often demonstrate an eosinophilia, especially cats. This is something to bear in mind when a cat with a palpable abdominal mass shows a marked eosinophilia.

(5) Alsatians (German shepherd dogs) and certain other large continental breeds frequently demonstrate quite marked eosinophilia in 'routine' blood sampling. This has sometimes been considered 'normal' for the breed but, in fact, this may not be the case. An allergic enteritis-type condition is very common in these dogs and it is quite possible that the 'normal' eosinophilia is in fact a reflection of subclinical disease.

(6) Oestrus. Eosinophilia has been noticed in a number of species during oestrus, particularly in bitches.

(7) Pregnancy/recent parturition. The canine placenta contains large numbers of eosinophils, and circulating eosinophilia is sometimes observed in association with the presence or recent presence of placentas *in utero*.

Case 3.1

A 2-year-old brown tabby domestic short hair cat was presented because of a raw, hairless area on the left side of the face. Examination revealed widespread erythematous skin lesions with broken hairs and a sparse hair coat. The haematology results shown below were received. What is the probable cause of the lesions?

PCV		0.34	
Hb		11.3 g/100 ml	
RBC count		$7.22 \times 10^{12}/l$	
MCV		47.1 fl	
MCHC		33.2 g/100 ml	
Total WBC count		$24.8 \times 10^9/l$	high
Band neutrophils	5%	$1.2 \times 10^9/l$	
Adult neutrophils	59%	$14.6 \times 10^9/l$	raised
Eosinophils	18%	$4.5 \times 10^9/l$	high
Basophils	5%	$1.2 \times 10^9/l$	high
Lymphocytes	10%	$2.5 \times 10^9/l$	
Monocytes	3%	$0.7 \times 10^9/l$	raised

Film comment. RBCs: normal
        WBCs: normal morphology
        Platelets: adequate

Comments

The eosinophilia and basophilia suggest an allergic reaction of some sort, and the facial lesion is likely to be an eosinophilic plaque. Although there is also evidence of inflammation and possibly infection, this is likely to be secondary. Flea infestation/flea allergic dermatitis is the commonest cause of this presentation, and although no fleas were seen on initial examination (perhaps due to the dark coat colour), coat brushings revealed flea faeces.

Eosinopenia

This refers to a decreased number of eosinophils in circulation, usually to below $0.1 \times 10^9/l$ or indeed where none at all are found during a differential white cell count. Although eosinopenia can be caused by adrenaline via a β-adrenergic reaction, the clinical causes of eosinopenia can nearly all be traced back to the action of corticosteroids. Glucocorticoids neutralize histamine and so reduce blood histamine levels. This causes eosinophils to remain in the bone marrow so that after those already in circulation have reached the end of their lifespan an eosinopenia develops which persists until blood histamine levels rise again. In addition, corticosteroids inhibit mast cell regranulation and so reduce histamine production even further, and prolonged exposure to corticosteroids will reduce bone marrow eosinophil production.

(1) Iatrogenic. Corticosteroid treatment is widely used in many disease situations, particularly where inflammation is involved. Patients being treated with corticosteroids (including, apparently, anabolic steroids as well as the more usual glucocorticoids) will naturally show an eosinopenia. It is most important to record such treatment on a haematology request form so that the laboratory knows how to interpret the results.

(2) Stress, including prolonged intensive athletic training. Acute stress causes increased catecholamine secretion and chronic stress causes increased corticosteroid secretion. Since both of these types of adrenal hormone cause eosinopenia, this is a common finding in stressed patients, for example greyhounds and racehorses in training, patients under anaesthesia, patients recently subjected to a stressful road journey, and patients stressed by severe pain or illness. Note also that most sight-hounds (greyhounds, whippets and related breeds) have lower eosinophil counts than other breeds of dog, even when not in training.

(3) Cushing's disease. This condition is essentially one of hyperadrenocorticism, i.e. overproduction of corticosteroids, particularly glucocorticoids. Most cases present with low (less than $0.3 \times 10^9/l$) or zero eosonophil counts, although if other features of the condition are strikingly present, the finding of a normal or even slightly increased count should not be taken as an absolute exclusion of the diagnosis.

Basophils

Morphology

Basophils again appear very similar to neutrophils, this time with the addition of dark blue cytoplasmic granules. These granules, although very prominent, are not so large or so numerous as those of eosinophils (see Plates 3 and 4d). Basophils are more often seen in some species than in others; for example, they are common in rabbit blood and quite often found in horse blood, but it is very rare indeed to see a basophil in a dog sample.

Function and kinetics

The basophil is closely related to the tissue mast cell and shares its function of releasing histamine-containing granules and thus initiating the inflammatory response (which is then modified and kept in balance by the eosinophils). Basophils are produced in the bone marrow and have a lifespan of about 10–12 days.

Basophilia

This refers to an increased number of circulating basophils, above about $0.5 \times 10^9/l$. It has been observed in hypothyroidism and during sensitization to an allergen or antigen, but in general basophils have been much less studied than other leucocytes (because there are so few of them around). Basophilia sometimes accompanies eosinophilia in the cat (and sometimes the horse) and appears to be part of the hypersensitivity reaction in this situation.

Basopenia

Since it is quite normal to find no basophils at all on a blood film the theoretical possibilities of basopenia are not worth considering in clinical situations.

Monocytes

Morphology

The monocyte is the largest of the circulating white cells. It has quite deeply staining blue or blue-grey cytoplasm which is rather granular and may be vacuolated (see Plates 2 and 5d). The shape of the nucleus is very variable, particularly between species, typical shapes being kidney-bean, band, clover leaf and trilobular. Those with kidney-bean and band-shaped nuclei are easily confused with metamyelocytes and band neutrophils, while young monocytes with round nuclei look very like lymphocytes.

Function and kinetics

Monocytes are formed in the bone marrow (where there is a small monocyte pool of about 2–3 times as many cells as are circulating); from there they move out into the blood where they spend about 2–3 days before moving into the tissues to become macrophages. There are about 400 times as many tissue macrophages as there are circulating monocytes and the total lifespan of the cells is about 3 months. The main function of the monocytes and macrophages is phagocytosis, particularly of larger items such as tissue debris and the more difficult pathogens such as fungi, protozoa and *Brucella* spp. These cells are also intimately involved in the immune system.

Monocytosis

This refers to an increased number of circulating monocytes, above about 0.5×10^9/l. The mechanisms controlling this response are not well under-stood, but monocytosis is traditionally associated with chronic disease, particularly chronic inflammatory conditions. A transient monocytosis may also be seen a few days after the start of an acute inflammatory condition. In dogs, unlike most other species, monocytosis is part of the 'steroid picture'. In general a slight to moderate monocytosis will accompany a neutrophilia where inflammation, infection and sepsis are present. Very marked monocytosis which is disproportionate to the degree of neutrophilia can sometimes be a pointer to the presence of neoplasia. However, this should be seen as merely an indication to investigate further; it is not a diagnostic finding. Note that the monocyte is the cell whose distribution is most affected by mechanical preparation of blood films, as opposed to manual film spreading (see p. 292). In mechanically spread films many more monocytes are seen, and the upper limit of normal is correspondingly higher (about 1.0×10^9/l).

Monocytopenia

This has been reported to occur in certain species (cats, horses, cattle) as part of the acute steroid response, but as it is not uncommon to find no monocytes at all in a blood film from a normal animal this possibility is not really worth considering when interpreting routine haematology results.

Lymphocytes

Development

Unlike the other blood cell types, the lymphocytes develop mainly outside the bone marrow, in the lymph nodes, spleen and gut-associated lymphoid tissues (and thymus of immature animals). This pathway involves about six to eight mitoses. A shorter pathway involving two or three mitoses also takes place in the bone marrow. The probable sequence of development is shown in Fig. 3.2.

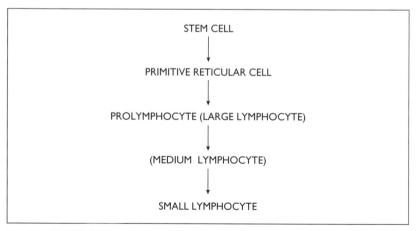

STEM CELL

PRIMITIVE RETICULAR CELL

PROLYMPHOCYTE (LARGE LYMPHOCYTE)

(MEDIUM LYMPHOCYTE)

SMALL LYMPHOCYTE

Fig. 3.2 Simplified representation of the probable stages of lymphocyte development.

Lymphocytes generally become smaller as they mature, and the division into large/medium/small or simply large/small is purely arbitrary. Prolymphocytes are distinguished by their vacuolated cytoplasm and the presence of appreciable nucleoli (see Plate 6d) and are uncommon in the normal blood of any species. In certain species (e.g. the dog) all of the circulating lymphocytes are normally small, and 'large lymphocyte' is essentially synonymous with pro-lymphocyte, while in other species (e.g. cow) large lymphocytes are often seen in blood films and are distinct from the vacuolated prolymphocytes. The term 'lymphoblast' is usually confined in a clinical context to neoplastic lymphocytes which often have very bizarre-shaped nuclei.

Morphology

Mature lymphocytes are the smallest of the circulating white cells. Their appearance varies somewhat between species (see Plates 2–5c), but the nucleus is usually round and evenly stained a medium to dark blue (not so darkly staining as the nucleus of a normoblast). Cytoplasm is very sparse and pale blue staining – it appears as a narrow ring around the nucleus or may even not be evident at all. Large lymphocytes have somewhat more cytoplasm. It is *not* possible to distinguish different functional types of lymphocytes (e.g. T and B cells) by morphology.

Function and kinetics

The primary functions of the lymphocytes are immunological, in humoral antibody formation and cell-mediated immunity, and detailed accounts of these will be found elsewhere. Investigations of lymphocyte function for diagnostic purposes are an essential component of management of HIV infections in man, but similar investigations in cats with HIV are not routinely undertaken.

The lymphocytes can be divided into two groups on the basis of lifespan, with short-lived lymphocytes surviving for only a few days and long-lived lymphocytes surviving, depending on the species, for years. Lymphocytes circulate freely from blood to lymph nodes to blood, and also through the splenic follicles and gut-associated lymphoid tissue, which makes it difficult to obtain accurate measurements of their lifespan. The number in the blood at any one time reflects a balance between cells leaving the circulation and cells entering the circulation, and so alterations in this number do not necessarily reflect a change in lymphopoiesis.

Lymphocytosis

This refers to an increased number of circulating lymphocytes. It is difficult to put a precise upper limit on lymphocyte numbers in different species, but about $9 \times 10^9/l$ in ruminants (where they are the predominant leucocyte), decreasing with age, and about $6 \times 10^9/l$ in monogastric species may serve as a guide. In the horse, circulating lymphocyte numbers (and hence total white cell numbers) decrease with age to a quite marked extent, so that an apparent leucopenia is fairly normal in old horses. With the exception of neoplastic conditions a clinical finding of lymphocytosis is fairly uncommon and interpretation is rather non-specific. A physiological lymphocytosis due to mobilization of cells sequestered in collapsed capillary beds can occur in the same way as for neutrophils, and is quite common in frightened cats. While it is possible to induce lymphocytosis by experimental means (e.g. injection of heparin or *Bordetella pertussis*), an immune response to a bacterial antigen, although it may stimulate lymphopoiesis, does *not* normally cause a significant increase in the number of circulating lymphocytes. Lymphocytosis is not usually a feature of viral infections, this is a misleading impression gathered by attempting to interpret relative (percentage) counts rather than absolute numerical counts – an absolute neutropenia will of course lead to an apparent relative lymphocytosis.

Leukaemia is a complex subject best approached through specialist oncology texts. It can manifest as either abnormally high numbers of circulating lymphocytes, or abnormal lymphocyte forms in circulation, or both. When the lymphocyte count is markedly elevated (with or without abnormal cells) the basic diagnosis is seldom in any real doubt (see Plate 11); however, confusion may occur where the count is only slightly elevated, or where abnormal cells are seen in the absence of an increased count, or where the cells are either too abnormal or too degenerate to recognize at all. In the first two situations (slightly elevated count of normal cells, or some abnormal cells the only abnormality), a repeat examination in about 5–7 days will usually provide a clearer picture. Genuinely bizarre, unrecognizable cells are virtually always neoplastic, but abnormally fast degeneration of white cells should also be regarded as potentially sinister. Although equine leucocytes regularly degenerate to unrecognizable forms within 18–24 hours of sample collection, this is not usual in the dog or cat. Thus the finding of many degenerate cells (see Plate 6b) in a sample which has been properly handled and not unduly delayed in transport to the laboratory may well be a warning of a potential leukaemia in a small animal. The solution is to make a blood film immediately the sample is collected and send that with the repeat sample – a wise precaution in any event, and an essential one if equine blood samples are being posted or retained for next-day analysis. Remember to check the FeLV status of all apparently leukaemic cats, even those which have been vaccinated against FeLV.

Lymphopenia

This refers to a decreased number of circulating lymphocytes, below about $1 \times 10^9/l$ in monogastric animals and about $3 \times 10^9/l$ in ruminants. This is more common than a lymphocytosis and usually reflects an actual decrease in lymphopoiesis.

(1) Steroid effects. Any of the reasons for increased circulating corticosteroids (stress, steroid therapy, Cushing's disease) will lead to a fairly marked lymphopenia.

(2) Infection. Lymphopenia often accompanies the neutropenia seen in acute viral infections, especially feline parvovirus ('panleucopenia'). However, a

Case 3.2

A client presented a cat which she had taken in as a stray 6 months previously. Originally she had believed the cat to be a half-grown kitten, but in spite of good quality feeding the animal had grown little, if at all, during the six months. On examination, body condition was lean and bodyweight was 2.5 kg. Mucous membranes were pale. The attached haematology results were received. What is the next test which should be requested?

PCV		0.24	
Hb		$7.3 \times$ g/100 ml	low
RBC count		$5.69 \times 10^{12}/l$	
MCV		47.1 fl	
MCHC		30.4 g/100 ml	
Total WBC count		$45.2 \times 10^9/l$	high
Band neutrophils	1%	$0.5 \times 10^9/l$	
Adult neutrophils	5%	$2.3 \times 10^9/l$	low
Eosinophils	0%	$0 \quad 10^9/l$	
Lymphocytes	93%	$42.0 \times 10^9/l$	high
Monocytes	1%	$0.5 \times 10^9/l$	

Film comment. RBCs: slightly regenerative, slightly hypochromic
WBCs: many lymphocytes are enlarged and atypical, with bizarre nuclei
Platelets: scarce

Comments

This cat is grossly leukaemic. Given the dubious origins, FeLV infection is very probable, and the next thing to do is check for FeLV antigen in the blood sample.

general leucopenia is also often present in overwhelming bacterial infections, particularly in the early stages and particularly in cattle.

(3) Neoplasia. Although 'leukaemia' describes an increased cell count and/or abnormal cells in circulation, the term 'aleukaemic leukaemia' is sometimes (confusingly) used for solid-organ lymphosarcomas, e.g. multicentric lymphosarcoma with enlargement of all lymph nodes. A small proportion of these cases (less than 20%) are also leukaemic, but in the majority of the remainder a lymphopenia (or low normal lymphocyte count) is seen. Neutropenia and anaemia are also common findings.

Neutrophil/lymphocyte ratios

It is generally good practice to consider each white cell type individually and not in relation to any of the others present; however, a few basic points regarding neutrophil/lymphocyte ratios are worth noting.

(1) In cats and dogs there are normally more neutrophils than lymphocytes in a proportion of about 70:30.

(2)   In ruminants this is normally reversed with the lymphocytes being the commoner cell, again in an approximate 70:30 ratio (i.e. 30:70 neutrophils/lymphocytes). The small number of neutrophils in cattle blood means that a neutrophilia may not necessarily lead to a frank leucocytosis (i.e. increased total white cell count) and may only be evident as a reversed neutrophil/lymphocyte ratio.

(3)   Horses are similar to other monogastric species in that the neutrophil predominates, but the ratio is often closer than in dogs and cats. To some extent this is age dependent, as lymphocyte numbers decline through adult life.

Steroid effects

Various effects of corticosteroids have been detailed in this chapter and in Chapter 1, and taken together they form what is known as a 'steroid picture' or 'stress picture'. While any of the causes of increased circulating corticosteroids will produce this effect it is true to say that it is practically certain to be present in a case of Cushing's disease. Thus the absence of a steroid picture is very useful in ruling out Cushing's disease, and once other possible causes of this effect have been ruled out (e.g. stress, anaesthesia, steroid administration) the presence of a steroid picture is very useful in building up a preliminary diagnosis of Cushing's disease. The steroid picture is as follows:

Red cells

PCV slightly raised or just around the top of the normal range for the species in question. In dogs and cats there may be slightly more juvenile erythrocyte forms than usual, especially in a chronic case.

White cells – total count

This may be either increased, decreased or normal, depending on the dose of steroids and particularly on the duration. During a short period of high level corticosteroid therapy total white blood cell count is generally high, but in chronic low level cases such as animals in athletic training and some longstanding Cushing's cases the count may be slightly low.

Differential white cell count

The basic findings are relative neutrophilia, eosinopenia and lymphopenia (plus monocytosis in dogs, monocytopenia in most other species). In absolute terms, neutrophil count is usually normal (but may be high where high doses of steroids are being administered), eosinophil count is usually under 0.3×10^9/l and often zero, lymphocyte count is almost always under 2.0×10^9/l (usually under 1.0×10^9/l), and in the dog monocyte count is generally $1.0-$

3.0×10^9/l. It is generally regarded as courteous when a blood sample is submitted to inform the laboratory that the patient is on steroids so that interpretation of this finding is facilitated.

Rare circulating cells

Occasionally cells of a type not normally found in circulation will be present on a blood film.

The cell most likely to be encountered in this situation is the mast cell. Mast cell tumours are usually discrete masses in the skin or elsewhere, but occasionally the condition of *systemic mastocytosis* (mast cell leukaemia) is encountered, usually in the cat. Sometimes many mast cells can be seen, but even one mast cell in a blood film is abnormal and indicative of mast cell neoplasia. The dark, deeply staining granules are almost unmistakable. Some publications have suggested that the proprietary rapid haematology stains may fail to stain mast cell granules, and that Leishman's stain must be used. However, practical experience indicates that this problem is uncommon, and many cases of systemic mastocytosis are picked up by chance when performing routine differential white cell counts using rapid stains.

Plasma cells in circulation have been reported in animals with multiple myeloma (see p. 74), but in practice this is extremely rare.

II

Clinical Biochemistry

Introduction to Clinical Biochemistry

Basic principles of plasma biochemistry

The plasma is basically extracellular fluid (ECF) on the move, with added protein to retain water in the circulation (by raising the osmotic pressure). It transports a large number of substances from sites of absorption or production to sites of utilization or excretion and contains many other substances which are essential in precise concentrations for the proper function of the ECF. Therefore, analysis of plasma samples can provide a variety of types of information.

Interpretation of plasma biochemistry results is really specific to each particular constituent, but there are certain basic principles which can be followed. An understanding of these is helpful when tackling the subject for the first time, and can be especially useful when trying to make sense of a puzzling or unusual result. The first thing to consider is the reason for the particular substance being present in the plasma. Is its primary purpose to be in the plasma (albumin, electrolytes)? Is it being taken to somewhere it is needed (glucose, hormones)? Is it a waste product on its way to being excreted (urea, creatinine, bilirubin)? Or is it present in the plasma accidentally (most enzymes)? The next thing to think about is where exactly is this substance coming from, and where is it going to – in other words, what are the mechanisms responsible for its addition to and removal from the plasma, both normal and abnormal, and how are they controlled? From there it is not difficult to work out the possible reasons for abnormal concentrations. Abnormally low concentrations may be due to decreased addition to the plasma (impaired synthesis, nutritional deficiency, poor absorption, lack of precursors, etc.) or to accelerated removal from the plasma (excessive demand, increased excretion, pathological losses, etc.). Abnormally high concentrations may be due to increased addition to the plasma (increased production or intake, pathological leakage from the intracellular compartment, etc.) or decreased removal from the plasma (decreased utilization, impaired excretion, etc.). Also, remember that a disturbance of the normal homeostatic mechanisms may be involved in many cases.

This sounds complicated, but with practice the train of thought becomes automatic. The interpretation of as many cases as possible from first principles is the best way to become proficient, particularly as regards remembering which of the theoretical possibilities outlined above are probable and which are impossible in relation to specific substances. With experience one also begins to recognize patterns of abnormality in certain groups of analytes and their relationship to particular conditions. Used correctly, this 'pattern recognition' approach can speed up assessment of laboratory reports considerably, and it can be argued that this is what the subject is all about. The 'steroid pattern' described in the previous chapter is one example, but this aspect is gone into more fully in Chapter 14.

The plasma constituents discussed here are those which are most commonly in routine use. Many more specialized tests are available for specific purposes (e.g. the more specialized hormone assays), but detailed coverage of these tests is more appropriate to texts which are dealing with the specific clinical conditions involved.

Plasma or serum?

Plasma is the supernatant obtained when a blood sample which has been taken into anticoagulant is centrifuged; serum is the equivalent from a sample which has been allowed to clot. In general, most biochemical tests can be performed on either plasma from a *heparinized* sample or on serum – there are a few particular exceptions with their own specific requirements. Heparinized samples are generally favoured by practices which own a centrifuge and routinely separate samples before despatch to the laboratory, because they can go straight into the centrifuge without delay and separate very easily – a huge advantage if a courier is just about to call or the post is just about to go. Plasma can form annoying little clots of cryoprotein when stored in the fridge, but this is not usually a major concern. Clotted blood, in contrast, *must* be left at room temperature until the clot has fully formed (can be around 2 hours) before any attempt is made to separate it. If clotted samples are centrifuged too soon the serum itself will clot solid, and this can often result in the entire sample being unusable. Also note that clotted blood must be collected into *glass* vials, or plastic vials which have been specially coated to be suitable for the purpose. Whole blood will stick to uncoated plastic as it clots, the clot will not retract, and the resulting serum will be haemolysed and of very poor quality – plastic vials should be reserved for storing already separated serum or plasma. However, if samples must be despatched to the laboratory unseparated, clotted blood (in the correct container) is just as good as heparinized, perhaps even slightly better (it is possible that once the clot has stabilized the blood is less likely to haemolyse in transit than unclotted blood).

The main thing to beware of is that there are a few tests which specifically require serum and cannot be performed on plasma (bile acids, insulin and a number of serology investigations, for example); therefore if one of these test is being requested *or might be required as a follow-up* it is essential either to provide a clotted or serum sample in addition to the heparinized plasma, or to send the whole sample as serum. There are no tests which specifically require heparinized plasma rather than serum, though heparinized plasma is preferable for potassium estimation. However, whichever is used, it is important to be aware that there is a distinction and not to speak of serum concentrations when the sample was actually plasma, or vice versa. Also, be aware that it is plasma which is actually in circulation in the animal; serum is an artificial preparation.

The Plasma Proteins

Normal total protein around 60–80 g/l (a little lower in dogs). Normal albumin around 25–35 g/l (dogs and cats lower than large animals).

Plasma contains a mixture of proteins – albumin, 'globulins' (immunoglobulins and other proteins loosely grouped under this name), enzymes, specific transfer proteins (e.g. transferrin), protein hormones and clotting factors. Because of this heterogeneity, molar concentrations cannot be given. Most are synthesized in the liver from amino acids. All have different specific functions but as a group they function to maintain the osmotic pressure of the plasma. Only the very largest, however, are completely trapped in the bloodstream. There is also a secondary circulation of proteins (especially albumin) out of the capillaries into the tissue fluids then back into the bloodstream via the lymph.

Total protein is usually measured by the biuret method, but refractometry is useful if an emergency result is required. Separation of protein fractions in the first instance is done by measuring albumin separately, and subtracting this from the total protein result to give the 'globulin' concentration. This is quick and cheap, but the bromocresol green (BCG) dye-binding albumin method is erratic on occasion and subject to interference, and the variation between laboratories can be considerable.

The *zinc sulphate turbidity* (ZST) test is a crude but quite effective precipitation method for measuring plasma immunoglobulin levels. It is used specifically to assess whether neonates have consumed and absorbed sufficient colostrum, and it is really only applicable to animals under 1 week old. A lower cut-off point of about 15 arbitrary ZST units is usually applied, and calves or foals with values of less than this are considered to be colostrum deficient. This test can be used as an initial screen, with more sophisticated immunological investigation available if required.

Other specific proteins recognized are the *acute phase proteins*, considered to be markers for acute inflammatory disease. Their relative importance varies between species, but the most important are α_1-antitrypsin, α_1-acid glycoprotein, C-reactive protein, α_2-macroglobulin, caeruloplasmin (α_2), haptoglobin (α_2) and fibrinogen (β). Specific assays for several of these proteins (particularly C-reactive protein, fibrinogen and haptoglobin) are sometimes used in the investigation of inflammatory conditions.

Increased total protein concentration

This has three main causes:

(1) Relative water deficiency. As proteins are not completely confined to the circulation, total plasma protein concentration is theoretically a poorer measure of dehydration than PCV, but in practice it has certain advantages. It is not affected by splenic contraction, thus avoiding the misinterpretation of excitement or stress as dehydration, and in dogs the normal range is much narrower than that of PCV which makes it easier to assess the extent of the dehydration on a single sample. (Note that when samples are collected with excessive venous stasis, e.g. drip bleeding from cephalic veins of dogs and cats, fluid and small molecules leave the plasma leading to an artefactual finding of raised protein concentrations.) When plasma protein concentrations increase due to a *relative* water deficiency all fractions, albumin and globulins, increase by approximately the same percentage. When there is an *absolute* increase in protein due to some other cause (below), only the globulin fractions increase while albumin remains unchanged or decreases.

(2) Chronic inflammatory and immune-mediated diseases can cause increases in globulin fractions, particularly the γ-globulins. These include cirrhosis of the liver, chronic subacute bacterial infections and autoimmune disease. In particular, feline infectious peritonitis (FIP) is often associated with markedly elevated total protein concentration almost always accompanied by low albumin concentration. However, confusion may arise because the same picture is often seen in cats with chronic stomatitis, simply as a result of the chronic inflammation. In general, where this protein picture is seen in a cat less than 4 years old with a clean mouth, suspect FIP, but in an old cat with a poor mouth, suspect the mouth (this is discussed in more detail on p. 193). Very high globulin concentrations are also seen in the neonate after consumption of colostrum, but this does not persist for long.

(3) Paraproteinaemia. This is a comparatively uncommon finding, almost always associated with a malignancy, where the proliferation of a single clone of immunoglobulin-producing cells leads to the appearance of an abnormally large amount of one single immunoglobulin. The condition most usually associated with this finding is a plasma cell (or multiple) myeloma, but occasionally lymphosarcoma or leukaemia are involved. However, certain parasitic conditions not often seen in the UK (most notably ehrlichiosis) can also produce paraproteinaemia, and once again this is a complication to beware of following the relaxation of the quarantine restrictions. Suspect a paraprotein most particularly when the total

protein is extremely elevated (sometimes up to 140 g/l) and the albumin markedly depressed (often 10 g/l or lower), also (especially in dogs) where what may look like a marked inflammatory response in the proteins is not mirrored in the white cell picture. There may also be evidence of bone marrow depression and renal dysfunction. Sometimes (though by no means always) the plasma is abnormally viscous and sticky.

Electrophoresis

This technique allows more detailed appreciation of the various globulin fractions. Protein fractions are separated on an agarose or polyacrylamide gel at pH 8.4–8.6. The dried and stained gel is then scanned by a densitometer to produce the characteristic electrophoretic trace. The numerous variations which can be recognized in the trace have led to many suggested diagnostic applications, most of which unfortunately are not reliable for clinical purposes. Any inflammatory response will produce increases in the inflammatory proteins, and the pattern will change (with the more prominent peaks moving towards the gamma region) as the condition becomes more chronic. However, this does not really help decide the cause of the inflammation, and in this situation the electrophoretic trace often leaves one no further forward than simply knowing that the globulin concentration is elevated.

The main application for the technique is where an elevated globulin concentration is found and there is genuine doubt as to whether this is simply inflammatory proteins or a paraproteinaemia (or occasionally, in the cat, FIP). In addition, samples demonstrating marked hyperviscosity should be electrophoresed even if the measured protein concentrations are relatively normal. Some example traces are shown in Fig. 4.1: (a) is a normal trace, while (b) is purely a curiosity – the horse has a genetic peculiarity causing it to produce albumins of two molecular weights, but this is of no clinical significance (there are also a couple of minor inflammatory proteins evident); note the multiple globulin peaks in the inflammatory reaction (c) compared with the single peak of the FIP case (d) and the paraproteins (e) and (f). Note also the much wider peak of the FIP case compared with the paraprotein, but appreciate that paraproteinaemia can occasionally manifest as a double peak (f), thought to be a feature of immunoglobulin light and heavy chains.

Decreased total protein and/or albumin concentration

This may be found in a variety of different clinical conditions:

(1)   Relative water excess. Overhydration is uncommon but may be produced iatrogenically. It is more common to find that a sample has been taken from a limb into which a drip is running, or even from the i/v cannula itself,

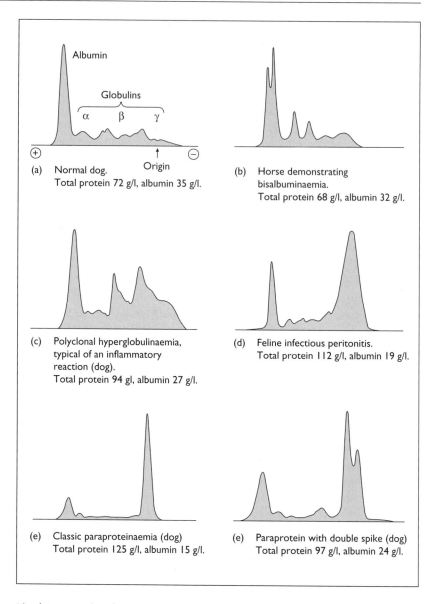

Fig. 4.1   Examples of serum protein electrophoretic traces.

which then appears falsely diluted. Again all fractions will change by the same percentage.

(2)   Excessive loss of protein. As albumin is one of the smallest of the plasma proteins it tends to be lost more readily than the others and so these conditions often present primarily as hypoalbuminaemia.

(a) Renal protein loss – nephrotic syndrome, glomerulonephritis, amyloidosis. This is easily confirmed by testing the urine for protein, but a concurrent cystitis may sometimes confuse the issue, when measurement of urine protein/creatinine ratio will clarify the situation (see p. 172). In protein-losing nephropathy the albumin is always markedly depressed but the globulin can often be normal or even somewhat raised, especially in glomerulonephritis.

(b) Intestinal protein loss (protein-losing enteropathy). In large animals, particularly horses, this is often associated with heavy parasite burdens. This is also the major toxic effect of phenylbutazone overdose in the horse (unlike other species which generally develop aplastic anaemia). In small animals some conditions to consider are lymphosarcoma, villous atrophy, colitis and eosinophilic enteritis. Severe cases of food toxicosis may also develop hypoproteinaemia.

In protein-losing enteropathy both albumin and globulin fractions are depressed, often markedly, and it is the first thing to suspect when a total protein concentration below about 50 g/l is encountered. In severe cases total protein can fall as low as 25 g/l. Most patients with this condition have diarrhoea, which makes diagnosis easy, but where a very low protein is seen without diarrhoea, and renal or liver pathology has been ruled out, suspect intestinal lymphosarcoma.

(c) Haemorrhage. When whole blood is being lost the loss of plasma proteins leads to a hypoproteinaemia in addition to the anaemia. This is the easiest way of assessing whether a regenerative anaemia is likely to be haemorrhagic or haemolytic (if the latter, plasma proteins will not be decreased).

(d) Burns. Extensive areas of burnt skin oozing serum will soon lead to hypoproteinaemia.

(3) Decreased protein synthesis.

(a) Dietary protein deficiency. This is remarkably common in farm animals under certain types of management regime.

(b) Malabsorption. There are various causes of this condition, e.g. exocrine pancreatic insufficiency (congenital or acquired), and various small intestinal disorders. In addition, in many cases of protein-losing enteropathy (above) there is also a degree of malabsorption complicating the issue.

(c) Liver failure. Albumin is the major liver-synthesized protein, and these cases usually present primarily as hypoalbuminaemia. As certain types of liver disease can be associated with hyperglobulinaemia then total protein concentrations may be more or less normal. Note that *liver failure* and *hepatocellular damage* are not synonymous and liver failure should not be rejected as a cause of hypoalbuminaemia just because liver enzymes are not elevated. Specialized liver function tests such as bile acid measurement are necessary. If liver failure is severe enough to lead to marked hypoalbuminaemia it is likely that there will also be hypoprothrombinaemia, something to bear in mind if contemplating liver biopsy.

(d) Viral conditions. Low plasma globulin with a *normal* albumin concentration is often a feature of respiratory virus infections in horses – this is often seen in conjunction with a neutropenia. Particularly striking hypoglobulinaemia may be part of the 'post-viral syndrome', when the horse can show no clinical signs apart from lack of energy or disappointing athletic performance. A prolonged period of rest may be required for full recovery, and it is wise not to push such a horse if it is unwilling to exercise. Levamisole (6.5 mg/kg/day orally for 2 weeks, or 5.5 mg/kg intramuscularly) is sometimes used to treat this condition, but the drug has no product licence for the horse.

Hypoalbuminaemia

Firstly, it is important to recognize that albumin is often slightly to moderately depressed in long-term illness, debility or chronic inflammatory conditions. Causes are a bit vague, but it is often a result of reaction to inflammation-

---

Case 4.1

A 9-year-old English bull terrier bitch was presented because she was 'getting fat', but eating very little. On examination she was, if anything, slightly thin, but had a markedly enlarged abdomen. A fluid thrill could be palpated, and paracentesis obtained a clear, colourless, non-viscous fluid which frothed very little on shaking. Given these plasma biochemistry findings, what is the next investigation to carry out?

Total protein	64 g/l	
Albumin	12 g/l	low
Globulin	52 g/l	raised
Calcium	1.37 mmol/l	low
Urea	14.2 mmol/l	raised
Creatinine	156 mmol/l	raised
ALT	46 iu/l	
ALP	219 iu/l	

Comments

The hypoalbuminaemia is consistent with the aspirated fluid being a true transudate. The raised globulin concentration and the apparent absence of diarrhoea argue against a protein-losing enteropathy, and the rest of the results suggest that a renal aetiology is more likely than a hepatic cause. Thus the provisional diagnosis is nephrotic syndrome, which should be confirmed by demonstrating a high urine protein concentration, or (preferably) urine protein/creatinine ratio.

induced increases in globulins – for this reason albumin is sometimes referred to as a 'negative acute phase protein'. This non-specific sort of reaction should be borne in mind at concentrations down to about 16 g/l in small animals (and Shetland ponies) and about 20 g/l in large animals. Below this, there is little doubt that a true hypoalbuminaemia is present.

Due to the major importance of albumin in retaining water in the plasma, hypoalbuminaemic patients are almost always oedematous and/or ascitic. This is frequently the major presenting sign, so that differential diagnosis of hypoalbuminaemia as such is important. Extensive burns are, of course, obvious, and haemorrhaging animals usually present primarily as anaemia. Dietary deficiencies are seldom serious enough to cause major oedema unless extreme malnutrition has occurred, and so the three main places to look are liver, kidney and gut. Renal protein loss is easy to demonstrate on a urine sample. Liver failure can be demonstrated by liver function tests. Malabsorption/protein-losing enteropathy cases are usually at least intermittently diarrhoeic, but this is not invariable, and after liver and kidney problems have been ruled out the possibility of specific intestinal disease should be investigated. Laboratory tests may help in certain conditions (see exocrine pancreatic dysfunction, p. 203, and intestinal dysfunction, p. 205), but in other cases these cannot provide a definite diagnosis and other diagnostic techniques such as radiography or endoscopy may prove more helpful.

Remember that hypoalbuminaemic patients heal very slowly and repeated wound breakdowns are common. For this reason, and because surgery of liver failure cases is generally contraindicated on other grounds (coagulation problems, poor anaesthetic tolerance), exploratory laparotomy should be regarded very much as a last resort, and certainly should not be considered before every possible non-invasive investigation has been carried out.

5 The Electrolytes

Sodium, potassium and chloride are the three electrolytes most commonly considered in veterinary medicine, while bicarbonate is measured much less frequently. These ions are all freely diffusible throughout the entire ECF (plasma, interstitial fluid, lymph). When there is a disturbance of electrolyte status this is invariably related in some way to a body fluid problem; hence the real subject at issue is fluid/electrolyte status and balance. Normal ECF (and plasma) electrolyte concentrations are necessary for the normal functioning of the electrical activities of the cell membranes and for the maintenance of the body fluid compartments at the correct volumes. The electrolytes are all normally present to vast excess in the diet, and in the healthy animal this excess is simply excreted via the kidney and/or gut. Dietary electrolyte deficiencies are quite difficult to organize on an experimental basis and are seldom encountered clinically; the normal animal's excretory capacity is such that even quite alarmingly excessive intakes do not lead to clinical problems unless *water* is restricted.

This means that clinical fluid/electrolyte problems are associated not with dietary factors but with abnormal fluid losses, and it is the amount *and composition* of the fluid being lost which will determine the direction of any electrolyte abnormalities seen. For example, if almost pure water alone is being lost from the body (as in trained human athletes during sweating, and panting dogs) then all plasma electrolyte concentrations will rise. If the fluid being lost is isotonic to the ECF with regard to electrolyte concentrations (as in sweating *horses*) then plasma electrolyte concentrations will not change even though an absolute deficiency may be developing. If the fluid being lost has a higher electrolyte concentration than the ECF (as during severe vomiting at least so far as potassium and chloride are concerned) then plasma electrolyte concentrations will fall.

It is difficult to consider each of the electrolytes in isolation, but the following are some of the conditions particularly associated with abnormal electrolyte concentrations.

Sodium

Normal plasma concentration about 135–155 mmol/l (horses tend to the low range, cats to the high).

Sodium is the electrolyte which is most intimately associated with water balance and most disturbances tend to be primarily fluid problems. Symptoms are generally related to changes in volume of body fluid compartments, particularly ICF/ECF volumes in the CNS.

Increase (hypernatraemia)

This will occur when loss of a low-sodium fluid occurs, as in vomiting, excessive panting, and sweating in humans. It is also seen when restricted water intake prevents normal sodium excretion – the classic example of this is salt poisoning in pigs. It might be expected that cases of Cushing's disease would be hypernatraemic on the basis of excessive secretion of mineralocorticoids, but in practice this does not really happen and the clinical problems are primarily associated with excessive glucocorticoids. Conn's syndrome (aldosterone-producing tumour of the adrenal gland) will cause hypernatraemia and has been recorded in the cat, but this is quite rare.

Hypernatraemia causes a variety of CNS signs – head-pressing, apparent blindness, coma (due to cellular dehydration in the CNS) – and plasma sodium concentrations greater than about 170 mmol/l are liable to prove fatal. The rate of change of plasma sodium concentration is crucial, and over-rapid correction of hypernatraemia will also cause CNS signs. This is because plasma osmolarity is restored faster than intracellular osmolarity and the brain cells therefore take up water and become oedematous.

However, beware of sample contamination producing erroneous results. Sodium is ubiquitous, and it doesn't take much salt to alter a plasma result. In addition, both fluoride (in glucose tubes) and citrate (in coagulation tubes) are incorporated into specimen containers as the sodium salts, and plasma from such tubes, or even contaminated by the contents of such tubes, will have a preposterously high sodium concentration.

Decrease (hyponatraemia)

This will occur when loss of a high-sodium fluid occurs – the most common instance of this is in renal failure when the kidney cannot concentrate the urine, and the fast urine flow through the tubules also prevents effective Na/K exchange in the loop of Henle and leads to the production of a high-sodium urine. It will also occur when loss of any sodium-containing fluid is replaced by a low-sodium fluid, for example water (by mouth) or i/v dextrose saline. The other major cause of hyponatraemia is *Addison's disease* (see p. 84) where the lack of mineralocorticoids (especially aldosterone) also leads to the production of very high-sodium urine. In this condition water loss is also enormous and severe hypovolaemia and circulatory collapse occur.

Potassium

Normal plasma concentration about 3.3–5.5 mmol/l.

Potassium is primarily an intracellular ion and concentrations in the ECF are low. It is less intimately connected with water balance than sodium, and most disturbances tend to be directly due to excessive losses or lack of excretion, irrespective of the state of hydration. Symptoms are generally related to impairment of electrical activity, particularly in the heart and skeletal muscles.

To obtain an accurate potassium result from a blood sample it is essential that haemolysis should be minimized and that the plasma (or serum, but plasma is preferred because the formation of a clot can cause potassium release from all cellular elements in the blood) should be separated from the cells within an absolute maximum of 8 hours from collection. This is because, once the Na/K pump on the erythrocyte membrane has exhausted the glucose present in the sample, potassium will passively diffuse from the intracellular to the extra-cellular space. In large animals, especially horses, the intraerythrocyte potassium concentration is very high, and apparent plasma levels incompatible with life (over about 11 mmol/l) can be reached quite easily. This sort of extreme artefact is not usually difficult to spot. More difficult is the situation in the dog and cat, where the intraerythrocyte potassium concentration is itself only about 10–12 mmol/l, and a sample left as whole blood for 24 hours may have a potassium concentration only about 1 mmol/l higher than the true value. It is only too easy to start trying to interpret this sort of result clinically, and many spurious diagnoses of Addison's disease have been reached by the unwary. *Never* post whole blood or keep it overnight if an accurate potassium result is required.

Note also that both EDTA and oxalate are included in specimen tubes as potassium salts, and samples collected into either of these anticoagulants will give preposterously high potassium readings. Heparinized or clotted samples which are contaminated with EDTA or oxalate will also give erroneously high results.

Increase (hyperkalaemia)

This can occur when loss of a low-potassium fluid is occurring, but increases are generally not very great and do not reach the danger level. The cause of significant hyperkalaemia is nearly always a failure of the kidney to excrete potassium. However, not all renal failure cases do have high plasma potassium concentrations. Fairly acute cases (e.g. nephrotoxicity) may indeed be hyper-kalaemic, but chronic renal failure cases soon begin to compensate and may even be hypokalaemic as a result of vomiting. The most important condition to consider when high plasma potassium concentrations are found is again

Addison's disease. These cases cannot excrete potassium due to aldosterone deficiency and it is the hyperkalaemia which leads to the classic ECG findings. In addition, note that prolonged use of potassium-sparing diuretics (e.g. spiro-nolactone, which is an aldosterone antagonist) can lead to hyperkalaemia. Severely dehydrated patients may sometimes be hyperkalaemic due to a serious decrease in renal perfusion leading to a failure of excretion, but as most of these cases are vomiting, hypokalaemia is more common.

When a plasma potassium of over 7 mmol/l is measured in a properly handled specimen, this should be regarded as an emergency as this level of ECF potassium concentration is liable to stop the heart (but remember, before you panic, that badly haemolysed plasma or plasma which has not been separated from the red cells until several hours after collection will have a falsely elevated potassium concentration; see above). Treatment is i/v administration of dextrose saline, which will dilute out the potassium and, by raising insulin, promote potassium uptake into the cells. However, if plasma sodium is low (as it often is in these cases) dextrose saline may be contraindicated as it is hypotonic for sodium, and isotonic saline should be used instead.

Addison's disease

Addison's disease is hypoadrenocorticism caused by (usually autoimmune) destruction of the adrenal cortices, and it is hypoaldosteronism (mineralo-corticoid deficiency) which is the principal clinical problem. Lack of aldosterone causes massive renal losses of sodium and water, together with retention of potassium, with resulting dehydration, hyponatraemia and hyperkalaemia. The condition is essentially confined to the dog (and man, where it was originally described as a complication of tuberculosis). Most cases occur in the young adult/middle-aged animal, and there are breed predispositions (including Springer Spaniels, Standard Poodles and Bearded Collies). First presentation (often in Addisonian crisis) is disproportionately common in unusually hot or cold weather. Clinical signs are often vague – malaise, depression, pallor (with poor capillary refill time), peripheral hypothermia, weak pulse, bradycardia, and sometimes vomiting. Patients are usually much more dehydrated than they look, and if electrolytes are not measured during initial investigation the pre-renal urea increase (see p. 104), or indeed the fact that a fair proportion of cases do progress to secondary renal failure, may lead to a mistaken diagnosis of primary renal disease. Be particularly suspicious of an apparent moderate renal dysfunction in a very depressed, relatively young dog. The finding of marked hyponatraemia and hyperkalaemia in the absence of *severe* renal dysfunction is virtually pathognomonic for Addison's disease.

Treatment of an Addisonian crisis is an emergency, but see p. 158 regarding timing of diagnostic sampling relative to treatment. Rehydration (isotonic saline or dextrose saline, see above) is the most important priority, and a corticosteroid (preferably cortisol, but soluble dexamethasone may suffice) should be added to the drip at about 2 mg/kg bwt. Once destroyed, the adrenal cortices do not recover, and when the immediate crisis is over and plasma sodium, potassium, urea and creatinine have returned to near normal, patients should be transferred to maintenance hormone replacement therapy which will be life-long. Fludrocortisone (Florinef: Squibb) is the mainstay; initial dose should be about 10 μg/kg b.i.d., but requirements can vary quite widely and this should be adjusted according to follow-up electrolyte estimations. Additional pred-nisolone (0.1 to 0.5 mg/kg) should be provided at times of stress (some patients require continuous low-dose prednisolone in addition to the fludrocortisone), and extra salt (1 to 5 g/day) incorporated in the diet or as salt tablets. Once stabilised on maintenance therapy, plasma sodium, potassium, urea and creatinine should be checked every 3–6 months and the régime adjusted where necessary.

Decrease (hypokalaemia)

This occurs most commonly due to persistent loss of a high-potassium fluid. Diarrhoea is considered to be the classic instance, but note that persistent *vomiting* even without diarrhoea will have a similar or even more marked effect. Hypokalaemia will also be seen in patients on long-term fluid therapy being given potassium-free fluids such as dextrose saline or isotonic saline. In addition, note that prolonged use of potassium-losing diuretics (e.g. frusemide) will lead to hypokalaemia and it is essential that plasma potassium be monitored in patients on this type of treatment (note also that it is essential to know which type of diuretic is being used as the administration of potassium supplements to patients on spironolactone can be disastrous). The involvement of hypo-kalaemia in the 'downer cow' syndrome has also been suspected. Symptoms include lethargy, poor muscle tone and cardiac irregularities. Hypokalaemia is also a potential complication when treating diabetes mellitus. Insulin promotes uptake of potassium into the cells, and patients receiving insulin (particularly during the initial stabilization period) should be monitored and supplemented as necessary.

The horse is an unusual case so far as plasma potassium is concerned in that concentrations may fall as low as 2.5 mmol/l in the resting animal with no ill effects; this occurs especially while eating hay, due to the secretion of large volumes of saliva. Horses also have a very high concentration of potassium in the sweat and this may lead to plasma potassium concentrations falling as low as 2.0 mmol/l after prolonged exercise, again with no apparent ill effects. *During* active exercise, however, plasma potassium is always higher (around 4 mmol/l) due to flux of plasma out of the active muscle cells.

The cat is also unusual in being much *more* susceptible to clinical hypo-kalaemia than other species. Although it is commonly believed that a carni-vorous diet is usually more than adequate in potassium (indeed, it has been said with some truth that there is a lethal dose of potassium in a hamburger!), middle-aged and elderly cats quite frequently demonstrate hypokalaemia. This phenomenon is often termed 'idiopathic hypokalaemia' and it is a different entity from Conn's syndrome in man (hyperaldosteronism). It appears it may be related to a rather low potassium content in some commercial feline diets in combination with mild renal insufficiency. Although the kidney's role in potassium homeostasis is usually seen as excreting the excess in that hamburger, and acute renal failure carries the risk of dangerous hyperkalaemia, mild chronic renal dysfunction may mean that the kidney is unable to conserve potassium if required. A more marked hypokalaemia is recognized as a hereditary problem in the Burmese breed. Affected kittens present at about 4–12 months of age and potassium levels are often very low (less than 2 mmol/l). True Conn's syndrome has also been reported in the cat.

Clinical signs are related to weakness of the large muscle groups, particularly those of the hindquarters and the dorsal neck. This causes a characteristic crouching gait and an inability to lift the head – especially obvious when an affected cat tries to look at something behind him – which may at first sight suggest a neurological problem. Unlikely though it may seem, some cats display these signs at plasma potassium concentrations as high as 3.8–3.9 mmol/l (probably because the actual ECF concentration inside these large muscle masses is considerably below this, and so the ICF potassium is also low). In the elderly idiopathic case signs usually resolve with oral potassium supplementation, but the problem in the Burmese can be more difficult to control.

In all other species a plasma potassium concentration of less than about 3.5 mmol/l should be considered significant, and less than 3.0 mmol/l is an action level. The oral route is preferable for replacement in potassium depleted animals as i/v potassium can be dangerous at the concentrations required (Ringer's/Hartmann's solution has 4.0 mmol/l which is quite safe and correct for short-term maintenance but will not improve an already hypokalaemic situation). However, hypokalaemic vomiting and/or diarrhoeic patients will require i/v therapy with Darrow's solution (30 mmol/l K^+) which should be given *slowly*. Alternatively, concentrated potassium chloride may be added to any other intravenous fluid preparation – one vial in a 500 ml bag achieves much the same potassium concentration. Anorectic animals may also require either oral or i/v potassium supplementation – this is particularly true in the cat.

Chloride

Normal plasma concentration about 100–115 mmol/l (up to 140 mmol/l in cats).

Chloride tends to be the least regarded of the electrolytes but can often give quite useful information. As an anion, its concentrations are affected by concentrations of the other main anion, bicarbonate. This means that in acidotic patients with low bicarbonate concentrations chloride is generally high, while in alkalotic patients with high bicarbonate concentrations chloride is generally low (in an effort to maintain the anion/cation balance). In the absence of significant acid/base disturbances plasma chloride concentration generally parallels that of sodium. Specific symptoms of chloride abnormalities (as distinct from sodium or acid/base disturbances) are not generally recognized.

Case 5.1

An elderly domestic short hair cat was presented because the owner thought he had had a fit. In the surgery he was ataxic, walked with a crouching gait, and appeared to be unable to raise his head. Neurological examination was unremarkable. What is the significance of the biochemistry findings?

Total protein	81 g/l	
Albumin	23 g/l	low
Globulin	58 g/l	raised
Sodium	149 mmol/l	
Potassium	3.2 mmol/l	low
Calcium	1.98 mmol/l	low
Urea	13.4 mmol/l	
Creatinine	163 mmol/l	

Comment

The proteins are unremarkable in an elderly cat, and the calcium is only marginally depressed. The most significant finding is the potassium, and this is a typical idiopathic hypokalaemia. Conn's syndrome is relatively rare, and usually presents with a marked hypernatraemia as well as severe hypokalaemia.

Increase (hyperchloraemia)

This occurs in acidosis (see above), and is also found in nearly all conditions where hypernatraemia occurs. Note that the assessment of the severity of dehydration by measuring chloride concentration (on the assumption that as water is lost chloride concentration will increase) is *not valid*.

Decrease (hypochloraemia)

This occurs in alkalosis (see above) and in addition is often found in conditions which are associated with hyponatraemia. Hypochloraemia without hyponatraemia can occur when significant volumes of a high chloride/low sodium fluid are being lost. This generally means hydrochloric acid, i.e. gastric secretions, and so persistent vomiting *just after eating* is one possible cause (but note that potassium is the main loss in vomiting on an empty stomach). Another situation is in certain types of colic in horses, where there is an obstruction high up in the gastrointestinal tract, and although fluid is not actually being lost, large volumes of chloride-containing fluid may pool in the stomach/upper small intestine. Note also that plasma chloride concentrations seem to fall quite markedly in excited/frightened horses for unknown reasons (post-sprint plasma chloride concentrations of 85–90 mmol/l are not uncommon in racehorses).

Treatment of chloride disturbances is primarily aimed at correcting the acid/base or sodium abnormality rather than specifically correcting the chloride concentration itself.

Total CO_2

Normal plasma concentration about 20–30 mmol/l (lower in cats).

Total CO_2 is the only measurement of direct relevance to acid/base status which can be carried out on ordinary venous plasma without the special procedures necessary for collecting blood for blood gas analysis. Most of the plasma total CO_2 is in fact bicarbonate (HCO_3). The use of this measurement on its own has its limitations, but it can be extremely useful in patients with a metabolic acid/base disturbance. In these cases this single measurement is often sufficient both to demonstrate the presence of acidosis or alkalosis and to give some idea of the severity. The availability of this test is thus very helpful when dealing with severely ill vomiting and/or diarrhoeic animals. Total CO_2 measurement alone is much less helpful in assessing respiratory acid/base disturbances.

Fluid therapy

The classic approach to fluid/electrolyte therapy involves assessment of sensible and insensible losses plus estimation of maintenance requirements, and the calculation of exact requirements for water (in ml) and each electrolyte (in mmol). This then has to be translated into so many ml of such-and-such a solution. This is certainly the correct way to proceed and the way it is done in human hospitals. However, practical considerations in veterinary practice mean that proper fluid therapy charts are very seldom kept, and without these it is easy for fluid therapy to degenerate into a very hit-or-miss state.

Volume of fluid is not usually the main problem. A diagnosis of fluid deficit is not difficult to make on the basis of skin elasticity, mucous membrane appearance, etc., and the practice of continuing to administer fluids until these signs are reversed, while not perfectly scientific, is usually reasonably effective. Laboratory measurements (PCV and particularly plasma proteins) will be of some help here in taking away much of the guesswork.

The much trickier problem is which fluid to administer. The commercially produced i/v fluids usually stocked in practice are:

(1) *Ringer's*: Na, K and Cl all the same as in ECF. For maintenance. (Ringer's is less usually stocked as many practices find they use Hartmann's more frequently.)

(2) *Hartmann's*: lactated Ringer's. Na, K and Cl all the same as in ECF, plus lactate (to provide bicarbonate). For maintenance and correction of acidosis.

(3) *Isotonic saline*: Na slightly higher than in ECF, Cl considerably higher than in ECF, no potassium. Will correct hyponatraemia but will also lower potassium, so care is needed if long-term use is envisaged. If too much sodium is administered this way actual dehydration can result as the excess is excreted.

(4) *Dextrose saline*: Na and Cl much lower than in ECF, no potassium, correct osmolarity of fluid attained by addition of dextrose (glucose). Provides fluid alone for cases which are dehydrated but have not lost electrolytes, will correct hypernatraemia and hyperkalaemia. The glucose is only there to provide the correct osmolarity for i/v administration – it is *negligible* as a source of calories. However, it will correct hypoglycaemia and is particularly useful in helping to correct hyperkalaemia in that as well as diluting out excess potassium it raises plasma insulin levels and so promotes potassium uptake into the cells. Note that over-fast administration will raise plasma glucose above the renal threshold and lead to an osmotic diuresis – this is undesirable as it may again lead to dehydration.

(5) *Darrow's*: Na and Cl lower than in ECF, K very much higher. For the treatment of hypokalaemia. Administration must be slow and over-administration avoided because if you hit the heart with too high a potassium concentration you will stop it.

Hartmann's or Ringer's are the safe choice in an emergency and for short-term maintenance, because they are closest to normal plasma concentrations for all electrolytes and thus cannot *cause* any harm. Even severely hyper-kalaemic Addison's cases have been saved by Hartmann's solution because even 4 mmol/l potassium will dilute out a plasma concentration of double that, and correction of the hypovolaemia is the most urgent consideration in these animals. However, these preparations cannot do much to correct any previously existing imbalance beyond simply diluting it out, and it is helpful to have some more rational basis for a decision.

Ideally, samples for electrolyte estimations should be collected before initiating fluid therapy, even if treatment is to be started before any results will be available. However, if sampling an animal on fluids, on no account should the blood be taken from the limb into which the drip is running – always perform another venepuncture, preferably using the jugular vein (the contralateral one if a jugular is already in use for the drip). Remember to ensure that the plasma will be separated in good time to allow an accurate potassium result (maximum delay 8 hours). Although results may be available quite quickly from a professional laboratory during normal working hours where a courier service is provided, delays are inevitable in the evenings and at weekends. This makes the acquisition of some means of measuring sodium and potassium in the practice side-room an attractive proposition. Modern ion specific electrodes are very reliable if properly maintained, but be wary of potentiometry or other 'dry-reagent' methods – these should be regarded as an emergency approximation.

Reassessment is also important in fluid therapy, and should be carried out fairly frequently – perhaps after every 500 ml bag in a medium-sized dog. It is not much good diagnosing hypokalaemia and treating correctly with Darrow's if this is carried out past the correction point and the patient allowed to become hyperkalaemic! Check state of hydration both clinically and by measuring PCV and/or total protein; check for hypo/hyperglycaemia (all these are very easy side-room tests), and check electrolyte concentrations if practical. Once plasma electrolytes are normal and stable, Hartmann's/Ringer's is initially best for maintenance, but regular monitoring should still be carried out so long as intravenous fluids are being administered. If an anorectic patient is on intravenous fluids for any length of time, potassium supplementation is likely to be required as described on p. 86. If hyperglycaemia occurs in a patient on a dextrose-containing fluid, switch to a glucose-free preparation, as the osmotic diuresis which occurs when the renal glucose threshold (about 10 mmol/l) is exceeded is counterproductive.

6

The Minerals

Calcium and phosphate are the two minerals which are of diagnostic import-ance in all species, while magnesium, copper, cobalt and selenium are only important in ruminants (except under very unusual circumstances). Like the electrolytes, the minerals are important in maintaining electrical activity of one sort or another and abnormalities often lead to symptoms involving either nervous signs or failure of muscle contraction. They are also, particularly calcium and phosphate, important structural elements, especially in bone. Unlike the electrolytes, correct dietary levels are very important in maintaining correct mineral balance and dietary deficiencies are very commonly, even usually, the underlying cause of mineral problems. The most important reg-ulation of calcium/phosphate metabolism is by parathyroid hormone and vitamin D, and calcitonin appears to be of little clinical relevance.

Calcium

Normal plasma concentration about 2–3 mmol/l (2.5–3.5 mmol/l in horses).

Calcium is of major importance in transmission at the neuromuscular junction and in the propagation of the contraction impulse within the muscle. It is also a major component of bone. About half of the plasma calcium is free, and this is the active proportion, while the other half is inactive, bound to albumin.

Increase (hypercalcaemia)

This is much less common than hypocalcaemia. Mild hypercalcaemia may be due to raised plasma albumin concentration (i.e. dehydration) or to excessive venous stasis during sample collection. Probably the commonest cause of marked hypercalcaemia seen in veterinary practice is the over-enthusiastic treatment of hypocalcaemic patients with calcium borogluconate (farmers frequently administer this themselves before seeking veterinary help); how-ever, genuine hypercalcaemia is almost always due to some type of hyper-parathyroidism. Primary hyperparathyroidism, usually due to an adenoma of the parathyroid gland, and primary pseudohyperparathyroidism, due to production of parathyroid hormone by a tumour of a completely different tissue, are clinically very similar. The commonest cause of primary pseudo-hyperparathyroidism is a perianal adenocarcinoma. Some lymphosarcomas, especially the mediastinal form, come second, but a wide variety of tumours have been implicated. Another consideration is where a tumour (such as a mammary carcinoma) is extensively invading the skeleton, where widespread bone lysis can lead to hypercalcaemia. Rarely, hypercalcaemia is also seen in cases of severe thyrotoxicosis. The main presenting sign of hypercalcaemia is usually polydipsia, as high circulating calcium concentrations interfere with the normal urinary concentrating mechanisms, and so cause polyuria.

Compared with other causes of polydipsia/polyuria, hypercalcaemia is rare, but it is good practice to screen plasma calcium concentration in all patients presenting with this sign as otherwise the small proportion of cases which do occur will be missed. Once hypercalcaemia has been established, radiographic search for the tumour is usually the most productive investigation. Apart from polydipsia, other clinical signs of hypercalcaemia are constipation and abdominal pain (due to depressed neuromuscular excitability), ECG changes and in extreme cases cardiac arrest.

Decrease (hypocalcaemia)

This is by far the more commonly encountered calcium abnormality, and may have several causes.

(1)   Hypoalbuminaemia. When plasma albumin is low, the protein-bound calcium fraction decreases. Hypocalcaemia is only moderate, and when the free active calcium concentration is unaffected this is asymptomatic. However, where the hypoalbuminaemia is due to albumin *loss*, loss of calcium bound to this albumin may lead to development of a genuine, symptomatic hypocalcaemia over a period of time.

(2)   Parturient paresis. 'Milk fever' in dairy cattle is extremely common, presenting as hypocalcaemic tetany shortly after calving. This is due to a combination of dietary factors, hormonal factors, and the excessively high demand for calcium imposed on dairy cows in early lactation. A similar syndrome occurs in some other species, particularly in sheep, usually before lambing. Bitches (and rarely cats) are usually affected a few weeks after whelping but the condition ('eclampsia' in this case) may occur any time during lactation or immediately pre-partum. Mares may be affected either about 10 days after foaling or 1 or 2 days after weaning.

(3)   Oxalate poisoning. This occurs in herbivores as a result of consuming large amounts of a plant high in potassium oxalate – a number of botanical specimens have been implicated. In cats it is a consequence of antifreeze poisoning, as ethylene glycol is metabolised to oxalate. Oxalate combines with calcium *in vivo* to produce insoluble calcium oxalate, which pre-cipitates out in the renal tubules and causes acute renal failure.

Case 6.1

Trading Standards Officers called a veterinary surgeon to attend a recumbent heifer, one of a group of 34 animals of mixed origins acquired at market by a dealer and being raised as beef store cattle. The heifer, a Friesian type, was in lateral recumbency with limbs and neck extended. Respiration was irregular, and there were intermittent tremors of the limbs. Body condition was poor.

Examination revealed the tag end of a retained placenta protruding from the vulval lips. Septicaemia was suspected and a blood sample collected for evidential purposes, but euthanasia was recommended on humane grounds. When the laboratory report was received the haematology was unremarkable. What is the significance of the biochemistry findings?

Total protein	84 g/l	
Albumin	38 g/l	
Globulin	46 g/l	
Calcium	1.04 mmol/l	low
Phosphate	0.78 mmol/l	low
Magnesium	1.25 mmol/l	
Copper	9.2 µmol/l	low
Urea	4.1 mmol/l	
Creatinine	166 µmol/l	raised

Comment

The most significant finding is the hypocalcaemia, and with hindsight this was a case of milk fever. The other abnormalities were not contributing to the clinical condition. The heifer had calved unexpectedly 4 days earlier, and was feeding the calf. Although milk fever is not normally associated with suckler cows, this was a dairy-type animal which had not been fed for pregnancy and lactation.

(4) Chronic renal failure, particularly in small animals. In these cases there is a failure to excrete phosphate, hyperphosphataemia (see below) and a consequent tendency for plasma calcium to fall. This in turn stimulates parathyroid hormone which increases release of calcium (and phosphate) from bone; the hypocalcaemia is corrected, but the hyperphosphataemia is aggravated. As a result this condition (secondary renal hyperparathyroidism) manifests primarily as hyperphosphataemia rather than hypocalcaemia.

(5) Acute pancreatitis. A proportion of acute pancreatitis cases develop hypocalcaemia and tetany, and this can occasionally be a useful aid to diagnosis. A number of suggestions have been put forward to explain this occurrence, including the precipitation of insoluble calcium 'soaps', but the full biochemical events are still not entirely clear. If this is treated by intravenous calcium administration during the acute phase most cases will recover as the pancreatitis resolves, but one case has been reported which remained hypocalcaemic and required permanent dihydrotachysterol therapy. This phenomenon should be watched for in a pancreatitis case as, untreated, it can prove fatal.

(6)   When performing thyroidectomies on hyperthyroid cats, great care must be taken to preserve the parathyroid glands and their associated blood supply. However, even with all due care, it is not uncommon for problems with hypocalcaemia to arise post-operatively. For this reason many surgeons prefer to operate on one side at a time, even where it is clear that a bilateral thyroidectomy will eventually be required. Cats should be observed post-operatively for signs of hypocalcaemia, and the calcium checked in suspicious cases. The most effective treatment is synthetic vitamin D (dihydroxytachysterol, AT-10), as the problem is one of calcium metabolism, not calcium deficiency, and oral calcium supplements on their own have relatively little effect. Patients on dihydroxytachysterol treatment should be monitored regularly, as it is quite easy to go a little too far and produce iatrogenic hypercalcaemia. Almost all cats with post-operative hypocalcaemia sort themselves out within a few weeks, and permanent treatment is not necessary.

(7)   Occasionally hypocalcaemia is seen in the adult dog (male or female) with a history of trembling, collapse or even fitting. The cause is thought to be autoimmune destruction of the parathyroid glands, but this has not been confirmed, and the syndrome is sometimes termed 'idiopathic hypoparathyroidism'. These cases also respond to dihydroxytachysterol.

(8)   Finally, note that many anticoagulants (e.g. EDTA, oxalate and citrate) act by removing calcium from solution. Calcium is undetectable in samples collected into any of these anticoagulants, and even contamination with a trace can lead to erroneously low results.

Phosphate

Normal plasma concentration about 1–2.5 mmol/l (but can be much higher in pigs).

Inorganic phosphate is of major importance in many metabolic pathways, in particular where high energy compounds are involved, and, like calcium, it is a major component of bone. Plasma concentrations are again controlled by parathyroid hormone and vitamin D, but while parathyroid hormone unreservedly acts to raise plasma calcium concentrations, its two modes of action tend to have opposite effects on plasma phosphate concentration.

(1)   It acts directly on osteoclasts to release bone salts into circulation, which increases both calcium and phosphate in plasma.

(2)   It acts on renal tubular cells to *increase* phosphate excretion; this tends to *lower* plasma phosphate concentration, which in turn (by a mass action effect) increases release of phosphate (and calcium) from bone.

Increase (hyperphosphataemia)

This is seen most commonly in cases of chronic renal failure, usually in small animals. There is a failure of the kidney to excrete phosphate which causes plasma phosphate concentrations to rise. This actually leads to *increased* parathyroid hormone secretion by way of a consequent tendency to hypo-calcaemia (see above); this increases release of phosphate from bone which aggravates the hyperphosphataemia. In this way a vicious circle of bone demineralization develops, known as secondary renal hyperparathyroidism, and patients develop gross skeletal abnormalities (classically 'rubber jaw' or osteodystrophia fibrosa in advanced cases).

Note that pigs are often observed to have high plasma inorganic phosphate concentrations, even up to 5 mmol/l or higher, with no evidence of clinical illness. This may be a dietary effect but has not been fully investigated.

The phosphate assay is particularly sensitive to haemolysis, and erroneously high results are inevitable if the sample is not clear.

Decrease (hypophosphataemia)

The classic case of hypophosphataemia in veterinary practice is the 'downer cow', defined as a cow which remains recumbent post-partum in spite of adequate treatment for hypocalcaemia. While there are a number of different problems involved here, a fair proportion of these cases are, in fact, hypo-phosphataemic. These cows are typically bright, eating, drinking, ruminating, urinating and defaecating normally, have no other medical or surgical problem (e.g. mastitis, metritis or fractures), but simply won't get up.

When apparent hypophosphataemia (asymptomatic) is picked up in a horse or small animal, the cause is probably recent stress or excitement. The mode of action of adrenaline is the activation of cell membrane adenyl cyclase, which then sequentially activates numerous enzyme systems to produce the target effect – be it sweating, glycogenolysis, lipolysis, etc. It has been suggested that this multiple enzyme phosphorylation places sufficient demand on the inorganic phosphate pool to cause an appreciable decrease in plasma phosphate concentration.

Nutritional calcium/phosphorus/vitamin D abnormalities, secondary nutritional hyperparathyroidism, rickets and osteitis fibrosa

In cases of simple dietary phosphorus deficiency, hypophosphataemia is to be expected. Apart from this, plasma calcium and phosphate concentrations in the above conditions are a very complex subject, full discussion of which is outwith the scope of this book. The main problem is that the homeostatic mechanisms, particularly parathyroid hormone, are remarkably effective and to a certain extent rather complex in action, and as a result plasma calcium and phosphate concentrations are very often normal even in animals quite far advanced in skeletal disease. Sometimes homeostatic mechanisms actually lead to plasma changes in the opposite direction to what might be expected. In particular, too low a dietary Ca/PO_4 ratio, i.e. a calcium deficiency or a relative phosphate excess, will lead to secondary nutritional hyperparathyroidism. This usually results eventually in a normal plasma calcium concentration, but the effect on plasma phosphate concentration is variable depending on which of the two effects of parathyroid hormone on phosphate metabolism predominates. This varies with species, age of animal, and stage of the disease. If the bone mobilization effect predominates, hyperphosphataemia will be seen; if the renal effect (promotion of phosphate excretion) predominates then hypophosphataemia may paradoxically occur. Sometimes even advanced cases show no plasma mineral abnormalities.

Other tests such as estimation of plasma parathyroid hormone may also prove helpful, but in general the biochemical diagnosis of nutritional calcium/phosphorus/vitamin D problems is difficult and much more headway is liable to be made by investigating the actual diet itself.

Clearance ratios (fractional excretion)

An alternative approach to this situation is to look at what is being excreted, i.e. renal clearance of the analyte in question. However, accurate volumetric 24-hour urine collections are required to obtain real 'clearance' results, and this is a practical impossibility in veterinary species. The correct procedure in human medicine is to ask the patient to empty the bladder at time zero and discard that urine, then collect all urine passed for the next 24 hours until at time $0 + 24$ hours the bladder is again emptied and that collection added to the pool. Analysis is carried out on the well-mixed pooled sample, and the total volume of the sample must also be accurately measured. Clearance of the substance in question is then calculated from the formula

$$\text{Clearance} = \frac{\text{urine concentration (mmol/l)} \times \text{urine flow rate (ml/min)}}{\text{plasma concentration (mmol/l)}}$$

To circumvent the obviously impossible task of replicating this procedure in animal patients, the concept of the 'clearance ratio' (or fractional excretion) has been developed. This involves collecting fairly simultaneous blood and urine samples (ideally, collect the blood sample and then collect a sample of the next urine passed by the patient) and measuring both the analyte in question and creatinine in both samples. A clearance ratio is then calculated by the following formula:

Clearance of X (%) =

$$\frac{[X] \text{ urine (mmol/l)}}{[X] \text{ plasma (mmol/l)}} \times \frac{[\text{creatinine}] \text{ plasma (mmol/l)}}{[\text{creatinine}] \text{ urine (mmol/l)}} \times 100$$

This is in effect a ratio of the clearance of the substance under investigation to the clearance of creatinine. The flow rate is thus cancelled out of the equation, and as creatinine clearance is assumed to be a constant, the final figure relates mainly to the clearance of the substance in question. In practice, marked diurnal variations in the excretion of most urine constituents (and more minor variations in creatinine excretion) make this spot measurement fairly useless for all analytes except phosphate. However, fractional excretion of phosphate has some value as a very approximate guide to glomerular filtration rate in renal failure – less than 10% is considered normal while more than 30% is said to indicate a patient in real trouble. The measurement has also been used as a nutritional investigation in horses.

Magnesium

Normal plasma concentration about 1–2 mmol/l.

Disorders of magnesium metabolism in monogastric species are very rare, but in ruminants (especially cattle) problems, particularly of magnesium deficiency, are common. Probably because of the rarity of magnesium problems among human patients this is a comparatively little understood mineral and information regarding mechanisms of homeostasis, etc., is scanty. Magnesium (like potassium) is an intracellular ion, and again like potassium the plasma concentration can remain within normal limits even in the face of marked depletion of the total body content.

Increase (hypermagnesaemia)

This is rare in any species and is usually seen in conjunction with other mineral abnormalities. The most usual cause is acute renal failure, when it accompanies hyperkalaemia. Clinically, hypermagnesaemia causes muscle hypotonia, but cases are unusual and it is little studied. Haemolysed samples will give falsely high results.

Decrease (hypomagnesaemia)

This is very common in cattle and seen also quite frequently in sheep. It is primarily due to dietary magnesium deficiency, but two forms are recognized depending on the suddenness of onset of the deficiency. 'Grass staggers' is seen most frequently in dairy cattle on first turning out on to spring grass. There is a sudden transition from a commercial ration, correctly balanced for minerals, to grass which may be superb in terms of energy and protein but is very poor in magnesium. Acutely convulsing cattle are seen, and response to i/v magnesium salts is dramatic. Plasma magnesium concentrations of clinical cases are very low (well below 0.5 mmol/l), but because of the suddenness of onset those of the unaffected members of the herd may be normal. When hypomagnesaemia affects sheep and calves it is usually the culmination of a fairly prolonged period of poor magnesium diet, and in this case screening of clinically healthy animals will often show subnormal plasma magnesium concentrations. Various husbandry techniques have been devised to combat these problems, such as intraruminal bullets of magnesium and pasture dusting.

When hypomagnesaemia occurs in monogastrics (this is very rare) it is usually the result of severe diarrhoea.

Copper

Normal plasma concentration about 15–30 μmol/l.

As with magnesium, disorders of copper metabolism are almost exclusively a ruminant problem, and again incorrect dietary intake is the primary problem in nearly all cases.

Increase (hypercupraemia, copper poisoning)

This is essentially a disease of housed sheep characterized by acute onset haemolytic anaemia (see p. 17). Sheep are particularly susceptible to excess dietary copper and it is quite difficult to formulate a ration for housed sheep which is sufficiently *low* in copper. Pig rations are particularly dangerous if accidentally fed to sheep. When sheep ingest excessive quantities of copper over a period of time plasma copper concentrations do not rise excessively because the copper is stored in the liver. However, the liver can take only so much copper and eventually there is a sudden release of the stored copper into the bloodstream. This may be spontaneous, but is often associated with handling stress such as blood sampling or vaccination. Plasma copper concentrations rise sharply and this directly causes lysis of the red cells. Symptoms are those of acute haemolytic anaemia – tachycardia, dyspnoea, jaundice, haemoglobinuria, pallor and sudden death. Thus a chronic intoxication situation results clinically in a very acute onset disease. While measurements of plasma copper concentration are of course diagnostic in clinical cases, rising to as much as 100 μmol/l in some cases (and the post-mortem finding of a copper-loaded liver is also pathognomonic), such measurements are of little value in predicting risk during the asymptomatic development of the condition. Elevated plasma aspartate aminotransferase (AST) levels have been reported in sheep at risk of copper poisoning (AST indicates, among other things, damage to or necrosis of liver cells) and liver biopsy is of course very useful, but considering the association of development of clinical disease with handling stress, the wisdom of embarking on this sort of procedure in at-risk sheep is very questionable.

Decrease (hypocupraemia, copper deficiency)

This is seen in both cattle and sheep and is usually associated with hill grazing on poor pasture. Symptoms in cattle are of weight loss and a failure to thrive, and a characteristic loss of pigment in the hair of dark coloured animals is noticeable (black animals look rusty, especially around the eyes). A microcytic hypochromic anaemia is also present due to a block in haem synthesis (see p. 26). Symptoms in sheep are similar, and in particular copper deficiency is associated with lambs being born incoordinated or developing incoordination during the first few weeks of life – 'swayback'.

Clinical symptoms of copper deficiency are usually associated with plasma copper concentrations below 10 μmol/l. However, similar low copper levels have also been found in animals which are apparently clinically healthy, and although such animals do grow better when given copper supplementation (thus demonstrating that they are in fact subclinically copper deficient), this can make it difficult to decide in some cases whether clinical symptoms are actually a direct result of copper deficiency or not.

Cobalt

Cobalt is a necessary cofactor for the formation of vitamin B_{12} (cobalamin). Monogastric species receive their vitamin B_{12} directly from the diet, and cobalt deficiency per se is a problem seen only in ruminants. In the ruminant, vitamin B_{12} in the diet cannot be directly utilized; instead microbial B_{12} from ruminal bacteria is absorbed in the small intestine. These ruminal bacteria themselves require cobalt for B_{12} synthesis; thus dietary cobalt deficiency in the ruminant manifests in a very similar way to pernicious anaemia in man (inability to absorb dietary B_{12}). Cattle and sheep on cobalt-deficient pastures (quite common in Scotland) are susceptible – affected animals show very poor growth rates, weight loss and emaciation even in the presence of apparently adequate grass, and there is a normocytic, normochromic anaemia (which may, however, be masked by dehydration). Clinical signs of cobalt deficiency are accompanied by low plasma cobalt and vitamin B_{12} concentrations. Numerical data are difficult to ascertain as plasma cobalt levels are normally so low that accurate measurement is extremely difficult. Treatment is by oral administration of cobalt or parenteral administration of vitamin B_{12}. Cobalt poisoning does not occur naturally as the toxic dose of cobalt compounds is about 100 times the requirement.

Selenium

This mineral is associated metabolically with vitamin E and is important for the correct functioning of muscle, both skeletal and cardiac. The development of 'white muscle disease' – muscular dystrophy – in cattle and sheep subjected to chronic dietary selenium deficiency is well known, but there is also some suspicion that certain myocardial problems in small animals may be associated with a selenium/vitamin E problem. While measurement of plasma selenium concentration by atomic absorption spectrophotometry is possible, it is more usual to assess selenium status by measuring the activity of glutathione peroxidase, a red blood cell enzyme which contains four selenium atoms in each enzyme molecule. Activity of this enzyme correlates well with plasma selenium concentration in the low and normal ranges. Glutathione peroxidase and its interpretation are discussed below in the chapter on clinical enzymology (p. 147).

7 The Nitrogenous Substances

Apart from the plasma proteins, the nitrogen-containing substances in the plasma which are of diagnostic importance are waste products involved in nitrogen excretion – these are urea, creatinine and ammonia. Uric acid is not usually considered to be diagnostically useful in mammalian veterinary medicine, but is important in avian and reptile investigations where it occupies essentially the same role as urea does in mammals.

Urea

Normal plasma concentration around 3–8 mmol/l (up to 15 mmol/l in cats and some cold-blooded horses).

Note that there is major potential for confusion when urea values in old units are encountered. There are two different gravimetric measurements of urea concentration, both expressed as mg/100 ml. One is straightforwardly mg of *urea* per 100 ml, the other is mg of *urea nitrogen* per 100 ml, referred to as BUN (blood urea nitrogen). The numbers involved in these two units are different (obviously a whole urea molecule weighs more than the two nitrogen atoms it contains) and so it is *essential* to know which is being used on a given occasion. The safest thing to do is to convert all figures to SI units (mmol of urea per litre) but even this requires the knowledge of which conversion factor to use (0.17 for urea units, 0.36 for BUN units), and this is not helped by an unfortunate tendency in some quarters to use the term BUN as a synonym for urea no matter which units are meant. If in doubt, American publications usually mean BUN when they say so, as do instruments of American origin, but British clinicians sometimes mean urea and even sometimes speak of 'BUN' in mmol/l, a contradiction in terms.

Urea is a nitrogenous waste product which is formed in the liver as the end product of amino acid breakdown (Fig. 7.1). After the urea has been formed in the liver it is transported in the plasma to the kidneys where it is excreted in the urine. This 'in transit' urea is what is being measured in a plasma sample, and thus the plasma urea concentration can be affected by a number of different factors (Fig. 7.2).

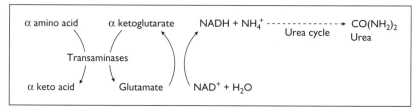

Fig. 7.1   Involvement of ammonia and urea in the deamination of amino acids.

Dietary factors

(1)   Excess dietary protein will lead to increased deamination and a rise in plasma urea concentration. Resulting concentrations are not *very* high, however – only about 7–10 mmol/l in most species. A particular instance of this situation is gastrointestinal haemorrhage, where the blood in the GI tract is digested as a 'meal of blood', with the same implications as any other high protein meal. (Obsessive licking of a bleeding wound or swallowing of blood from epistaxis will also cause this effect.) The finding of a raised urea concentration in an anaemic patient should be followed up by checking the faeces for occult blood (see p. 173). Nevertheless, the converse is not necessarily true, and gastrointestinal haemorrhage cannot be excluded simply on the basis of a normal plasma urea concentration.

(2)   Poor quality dietary protein can have the same effect – the non-essential amino acids will be deaminated in the absence of the essential amino acids, leading to slightly raised plasma urea concentrations.

(3)   Carbohydrate deficiency. Where there is insufficient energy in the diet, body stores of protein (initially labile protein stores in the liver) will be deaminated for their carbon skeletons. In cases of real starvation, especially where there is also some dehydration, this can send plasma urea concentrations up to 15 or even 20 mmol/l.

(4)   Marginal or low dietary protein levels will lead to a reduced plasma urea concentration of around 1–3 mmol/l, but see point (2) above.

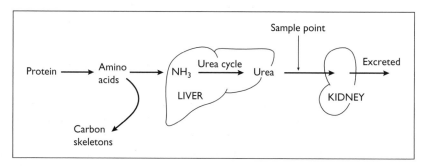

Fig. 7.2   Protein catabolism and urea excretion.

These dietary effects are the reason for including urea in ruminant 'metabolic profiles', but the interpretation is not completely straightforward and has to be considered along with plasma protein concentrations and other factors.

Other metabolic effects

(1) Gross sepsis. It is noticeable that many animals which are forming large amounts of pus demonstrate depressed urea levels, and this is most striking in bitches with pyometra (in the absence of renal impairment, obviously). The cause of this is not certain, but it may be a metabolic effect of sequestering (or losing from the body) large amounts of a highly proteinaceous material leading to a negative nitrogen balance and so to decreased synthesis of urea. However, once again one cannot exclude pyometra or other septic lesion solely on the basis of a normal urea concentration.

(2) Hormonal abnormalities. Certain endocrine disturbances, especially Cushing's disease, tend to depress urea concentration. It has been suggested that this is a consequence of the associated polyuria causing a 'wash-out' of more urea than would normally be excreted by the kidney; however, it is also possible that an anabolic effect of the endocrine abnormality may be responsible for an alteration in nitrogen balance. Treatment with anabolic steroids produces the same effect.

(3) Breed effects. In addition to the tendency of ponies and heavy horse breeds to have higher urea concentrations than hot-blooded horses, it is striking that a high proportion of Yorkshire terriers (particularly middle-aged and older individuals) demonstrate urea concentrations of up to about 15 mmol/l for no readily apparent reason. Whether this is a metabolic effect or a reflection of a high incidence of clinically inapparent congestive heart failure in this breed is not known. Yorkies in renal failure also frequently show disproportionately high urea concentrations relative to creatinine.

(4) Catabolic states. When there is increased breakdown of protein within the body the urea concentration can rise to as much as 20–30 mmol/l. This is most commonly seen in cases of neoplasia, where a possibly necrotizing tumour can combine with the adverse effects of neoplasia on the metabolism as a whole to increase protein catabolism substantially.

Failure of the urea cycle (hyperammonaemia)

The purpose of the urea cycle is to convert the toxic ammonium ions to the innocuous urea molecule for excretion. Failure leads to a build-up of ammonia in the body, accompanied by low plasma urea concentrations of around 0.5–2.5 mmol/l. The excess ammonia leads to a variety of bizarre CNS signs (fits, head-pressing, aggression, coma, mental retardation in children). However, note that urea is not reliable on its own for the diagnosis of these conditions. Some animals have naturally very low urea concentrations due to individual metabolic quirks, and some genuinely hyperammonaemic patients have normal or slightly raised urea concentrations due to minor renal problems. A low urea in an otherwise well animal may safely be ignored, while a genuine suspicion of hyperammonaemia should never be set aside purely on the basis that urea concentration is not low.

Renal insufficiency

This leads to a failure of urea excretion and so to elevated plasma urea concentrations:

(1) Poor renal perfusion. This can be caused either by fairly severe dehydration or by cardiac insufficiency. Where there is nothing actually wrong with the kidney itself the resulting plasma urea concentrations are around 15–35 mmol/l depending on the severity of the perfusion deficit. As the condition improves plasma urea will fall, and this can be a very useful way of monitoring the response to treatment of chronic heart failure cases. However, note that where poor perfusion has caused severe enough or prolonged enough renal hypoxia then primary renal failure can develop as a consequence – in these cases plasma urea concentration will go on rising above 35 mmol/l. In this 'pre-renal' situation plasma creatinine concentration either remains normal or increases proportionately less than urea concentration as compared to primary renal dysfunction (see point (2) below). Although creatinine concentration will become elevated if a consequent renal problem develops, the proportional preponderance of urea typical of the pre-renal aetiology tends to be maintained.

(2) Renal failure. The diagnosis of renal failure is the commonest reason for measuring plasma urea concentrations, especially in small animals where progressive chronic interstitial nephritis is common. Plasma urea may be anywhere from the high normal range to over 100 mmol/l depending on the severity of the condition. In primary renal failure plasma creatinine concentration usually increases in proportion to the urea concentration, but at about $\frac{1}{100}$th of the value (300 μmol/l creatinine usually accompanies 30 mmol/l urea, and so on). Due to the variety of pathological conditions which may be involved it is dangerous to place too much stress on urea as a prognostic indicator, particularly when the diagnosis has just been made, but some general points can be made. In acute onset cases (such as nephrotoxicity) or cases where the condition may be reversible (such as pyelonephritis) it is worth attempting treatment even if the urea is quite seriously elevated. Treatment should be aimed at restoring normal hydration and electrolyte balance (see electrolytes, above) in addition to treating the cause of the problem (e.g. antibiotics for pyelonephritis). In chronic cases the prognosis depends on the severity of the condition. Where the urea is only slightly elevated (under 20 mmol/l) the chances of

response to dietary management are quite good – they deteriorate with increasing plasma urea concentration until when the urea is over 60 mmol/l the condition is hopeless (short of a kidney transplant) and euthanasia will become inevitable on clinical grounds within a fairly short time.

Treatment is primarily by feeding low protein, low potassium, low magnesium, low phosphate diets, thus reducing the excretory load on the kidney – free access to water is also essential as these patients usually cannot concentrate their urine to conserve water and will become dangerously dehydrated if it is restricted. Anabolic steroids also have a role; however, treatment with both special diet and anabolic steroids does not usually produce twice the benefit of either therapy alone.

(3) Urethral obstruction. This can lead to an acute onset renal failure as a result of back-pressure to the kidney and plasma urea concentrations may reach 60 mmol/l or higher. This is not difficult to diagnose on clinical grounds (enlarged, painful bladder; constant straining with little or no urine being passed) and is usually reversible if the obstruction is successfully relieved.

(4) Ruptured bladder. Strictly speaking this is excretory insufficiency rather than renal insufficiency. It is a fairly common sequel to abdominal trauma

Table 7.1 Summary of causes of variation in plasma urea concentration

Increase	**Decrease**
'Pre-renal'	Dietary factors
Dietary factors	(a) Protein deficiency
(a) Increased protein intake	
(b) Intestinal bleeding or blood	Metabolic factors
ingestion	(a) Idiopathic
(c) Poor quality dietary protein	(b) Gross sepsis
(d) Carbohydrate deficiency	(c) Hormonal (anabolic steroid
	effects)
Metabolic and breed factors	(d) Failure of urea cycle
(a) Cold-blooded horses, Yorkshire	(i) Inborn error of metabolism
terriers	(ii) Congenital portocaval shunt
(b) Catabolic states (e.g. neoplasia)	(iii) End-stage liver, often with
	acquired shunt
Poor renal perfusion	
(a) Congestive heart failure	
(b) Hypovolaemia	
(i) Simple dehydration	
(ii) Addison's disease	
'Renal'	
Renal dysfunction	
'Post-renal'	
Urethral obstruction	
Ruptured bladder	

and leads to the presence of free urine in the abdominal cavity. This leads to plasma urea concentrations rising fairly quickly to over 100 mmol/l. Obviously this condition is reversible if surgical repair of the bladder can be effected, but anaesthesia of a severely uraemic patient can be very risky, and prognosis is often poor once this stage has been reached. Peritoneal dialysis prior to surgery can improve the success rates markedly.

It can therefore be seen that renal failure is in fact only one of a wide variety of conditions which can affect plasma urea concentrations. It is therefore important to keep all possibilities in mind until a definite diagnosis has been reached and to consider what other more specific tests will help to sort out the situation in each individual case. In particular, beware of misdiagnosing a cardiac case as renal failure on the basis of an elevated urea concentration.

Case 7.1

A 10-year-old German shepherd dog was presented in a semi-collapsed state with a history of having been missing for 24 hours after slipping his lead. Emergency tests in the practice side-room produced these results. What are the main possibilities and what should be done next?

Total protein	78 g/l	
Sodium	152 mmol/l	
Potassium	8.3 mmol/l	high
Urea	>45 mmol/l	high
Glucose	6.7 mmol/l	raised

Comment

The main concerns are Addisonian crisis, acute renal failure and ruptured bladder. Addison's disease is less likely, considering the relatively high sodium concentration and the absence of evidence of dehydration, but cannot be excluded. Priorities are initiation of appropriate fluid therapy and establishing whether or not the bladder is intact. The glucose is just a stress effect.

Further examination revealed road dirt in the coat and several torn claws. A urinary catheter was passed without difficulty but only a few drops of urine were obtained. Paracentesis yielded a clear, yellow-tinged low-protein fluid. When the laboratory report was received it confirmed the electrolyte results, gave urea as 53.6 mmol/l and creatinine as 1137 μmol/l (consistent with a post-renal phenomenon), and confirmed the abdominal fluid to be urine. Cortisol concentration was 743 nmol/l, which conclusively excluded Addison's disease.

Creatinine

Normal plasma concentration under about 150 μmol/l (with species variations). The main species variations are as follows: most breeds of dog, up to 120 μmol/l; greyhounds and other sight-hounds, also cattle and sheep, up to 150 μmol/l; cats and horses, up to 180 μmol/l.

Creatinine, like urea, is a nitrogenous waste product *en route* to the kidneys, but it is a product not of amino acid breakdown but of breakdown of creatine. Creatine is a substance present in the muscle which is involved in high energy metabolism, particularly in stabilizing high energy phosphate bonds not required for immediate use (see Fig. 7.3). This reaction is reversible and creatine is not automatically excreted just because it isn't needed at a particular time. There is simply a constant slow catabolism of creatine at a rate which is directly proportional to the individual's muscle mass; in effect there is a constant inflow of creatinine to the plasma which is unaffected by any change in muscle activity or muscle damage. Thus changes in plasma creatinine concentration are to all intents and purposes entirely due to changes in creatinine *excretion*, i.e. they reflect *renal* function. (Compare the related enzyme creatine kinase (CK) which has a similar name and is metabolically related to creatinine, but which is used in the plasma as an index of muscle damage – in clinical biochemistry, the two substances are unrelated.) Note, however, that there is a correlation between muscle mass and creatinine concentration. The species with the higher reference values are those with a greater proportion of muscle to total body mass, and within a species a particularly muscular individual might have a normal value somewhat above the reference limit.

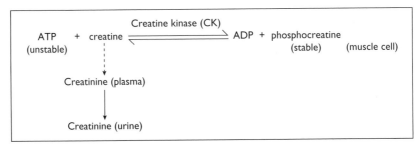

Fig. 7.3   Function of creatine in the storage of high energy P_i groups within the muscle.

Thus, like urea, plasma creatinine is used to investigate kidney disease. It behaves somewhat differently from urea, and measurement of both substances is normal practice in order to gain maximum information about renal function.

(1)   Plasma creatinine concentration is unaffected by diet, or by anything affecting liver or urea cycle metabolism.

(2)   It tends to increase more quickly than urea at the start of a disease and to decrease more quickly when an improvement takes place – thus measuring both plasma creatinine and urea can give some information on the time-course and progress of the disease.

(3)   It tends to show rather smaller alterations from normal, relative to urea, when there is pre-renal interference with renal function (i.e. heart failure or dehydration), and to show rather greater relative increases when there is a major primary failure of renal function – in other words it is a more sensitive indicator of renal function than urea, and a better prognostic indicator.

Other points to bear in mind regarding creatinine are that it is rather more labile than most substrate (i.e. non-enzyme) analytes and so a result from a sample several days old may not be absolutely accurate, and that it is subject to some assay interference. The most commonly used method, the Jaffé alkaline picrate reaction, has problems with bilirubin interference, and results from jaundiced samples can vary substantially from the true creatinine value. Creatininase methods (less commonly used) do not suffer from this problem. Creatinine methods can also be subject to some drug interference, most notably from cephalosporin antibiotics.

Interpretation of plasma creatinine results is fairly straightforward – decreases are not clinically significant; increases of up to around 250 µmol/l *may* be pre-renal (dehydration or heart failure); over this figure the kidneys are almost certainly involved (unless a ruptured bladder or urethral obstruction is present), and once plasma creatinine has risen above 500 µmol/l things are getting serious. Concentrations of over 1000 µmol/l (1 mmol/l) are seen in severe acute renal failure, the terminal stages of chronic renal failure, and in cases of ruptured bladder and urethral obstruction.

The practice of measuring both urea and creatinine together allows maximum information to be obtained – the combination is more than the sum of the parts. In particular it allows the pre-renal increases in urea concentration to be differentiated from renal conditions, and metabolic and circulatory effects to be recognized without ambiguity.

Ammonia

Normal plasma concentration under about 60 µmol/l in most species.

Note that ammonia concentration is very unstable in blood and plasma samples. The problem is that urea begins to break down to ammonia after the sample has been collected: this is not sufficient to cause a problem with urea measurement as only a small fraction of the total urea actually breaks down, but it is enough to elevate the ammonia concentration considerably and give the erroneous impression of hyperammonaemia in a genuinely normal sample (the breakdown of 0.1 mmol of urea will produce 200 µmol of ammonia). To avoid this, samples must be taken into *EDTA* (not heparin), *immediately* placed in ice and centrifuged, and the plasma separated within 30 minutes of collection. Plasma must be kept refrigerated and analysed within 3 hours, or it may be deep frozen ($-20°C$) and analysed within 3 days. It is therefore possible to have this test done externally if a centrifuge is available and the plasma can be delivered by hand to the laboratory, but posting deep-frozen samples is not really feasible and most cases have to be referred for sampling to a centre where the test can be performed on the spot.

Ammonia is essentially the substance which is one stage before urea in amino acid catabolism/nitrogen excretion (see Fig. 7.2). Failure of the urea cycle leads to a build-up of ammonia in the plasma in the presence of low plasma urea concentrations. Anything which causes high plasma urea will also cause a high plasma ammonia concentration, due to imbalance of the urea cycle. High ammonia is therefore of no diagnostic significance in uraemic patients.

There are several possible causes of hyperammonaemia.

(1) Inborn error of urea cycle metabolism. Congenital condition affecting young animals (or at any rate with a history of problems almost from birth). Clinical signs are bizarre CNS disturbances – aggression, sometimes related to food intake; recurrent episodes of coma; excessive stupidity (often diagnosed in children as mental handicap). The only biochemical abnormalities are the ammonia and urea findings (and the presence of orotic acid, the abnormal metabolite formed as a side branch when the urea cycle is blocked); there are no indications of any of the liver's other metabolic tasks being affected. Portal angiography, if performed, is normal.

Many cases respond well to low-protein diet alone. Nowadays children are treated orally with sodium benzoate (0.1 g/kg/day given last thing at night) which bypasses the blocked urea cycle and creates an alternative pathway for nitrogen to be excreted as hippuric acid. This is extremely effective in human patients, but veterinary experience is limited. A low-protein diet with supplementation of the essential amino acids is also recommended; in veterinary terms this usually means cottage cheese and rice. Also, antibiotic treatment (e.g. neomycin) to reduce the production of ammonia by enteric bacteria has been recommended.

(2) Congenital portosystemic shunt (patent ductus venosus or other vascular abnormality linking the portal and peripheral venous systems). Again these are young animals which are affected from birth, and in this case the defect is usually so severe that most cases present in the first year of life. Clinical signs are similar to inborn error cases, but in addition to the ammonia/urea abnormalities there is progressive impairment of other liver functions – hypoalbuminaemia, hypoprothrombinaemia, hypercholesterolaemia, raised plasma aminotransferase and alkaline phosphatase activities. This condition is best diagnosed by dynamic bile acid testing, and is dealt with under that heading (see p. 130).

(3) End-stage liver failure. When liver disease is reaching its terminal stages all of the liver's functions tend to fail, including the urea cycle. This is particularly true of cases where an acquired portosystemic shunt has developed. Again there will be clear evidence of general liver function impairment: hypoalbuminaemia and hypoprothrombinaemia tend to be severe, jaundice is usually evident, but transaminase levels may not be raised as there is often no real hepatic tissue left to release any enzymes. Again, bile acid measurements are the most practical method of investigating this condition (see p. 129). Angiography (not usually necessary or advisable) will demonstrate the multiple convoluted vessels of an acquired shunt in the mesentery. Short of a liver transplant, prognosis is hopeless. Whether or not the CNS signs typical of hyperammonaemia are seen in

an end-stage liver case depends to a large extent on the exact nature of the pathology and how seriously the urea cycle is affected compared with other functions. Horses in the terminal stages of ragwort poisoning often show head-pressing and blindness as a result of hyperammonaemia.

(4)   Young Irish wolfhound puppies demonstrate a benign, asymptomatic hyperammonaemia in the first few months of life, but ammonia concentrations are normal in the adult dogs. This has important implications for the investigation of congenital portosystemic shunts, which are not uncommon in this breed. Bile acid measurements are the test of choice in this situation (see p. 131).

Carbohydrate Metabolism

Glucose

Normal fasting plasma concentration about 4–6 mmol/l in monogastrics, 3–5 mmol/l in ruminants.

Note that these are *plasma* glucose concentrations. Older practice was to measure glucose in whole blood, without centrifugation, which gave values about 0.5 mmol/l less than this (depending on the PCV) because the intra-erythrocyte glucose concentration is significantly lower than the plasma concentration. The actual plasma concentration is more consistent and more meaningful, but beware of older publications referring to 'blood glucose'. (It can sometimes be difficult to know whether blood or plasma glucose is meant as sometimes the term 'blood glucose' is used loosely, meaning either.)

Glucose measurement has a specific sample requirement – blood must be collected into tubes containing fluoride (usually with oxalate as the anti-coagulant). Fluoride blocks glycolysis in the red cells, thus preventing consumption of glucose in the sample which would otherwise be significantly reduced within 30 minutes. Swift separation of non-fluoride plasma from the red cells can extend this time somewhat, but this is not reliable as bacteria can also consume glucose, and fluoride containers should be routinely used for glucose measurement. However, fluoride plasma is not suitable for any other analyses (including insulin and fructosamine).

An adequately high plasma glucose concentration is essential for normal brain function, and the body goes to quite elaborate lengths to ensure that this is maintained. As a result the glucose in the plasma at any particular time may come from one or more of a number of sources, depending on the current state of carbohydrate metabolism. In the post-absorptive phase, glucose is being transported from its site of uptake in the gut to the sites of glycogen storage, principally the liver and muscles. In the fasting animal plasma glucose concentrations are maintained by mobilizing carbohydrates from anywhere they can be found – normally hepatic glycogenolysis predominates, with some lipolysis and gluconeogenesis, but if starvation is prolonged lipolysis and even proteinolysis become more important. There is complex and tight feedback and hormonal control over these pathways to ensure a reasonably constant plasma glucose concentration no matter what the current state of feasting or fasting. In normal day-to-day circumstances glucagon and growth hormone are responsible for maintaining an adequate level, while in abnormal states such as prolonged fasting or stress the glucocorticoids and adrenaline are particularly important. In contrast to the multiple agents acting to increase plasma glucose concentration, there is only one hormone which decreases it: insulin (Fig. 8.1). Thus hyperglycaemia (which is less dangerous for the animal in the short term) is quite common and causes are various, while hypoglycaemia (which is potentially life-threatening) is less commonly encountered.

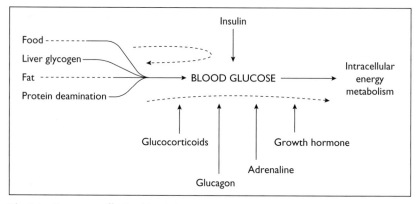

Fig. 8.1   Hormones affecting blood glucose concentration.

Renal glucose threshold

The kidney normally deals with glucose by allowing all the plasma glucose to be filtered and then reabsorbing it in the proximal tubule. However, the proximal tubular reabsorptive capacity is limited and at glucose loads approximating to a plasma glucose concentration of about 10 mmol/l reabsorption will not be complete and some glucose will appear in the urine. This *plasma* glucose concentration above which glycosuria occurs is the *renal* glucose threshold. The finding of glycosuria simply means that this plasma concentration has been exceeded during the period before the urine sample was collected and the quantitative relationship between plasma and urine glucose concentrations is very poor. Renal glucose thresholds below 10 mmol/l are seen in some normal individuals, especially in neonates and during pregnancy, and in proximal tubular defects (e.g. Fanconi syndrome) glucose reabsorption is poor and glycosuria is seen without hyperglycaemia. In some long-standing cases of diabetes mellitus the renal glucose threshold may rise, leading to absence of classical polydipsia/polyuria symptoms while plasma glucose is still uncontrolled enough to admit the risks of cataracts, fatty liver, etc. Another reason for the absence of glycosuria in the presence of hyperglycaemia is the presence of a renal problem with a reduction in glomerular filtration rate. The proximal tubule glucose load is hence much lower and complete reabsorption is possible. Again, other hyperglycaemia-related problems may be present without polydipsia/polyuria. Thus measurement of urine glucose is a very blunt instrument, and measurement of plasma glucose is essential to get any real idea of what is going on.

Increase (hyperglycaemia)

This can vary in severity from the mild hyperglycaemia occurring after a meal to very extreme hyperglycaemia found in uncontrolled diabetes mellitus, and an appreciation of the significance of the various degrees of severity is important for interpretation.

Non-diabetic hyperglycaemia

(1) After a high-carbohydrate meal. This is the 'post-absorptive' peak in plasma glucose concentration. The levels reached depend on a number of factors including the carbohydrate load consumed, but it is unusual for them to be much above 7 mmol/l.

(2) Sprint exercise. This involves a high level of adrenaline secretion, and plasma glucose levels of around 15 mmol/l are common in racehorses and greyhounds immediately after racing.

(3) 'Stress', particularly severe and/or acute stress. Situations include animals in severe pain, intractable animals which have been forcibly restrained, and large animals which have just undergone a road (or rail, sea or air) journey. Animals under anaesthesia also come into this category. Both adrenaline and the glucocorticoids are involved here, with adrenaline having the more marked effect. As with exercise, plasma glucose concentrations can reach 15 mmol/l, but levels of around 8–10 mmol/l are more usual. Cats, however, are a particular problem. Stress hyperglycaemia not infrequently reaches 20 mmol/l, which can cause real difficulty in differentiating this from diabetes mellitus.

(4) Other causes of raised glucocorticoid activity, e.g. treatment with glucocorticoids or Cushing's disease. This type of situation tends to be more long-term than the stress situations mentioned above and the counter-effects of insulin may completely mask the tendency to hyperglycaemia. However, plasma glucose concentrations of around 6–8 mmol/l are sometimes seen. Cushing's disease can also progress to type II (insulin resistant) diabetes mellitus, especially in horses and cats, and a similar consequence can arise from prolonged steroid administration.

(5) Treatment with glucose-containing i/v fluids. The most commonly used preparation in this class is dextrose saline (see fluid therapy, p. 89), but a number of i/v preparations contain dextrose or glucose. The primary

reason for the inclusion of the dextrose is to provide an infusion which is hypotonic for the electrolytes with the correct osmolarity for i/v administration. Naturally, the use of such preparations will raise plasma glucose. Ideally, since the purpose of administration is usually to correct dehydration, the speed of infusion should not be so fast as to raise the plasma glucose concentration above the renal threshold, as this will lead to an osmotic diuresis and further water loss. However, levels of 20 or even 25 mmol/l are quite possible as a result of over-enthusiastic administration of dextrose saline. Therefore, beware of the trap of diagnosing diabetes mellitus from a blood sample collected during or just after such treatment.

Diabetes mellitus

This is a common condition in both the dog and cat, and is not unusual in elderly horses. There are occasional reports of cases in other species such as rabbits. It is due to absolute or *relative* insulin deficiency, and can be divided into several categories based on the well-established classifications employed in human medicine:

Type I (insulin dependent) diabetes

In these patients there is essentially no insulin secretion. Presentation is often acute, and ketoacidosis is common. It tends to occur in younger animals but can happen at any age. In man this is known to be an autoimmune condition, with antibodies which react against the β-cells of the pancreas, and it is likely that the same is true of the dog. Occasionally recurrent attacks of pancreatitis may produce the same syndrome, however. Type I diabetes is uncommon in animals other than the dog.

Type II diabetes

Primary type II diabetes mellitus occurs when insulin secretion is simply inadequate to maintain normal blood glucose concentrations. It tends to occur in middle-aged and older animals, and there is often an association with obesity. As insulin is still actually present in these patients, type II generally presents less acutely than type I and ketoacidosis is less likely. Although this type of diabetes is often termed 'non-insulin-dependent', and insulin is not usually required to prevent ketosis, many patients do require insulin to maintain normal blood glucose concentrations. Perhaps because the disease is still generally diagnosed later in animals than in man, only a minority of veterinary patients tend to be controllable with diet (with or without oral hypoglycaemics) alone.

Secondary type II diabetes mellitus occurs as a result of some other hormonal factor which causes resistance to the action of insulin – either as a result of another endocrine condition where insulin is antagonized by a hormone or hormones with opposing activity, or of treatment with such a hormone. Insulin resistance can be very marked in these cases.

In the dog, type II diabetes becomes a problem in a proportion of cases of Cushing's disease (cortisol is a powerful insulin antagonist), and usually resolves with successful treatment of the Cushing's. Another common canine scenario is the bitch who becomes diabetic shortly after oestrus, due to a similar effect of progesterone (acting via growth hormone). This is an important condition to be aware of, as the presentation (malaise and polydipsia in the weeks following oestrus) makes it easy to confuse with a pyometra. If these bitches are spayed as soon as possible the diabetes often resolves within a few weeks. Gestational diabetes mellitus such as occurs in women is not recognized in animals; however, entire females who become diabetic for any reason should normally be spayed, as problems with control almost inevitably arise in association with oestrus.

Cats are particularly prone to develop iatrogenic type II diabetes as a result of powerful anti-inflammatory steroids being used to control a flea allergy – megestrol acetate (Ovarid: Schering-Plough) is often associated with this condition, as is methylprednisolone acetate (Depomedrone: Pharmacia & Upjohn), and more frequent dosing with a short-acting preparation such as prednisolone may be preferable as it can at least be withdrawn more quickly if a problem develops. Obsessive attention to parasite control is also advisable to minimize the dose of anti-inflammatory required. Nevertheless, iatrogenic diabetes usually resolves within a few weeks once the offending steroid is withdrawn.

When insulin-resistant diabetes occurs in a cat in the absence of any steroid administration, the two main conditions to consider are Cushing's disease and acromegaly (oversecretion of growth hormone) – not necessarily in that order. Cushing's disease is very much less common in the cat than in the dog, and (again unlike the dog) most cases actually present as insulin-resistant diabetes. However, acromegaly has a very similar clinical presentation and may, in fact, be the more common of the two conditions in this species. It is confirmed by demonstrating an increased concentration of IGF-1 (insulin-like growth factor).

The cat is the one species where apparently idiopathic type II diabetes does occasionally appear to resolve spontaneously – a cat which has been on insulin treatment will suddenly become hypoglycaemic, and once the dust has settled it is realized that normal blood glucose concentrations are being maintained without any treatment at all. It may be that this is associated with the disappearance of some insulin antagonist, but the mechanism is not well understood. Note also that while diabetes mellitus is commoner in bitches than in dogs, in the cat the condition is commoner in the male.

In the horse, almost all cases of diabetes mellitus are secondary to equine Cushing's disease (see p. 156).

Diagnosis of diabetes mellitus

Urine glucose measurement is an *extremely* blunt instrument. It has some use as a screening test in human medicine because of the extreme ease of sample collection. In veterinary medicine, where sample collection is much less straightforward, this is not a sensible initial investigation. Blood sampling is both easier and a much more precise tool, and there is no excuse at all for a laboratory request for a routine profile 'excluding glucose', with the comment 'diabetes suspected, but so far unable to obtain urine sample'.

In man, diagnosis of diabetes is highly standardized, with rigid guidelines issued by the World Health Organization. These guidelines are not directly applicable to veterinary cases; nevertheless, it is useful to be aware of the protocol (summarized here).

(1)   Random plasma glucose: 5.5 mmol/l or less, not diabetic; 11.1 mmol/l or over, diabetic (two separate results necessary in asymptomatic patients); 5.6–11.0 mmol/l, investigate further.

(2)   Fasting plasma glucose (15-hour fast): less than 6.1 mmol/l, not diabetic; 7.0 mmol/l or more, diabetic; 6.1–6.9 mmol/l ('impaired fasting glycaemia'), investigate further.

(3)   Oral glucose tolerance test, following overnight fast. The traditional five-sample test is now considered to be obsolete, and the critical value is the glucose concentration 2 hours after an oral glucose load of 75 g (nominally 1 g/kg) anhydrous glucose (82.5 g glucose monohydrate): less than 7.8 mmol/l, not diabetic; 11.1 mmol/l or over, diabetic; 7.8–11.0 mmol/l, 'impaired glucose tolerance' diagnosed, but not (yet?) diabetes as such.

Other results such as urine dipstix tests, glycated haemoglobin or fructosamine are regarded as suggestive, but not reliable for diagnostic purposes. In addition, analysis is required to be performed only by accredited laboratories and the use of pocket glucose meters is regarded as inappropriate in this context.

The very prescriptive nature of these guidelines is mainly designed to avoid missing mild, relatively asymptomatic type II diabetes, which is common in man, and which has a much more favourable long-term outlook if diagnosed and managed in its early stages. This is not such an issue in the veterinary field, when patients have often been symptomatic for some time before presentation and many animals present little diagnostic challenge. Nevertheless, diabetes management in animals does tend to catch up with advances in human medicine eventually, and it is possible that similar criteria may be adopted, at least in canine medicine, in the future.

The classic presentation of diabetes mellitus in the dog (and often also in the cat) is the middle-aged patient presented with a history of polydipsia and weight loss, often from a previously overweight condition. Blood glucose on a glucose meter is over 20 mmol/l and there is marked glycosuria (at least 3+ on the dipstick), possibly with a positive ketone result also. Pragmatically speaking, there is no doubt about the diagnosis in these cases.

The main difficulty encountered is when doubt arises as to whether a moderate hyperglycaemia is genuinely due to diabetes, or is simply a stress hyperglycaemia. This is a particular problem in the cat, where frightened, needle-shy individuals can occasionally produce glucose levels as high as 20–22 mmol/l at a particularly fraught sampling session. In dogs, stress hyperglycaemia rarely goes above 10–12 mmol/l. Some clarification may be gained by attempting to ascertain whether the hyperglycaemia is transient or has been persistent. If a urine sample can be obtained a *marked* glycosuria is very suggestive of diabetes, as it indicates persistent hyperglycaemia for at least several hours, though a trace to 1+ glucose should be regarded with caution as stress hyperglycaemia can exceed the renal glucose threshold. It may be helpful to ask the owners of a very stressed cat to obtain a urine sample at home, when the cat is (hopefully) relaxed. Fructosamine can also be very helpful (see p. 123). Fructosamine concentration is directly proportional to the average blood glucose level over about the 2 weeks preceding sampling – a markedly elevated result is diagnostic, but once again a minor deviation from normal must be treated with caution. In addition, a very recent-onset diabetes mellitus may be associated with an unremarkable fructosamine concentration. Finally, in monogastrics the only realistic cause of ketosis is diabetes mellitus, and demonstration of ketosis is conclusive. This is readily appreciable from a urine sample, or if urine is unobtainable a spot of plasma may be used on the ketone patch of a urine dipstick. However, many type II diabetics are not ketotic when presented.

Insulin measurement may be helpful, but it is mainly useful for distinguishing between type I (no measurable insulin) and type II (insulin present, either in inadequate amounts or being antagonized by another hormone) diabetes.

Monitoring the diabetic patient

Initial stabilization

It is overwhelmingly preferable to admit diabetic animals and stabilize them as in-patients. Blood glucose is the only practical test, and it should be performed frequently – at least every 2 hours while insulin dosage is being adjusted. If insulin injections are being given in the evening, it is necessary to arrange for this to continue during at least the early part of the night. Fortunately the pocket glucose meters marketed for human diabetic monitoring work quite satisfactorily in animals, and are ideal for this purpose. Unfortunately, the finger-prick capillary blood sampling systems marketed with them do not. However, repeated jugular venepuncture can be avoided by using a fine insulin needle and syringe to aspirate a drop or two of blood from the cephalic vein (the needle is so fine that there is usually no withdrawal reflex, and the vein seldom if ever 'blows'), or the capillary blood sampling systems which have recently come on to the market for animals may be investigated.

Quite apart from the difficulty of collecting urine from dogs and cats, urine glucose measurements are totally inadequate for this purpose – all a positive result tells you is that the blood glucose has been over the renal glucose threshold at some point during the preceding few hours, which is nowhere near enough information to allow the optimum insulin regime to be achieved. Urine glucose measurements as an adjunct to blood glucose monitoring add little extra information.

Glycated protein measurements change slowly in response to changes in blood glucose, and their place is in long-term monitoring, not initial stabilization.

Insulin resistance is recognized when a high dose of insulin – perhaps as much as twice the dose which would be expected for the animal's body weight – fails to have any effect on blood glucose concentration. The typical case has a blood glucose of around 25 mmol/l virtually constantly, and there is no appreciable fall following insulin injection. In these cases, it is then necessary to start looking for the insulin antagonist (Cushing's disease being the most obvious candidate). This is in contrast to insulin-responsive patients, where the glucose does fall appreciably after insulin injection, and the main problem may be that it doesn't fall far enough or increases again much too soon. These animals simply need further adjustment of the insulin regime – a longer-acting preparation or twice-daily injections may have to be considered.

Monitoring the stabilized diabetic

Once again, urine glucose measurement is a blunt instrument. Its only remaining application in human medicine is in the monitoring of elderly patients with mild type II diabetes who are not on insulin treatment. Younger patients and all patients on insulin are trained in blood glucose monitoring. In type I diabetes the incidence of long-term complications can be significantly reduced by very tight control, with insulin dose being frequently and carefully adjusted on the basis of multiple daily blood glucose measurements – occasional hypoglycaemic episodes are accepted as a fair trade-off for better long-term health. Milder type II diabetics may in contrast perform a check only two or three times a week.

The objectives of diabetic control in animals are not necessarily the same: in particular, owners usually prefer to avoid hypoglycaemic episodes, and somewhat more lax control may be preferable in the interests of the quality of life of all concerned. Nevertheless, it is advantageous to keep hyperglycaemia to a minimum, and once again urine glucose monitoring is not a particularly satisfactory approach.

In contrast to human patients, the routine with diabetic animals is generally to keep to the insulin regime which has been drawn up following the initial stabilization period, at least until the next scheduled reassessment. The question is, how much home monitoring by the owner is then necessary? Measurement of 24-hour water intake is very useful and should be carried out two or three times a week. The main problem with blood glucose measurement is sample collection; however, if this can be overcome and the owner is able to collect a drop of blood for a glucose meter (or even to read the blood glucose strip by eye) then doing this even a couple of times a week can be very useful. In addition, the ability of the owner to perform a blood glucose measurement can be crucial if a hypoglycaemic episode is suspected. Urine sample collection can be at least as problematical as capillary blood sampling, and often significantly less pleasant for the owner. In addition, as the only thing a urine sample can demonstrate is that the blood glucose has been over the renal glucose threshold in the preceding few hours, one would expect all urine measurements in a well-stabilized patient to be negative. It may be useful to encourage perhaps a weekly urine check if home blood testing cannot be undertaken, but obsessive daily monitoring is unpleasant, onerous and not really necessary. The owner should be instructed as to what level of water intake or spot blood or urine glucose result should be considered grounds for seeking early veterinary advice; otherwise an appointment is made for a routine reassessment after an appropriate time.

The mainstay of diabetic monitoring is the regular assessment in the veterinary practice. The frequency of this may vary according to how stable the patient appears to be, but every 3 months is probably the minimum. The patient is admitted first thing in the morning, and the owner's diary of water intake and any blood or urine measurements made since the previous assessment is inspected. All meals, exercise and insulin are given as normal and blood glucose is measured every 2 hours, continuing as far into the evening as practical. A blood sample is also collected for fructosamine or glycated haemoglobin measurement, and perhaps also routine biochemistry to check liver enzymes, etc. If all is well, the same regime may be continued until the next assessment, but if a problem emerges then a decision can be taken as to how much readjustment of the regime is required.

The advantages of this approach are that it does not place an intolerable burden on the animal's owner, and yet it allows diabetic control to be achieved at a level which will promote a good quality of life for the patient with minimum risk of complications due to persistent hyperglycaemia.

Decrease (hypoglycaemia)

As cerebral metabolism is dependent on glucose as its sole fuel source, hypoglycaemia produces symptoms similar to cerebral anoxia – faintness, dizziness, sometimes convulsing fits, sometimes coma. This condition is highly dangerous and so prompt recognition and correction are vital. In most species plasma glucose concentrations of under 3 mmol/l are nearly always associated with recognizable symptoms, but horses seem much more tolerant of hypoglycaemia, and plasma glucose concentrations as low as 2 mmol/l may be quite without effect. However, beware of spurious 'hypoglycaemia' when samples are not in the correct anticoagulant. Fluoride must always be used when a glucose concentration is required.

(1) Insulin-induced hypoglycaemia.

  (a) Overdosage of diabetic patient is the most common – a dog may fail to eat after insulin has been given, or the dose may be given twice in error. Now that a single standard concentration is in use for insulin preparations, administration of the wrong preparation is not a danger.

  (b) Insulinoma. This is a tumour of the islet cells of the pancreas and is not uncommon in dogs. Symptoms may be mistaken for primary CNS disease. Diagnosis is confirmed by demonstrating a high insulin/glucose ratio on a *fasting* blood sample (see p. 165). Although insulinomas are usually benign in man, most such tumours in dogs are malignant, and surgical outcome is often disappointing. However, severity of presentation can vary considerably, and more mildly affected individuals may be managed symptomatically, using prednisolone to promote gluconeogenesis and feeding frequent, high-carbohydrate meals. Development of obesity is an almost unavoidable complication.

  (c) Islet cell hyperplasia, non-malignant. This is uncommon, but may occur as a result of prolonged steroid exposure.

  (d) Not strictly insulin-induced, but hypoglycaemia has been recorded in dogs as a result of consuming their diabetic owner's oral hypoglycaemic tablets.

(2) Fasting hypoglycaemia.

  (a) Acetonaemia (cattle)/pregnancy toxaemia (sheep). This is a condition confined to ruminants and is a consequence of the unusual

---

Case 8.1

A 12-year-old cairn terrier spayed bitch was presented having had several short 'fits' over the preceding few days. The owner reported that she had been increasingly reluctant to exercise for about 2 months. On examination she was clinically normal, though overweight. The following biochemistry results were obtained. What is the likely cause of the fits and how could that be confirmed?

Sodium	147 mmol/l	
Potassium	5.2 mmol/l	
Calcium	2.28 mmol/l	
Glucose	2.8 mmol/l	low
Urea	4.6 mmol/l	
Creatinine	63 µmol/l	

Comment

Insulinoma. Hypoglycaemia is the only abnormality, and this is marked. Although idiopathic hypoglycaemia can occur in small dogs, the age and the history of weight gain and exercise intolerance are very suggestive of insulinoma. Confirmation is by demonstrating a high insulin/glucose ratio on a *fasted* sample.

routes of carbohydrate metabolism in these species. In the ruminant ingested carbohydrate is not absorbed as such but as bacterially produced volatile free fatty acids which are then transformed back to glucose by gluconeogenesis if necessary. This leaves these species susceptible to hypoglycaemia which tends to occur in association with late pregnancy (sheep)/early to peak lactation (cattle). At these times metabolic demand is maximal (maintenance of near-term twin or triplet fetuses or high milk production), and tends to be channelled to fetal rather than maternal benefit, and so maternal hypoglycaemia with ketosis develops (see p. 124). Note that clincial onset of hypoglycaemia and ketosis can be very rapid, and screening of clinically well animals is a poor guide to future, or indeed imminent, risk. Hypoglycaemia as a result of prolonged starvation does not occur in monogastrics.

(b) Idiopathic hypoglycaemia of toy breeds of dogs. This is a condition characterized by recurrent episodes of fainting associated with fasting and/or exercise. Insulinoma is not involved and very profound hypoglycaemia due to this cause is uncommon.

(c) Hypoglycaemia of acute illness. Occasionally a patient will present severely ill with a non-metabolic condition, and hypoglycaemia is discovered almost as an incidental finding. Such patients require glucose as part of their fluid therapy, but blood glucose will return to normal once the immediate crisis is over.

(3) Reactive hypoglycaemia-type conditions are considered in man but seldom recognized in animals.

(a) Functional hypoglycaemia. In normal individuals the peak in plasma glucose concentration seen after a meal is followed by a temporary swing below fasting levels. In individuals particularly sensitive to glucose this swing may be exaggerated enough to produce a genuine hypoglycaemia. Symptoms are not usually severe. Confirmation of functional hypoglycaemia is by demonstration of a 'lag storage' glucose tolerance curve where the post-prandial peak appears early and may be unusually high for a non-diabetic, and is then followed by an exaggerated fall below normal levels.

(b) Alcohol-induced hypoglycaemia.

(4) 'Glucose meter non-hypoglycaemia' is recognized in man when a non-diabetic individual uses someone else's glucose meter to check their own blood glucose, perhaps following an attack of giddiness, and then presents complaining of hypoglycaemia. Subsequent investigation almost always demonstrates this to be spurious. The same thing happens in veterinary medicine, in particular when a practice uses a reflectance meter as part of a routine work-up of a non-diabetic case. All apparent hypoglycaemias in non-diabetic animals reported by reflectance meters should be confirmed by the professional laboratory.

Table 8.1 Summary of causes of variation in plasma glucose concentration

Increase	Decrease
Food (post-absorptive state)	Insulin overdose
Intensive exercise, including	Insulinoma
struggling against restraint	Consumption of oral hypoglycaemic tablets
'Stress', including fear	Acute illness (transient)
Glucocorticoid treatment	Idiopathic/functional hypoglycaemia
Cushing's disease	Carbohydrate deficiency (ruminants)
Intravenous glucose/dextrose	Sample not in fluoride
Diabetes mellitus	Spurious glucose meter result

Glucose tolerance/absorption tests

The classic glucose tolerance test was never widely used in veterinary medicine, with most diagnoses of diabetes mellitus, renal glycosuria and related conditions being adequately decided without it. The one situation where it remains of some value is as an *absorption* test, when investigating suspected intestinal malabsorption, usually in the horse. The horse should have had no concentrate feed for at least 5 hours before the test; ideally the test is carried out in the morning before any feed is given. A baseline blood sample is collected (using fluoride/oxalate), then a standard dose of 1 g/kg anhydrous glucose (1.1 g/kg glucose monohydrate) dissolved in about 2 litres of water is administered by stomach tube. Serial blood samples are then collected every 30 minutes for 2 hours. Note that it is vitally important to avoid any excitement or stress to the patient throughout this procedure. A normal horse will show a peak in plasma glucose of over 6 mmol/l approximately 60 minutes after glucose administration. A 'flat curve', with very little change in glucose concentration over the period of the test and the level failing to rise above 5 mmol/l, is suggestive of possible malabsorption.

Glycated (glycosylated) proteins

Blood or plasma glucose measurements only reveal the glucose concentration at the time the sample was collected, and may not be especially representative of the overall level of control. However, glucose reacts with free amino groups on virtually all proteins to form covalent glycated proteins, and the extent of the glycation depends on both the half-life of the protein in question and the average glucose concentration to which it has been exposed over this period. It has been suggested that glycation of structural proteins (e.g. the protein of the lens of the eye) may be responsible for some of the long-term complications of diabetes mellitus. Measurement of glycated protein concentrations allows assessment of glycaemic control over a period roughly corresponding to the lifespan of the protein in question.

Fructosamine

Normal non-diabetic animals under about 300 μmol/l.

Fructosamines are ketoamine compounds formed when glucose reacts with amino groups on plasma proteins, mainly albumin. Plasma fructosamine concentration is essentially a measure of the average blood glucose concentration over the lifespan of these proteins, which is about 2 weeks. Its main use is in the monitoring of diabetic patients on treatment, and it can also be a useful aid to diagnosis of diabetes mellitus.

Fructosamine has fallen out of favour in human diabetes monitoring, with glycated haemoglobin being the test of choice. Nevertheless, fructosamine is technically simpler to analyse, and given the somewhat less stringent diabetic control in operation in veterinary circumstances, the test is frequently perfectly adequate for practical purposes. While a normal animal will have a fructosamine concentration of less than 300 μmol/l, less than 400 μmol/l is generally considered to be a reasonable goal in a diabetic patient on treatment. However, it must be borne in mind that fructosamine estimation is only a part of diabetic monitoring, and results must be assessed together with data on water intake and spot blood (and urine, if used) glucose measurements when deciding if control is adequate. In addition, there is far less information available regarding correlation between measured parameters of glycaemic control and occurrence of long-term health problems for animals than there is for human patients, and so precise goals cannot really be quoted.

Fructosamine can also be used to help with the initial diagnosis of diabetes mellitus, when it is unclear whether a moderate hyperglycaemia is genuinely due to diabetes or is simply a stress response. When the result is clear-cut it can be extremely useful, but intermediate values (around 300–400 μmol/l) should be interpreted with caution.

The use of fructosamine to investigate or confirm a tendency to hypoglycaemia (for example in pregnancy toxaemia in sheep or insulinoma in dogs) is not well characterized. It should also be recognized that disturbances in plasma protein metabolism will affect fructosamine concentrations, and animals with prolonged hypo- or hyperproteinaemia may have values outside the reference limits for that reason alone.

Glycated haemoglobin

Normally around 5–10% of whole blood haemoglobin.

Once formed, glycated haemoglobin stays within the red cell for its lifetime – in the dog, this translates to a measure of average plasma glucose over about the previous 3 months. Several glycated derivatives of haemoglobin are recognized, collectively termed HbA_1, with the principal complex being HbA_{1c}. In man, assays are available for both total HbA_1 and HbA_{1c}, but the latter is the only measure for which good data are available relating it to the risk of subsequent diabetic complications and it is the preferred method for monitoring glycaemic control. Nevertheless, difficulties with inter-laboratory variation in methodology and reporting conventions are still being ironed out.

Glycated haemoglobin methods have been validated for the dog, but in general the techniques are more complex than fructosamine measurement, and the assay is still not widely used. In addition, it is perhaps less useful than fructosamine in the initial investigation of suspected diabetes due to the longer half-life – there is a greater possibility of a recent-onset diabetes being missed by this method. Nevertheless, HbA_{1c} is now firmly established as the test of choice for diabetic monitoring in man, and as veterinary medicine tends to catch up with advances in human diabetology in the end, it is likely that this method will be more widely employed in the future.

'Ketone bodies' (acetone, acetoacetate and betahydroxybutyrate)

Normal plasma β-OH butyrate concentration under 1 mmol/l – often undetectable.

Older methods of measurement of ketones generally were sensitive only to acetone but nowadays assays specific for β-OH butyrate are most commonly used. All values given here are for β-OH butyrate.

Ketosis develops due to a deficiency of glucose passing through the glycolytic pathway in the cells. Lack of the products of glycolysis prevents the Krebs' cycle from functioning. At the same time fatty acids are being utilized as an alternative body fuel and the ketone bodies are formed as an abnormal by-product of fatty acid catabolism due to the blocked Krebs' cycle. There are two main situations where this occurs.

(1)   Diabetic ketoacidosis. In uncontrolled type 1 diabetes where insulin activity is almost zero, virtually no glucose can enter the cells. This precipitates the above sequence of events even in the presence of a high plasma glucose level. This situation often accompanies diabetic coma and so it is essential to differentiate this from hypoglycaemia as treatment for the wrong condition is obviously disastrous. Before treatment this is usually accompanied by hyperkalaemia, but treatment with insulin will reduce plasma potassium concentration markedly and severe hypokalaemia can result.

(2)   Absolute carbohydrate deficiency. This is most commonly seen in cattle and sheep with acetonaemia and pregnancy toxaemia (see p. 120), and is usually associated with hypoglycaemia. In severely affected animals plasma β-OH butyrate can be well above 10 mmol/l. Due to the unusual carbohydrate metabolism of ruminants, oral glucose administration is ineffective in raising plasma glucose concentration and reversing ketosis. Treatment therefore consists of oral administration of gluconeogenic substrates, e.g. propylene glycol. Glucocorticoids are also very effective in promoting gluconeogenesis and are routinely used in cattle for this

Case 8.2

A flock of Border Leicester ewes was almost due to be moved from winter grazing, when three were found dead in the field one morning. When the veterinary surgeon called, another ewe was seen to be recumbent. A blood sample from that ewe gave the following results. What is the diagnosis, and what should have been done to prevent this occurrence?

Calcium	2.34 mmol/l	
Phosphate	1.11 mmol/l	
Magnesium	0.98 mmol/l	
Copper	10.3 μmol/l	
Glucose	1.2 mmol/l	low
β-OH butyrate	8.6 mmol/l	high
GDH	53 iu/l	raised
γGT	84 iu/l	raised

Comment

Pregnancy toxaemia. The hypoglycaemia and ketosis reveal severe carbohydrate deficiency, a major risk to sheep in late pregnancy especially when carrying multiple fetuses. In this case the farmer had not separated out ewes scanned as carrying triplets for additional feeding, and all the affected individuals were found to have three fetuses *in utero*.

purpose. However, sheep are affected before parturition and the administration of corticosteroids to a pregnant animal will induce abortion. This will be beneficial to the ewe, but unless gestation is very advanced the lambs will be lost, and so this tends to be a treatment of last resort in this species.

Ketosis due to starvation in monogastrics is seldom encountered, but it is recognized in man, particularly in hunger strikers and occasionally in anorexia nervosa.

In ketotic animals ketones are readily detected in the urine by ordinary dipstix. When urine is unavailable a spot of plasma (*not* blood) or milk may be applied to the ketone block of a urine dipstick. However, this is a less sensitive method as ketone concentrations in these fluids are lower than in urine, sometimes below the sensitivity of the strip. Rothera's powder has been used for many years to test for ketones in milk and appears to be more sensitive. Many people can actually smell the ketones in the animal's breath.

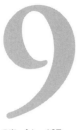

Bilirubin and Fat Metabolism

Bilirubin

Normal plasma concentration under about 2 μmol/l (or a little higher in ruminants) but in horses the normal can be up to 50 μmol/l.

Bilirubin is a by-product of haem breakdown. In its initial form it is not water-soluble and when in the plasma it is bound to albumin. It is transported via the reticulo-endothelial system to the liver where it is rendered soluble by conjugation with glucuronic acid and other substances. The bilirubin conjugate is excreted in the bile, and it and its associated pigments (mainly stercobilin) are responsible for the characteristic brown colour of faeces. On laboratory request forms 'total bilirubin' means just that. '*Direct* bilirubin' is *conjugated* bilirubin, and the unconjugated (or indirect) bilirubin is calculated by subtraction from the total. However, the fractionation of bilirubin into conjugated and unconjugated components is more of a pretty story than a useful diagnostic measurement. In practice, once an elevated bilirubin concentration has been established, it is more constructive to approach the individual possibilities directly (haematology for suspected haemolytic disease, other liver function tests for suspected hepato-biliary conditions).

Increased plasma bilirubin concentrations can be due to the following:

(1) Fasting hyperbilirubinaemia. The horse is the only species in which this is readily appreciable. In a starved or anorectic horse plasma bilirubin concentration can increase to around 100 μmol/l in the absence of any haemolytic or hepato-biliary abnormality. It may be due to the fact that free fatty acids, which increase in the plasma during fasting in horses, compete with bilirubin for uptake into liver cells. Thus far, this phenomenon is benign, but a proportion of animals will progress to develop clinical hyperlipidaemia (see p. 133). The jaundice which can develop in the anorectic cat is not quite the same, being generally related to the development of hepatic lipidosis.

(2) Intravascular haemolysis. Due to the efficiency of the normal reticulo-endothelial–hepato-biliary system it is quite possible for a slight to

moderate degree of haemolysis to be associated with no real increase in plasma bilirubin concentration. However, with increasing severity of haemolysis the excretory capacity is overloaded and hyperbilirubinaemia (jaundice) develops. This is usually not particularly severe, about 10–20 μmol/l depending on the severity of the haemolysis, and higher levels of bilirubin are usually accompanied by evidence of free haemoglobin in the plasma. The patient will be anaemic, and there will be evidence of red cell regeneration (except in horses, and when the onset of the condition is so recent that there has not been time for a regenerative response to occur).

(3)   Liver failure. Due to the number of different functions performed by the liver, failure of this organ can present as a variety of different clinical syndromes. In general, failure of the conjugatory/excretory functions occurs, often transiently, in cases of severe acute hepatitis, and as one of the later events in progressive generalized liver failure. Plasma bilirubin concentration can increase to around 300 μmol/l or more. Most cases, particularly of hepatitis, show increased plasma activities of liver enzymes, with activities of those enzymes associated with the liver parenchyma (especially the transaminases) being much higher than that of alkaline phosphatase. However, some cases of terminal cirrhosis or tumour infiltration of the liver have normal or even low plasma enzyme levels. Also, some cases of liver failure have an associated haemorrhagic anaemia (see pp. 20 & 43), and if there is any doubt in a jaundiced, anaemic patient then bile acid measurement is the test of choice to clarify the situation. In general, a jaundiced animal which presents acutely ill with pyrexia and vomiting is probably suffering from an acute hepatitis and recovery is usually uneventful no matter how astronomical the bilirubin concentration, while a gradual onset of jaundice with progressive weight loss and inappetance is a much more sinister scenario.

(4)   Obstructive biliary disease. This may be intrahepatic or post-hepatic obstruction – tumours are probably the most common cause. In cases of complete obstruction, plasma bilirubin concentrations can go very high – over 600 μmol/l – and the faeces will be pale due to the absence of stercobilin. In the early stages of the condition plasma activities of the liver parenchymal enzymes are usually normal, but alkaline phosphatase (ALP), which is both excreted in the bile and produced by the cells of the bile duct canaliculi, will show a very markedly raised plasma activity. In the later stages the 'damming back' effect of the bile will lead to actual liver damage and at this point plasma levels of the other liver enzymes will increase (though these increases are never as spectacular as that of ALP, which can easily exceed 10 000 iu/l in cases of obstructive jaundice). Again plasma bile acid concentrations will be high but plasma ammonia concentration may be normal.

Jaundice

This can be a deceptive clinical sign, as sick animals (especially horses and cattle) often seem to look yellow when, in fact, plasma bilirubin concentrations are normal – conversely some cases of hyperbilirubinaemia do not look particularly jaundiced. Accordingly, all cases of suspected jaundice should have plasma bilirubin actually *measured* (although in species other than horses and cattle the absence of a yellow colour in the plasma may be sufficient to rule out an increased bilirubin concentration). It should also be borne in mind that haemolysis tends to produce no more than a pale primrose shade in the mucous membranes, as a relatively mild jaundice combines with the pallor of anaemia. When very marked 'glow-in-the-dark' icterus is seen, haemolysis is the least likely cause and hepato-biliary disease should be suspected. See p. 171 regarding the significance of positive urine bilirubin results.

Bile acids

Normal plasma concentration under about 15 μmol/l. However, note that the test is invalid in the Maltese dog, which has a substance in the plasma which interferes with the usual bile acid assay method, giving spuriously high results.

The bile acid assay can only be performed on serum; heparinized (or other) plasma is unsuitable.

Bile acids (principally cholic acid, deoxycholic acid, chenodeoxycholic acid and lithocholic acid) are synthesized in the liver, conjugated and excreted in the bile in a similar way to bilirubin, and excreted into the duodenum where they assist in the digestion of fat. Subsequently they are reabsorbed in the distal small intestine and returned to the liver via the portal vein. Increased serum concentrations of bile acids occur in hepatic and biliary disease. The test provides a more sensitive indicator of impaired hepatic anion transport than bilirubin, with the additional advantage of being unaffected by haemolytic disease or fasting hyperbilirubinaemia.

The principal application of bile acid measurement is as a test for impaired hepatic anion transport when bilirubin is not elevated, for example when liver dysfunction is suspected on clinical grounds or because plasma liver enzymes are elevated. It is seldom necessary to measure bile acids in a jaundiced patient. However, it is occasionally necessary to distinguish genuine liver dysfunction from other causes of hyperbilirubinaemia – while most cases of haemolytic disease are not difficult to diagnose by other methods, doubt may arise when a patient with apparent liver disease is also anaemic; also (primarily in the cat) a jaundice which is due to a secondary hepatic problem (hepatic lipidosis secondary to anorexia, or feline infectious peritonitis (FIP) for example) tends to be associated with a lower bile acid concentration than would normally accompany jaundice due to primary liver disease. In addition, bile acid measurement is essential when investigating liver disease in the horse, as the high bilirubin concentration in normal individuals and the marked degree of fasting hyperbilirubinaemia seen in that species mean that bilirubin measurement is of very little value.

As a general guide, bile acid concentrations up to about 30–40 μmol/l may be seen in association with the somewhat impaired liver function which can occur secondary to a variety of conditions, while concentrations over about 50 μmol/l indicate probable primary hepatic dysfunction. If bile acids are measured in animals with severe hepatic or post-hepatic jaundice, concentrations in excess of 500 μmol/l may be observed.

Portosystemic shunts

This term describes any situation where there is a direct vascular connection between the portal and peripheral venous circulation, allowing portal blood to flow directly to the vena cava without passing through the liver. It may be congenital, either due to non-closure of the ductus venosus in the first few days of life, or to the existence of an abnormal vessel joining the two circulations (either within or outside the liver), or acquired. Congenital portosystemic shunts are usually a single vessel, while acquired shunts involve multiple connections. An acquired shunt develops secondary to severe, progressive liver disease (often cirrhosis), when it becomes gradually more difficult for the portal blood to flow through the liver. Blood pressure in the portal vein increases and multiple collateral circulation develops – abnormally large, convoluted vessels can be seen in the mesentery at exploratory laparotomy. Clinical signs are those of 'hepatic encephalopathy' – headpressing, obsessive behaviour and sometimes fits – due to concurrent hyperammonaemia (see pp. 103 and 109). In congenital cases clinical signs often develop soon after weaning, but it is not unusual for patients to present up to 2 years of age – in these cases stunted growth is often a feature. Acquired shunts may present at any age, but signs of severe liver impairment are usually quite obvious in these patients. Congenital portosystemic shunts are an inherited defect in some breeds of dog – the Irish wolfhound (where the problem is a patent ductus venosus) is the best studied, but other related breeds such as the Scottish deerhound, and some terrier breeds (the cairn and the West Highland White) have also been implicated. However, sporadic, non-inherited shunts may occur in any breed.

In a normal individual the enterohepatic recirculation of bile acids does not involve the peripheral circulation. In the 1 or 2 hours after a meal there is a marked increase in the bile acid concentration of portal venous blood due to the reabsorption of the bile secreted as part of the digestive process. However, as this blood is delivered directly to the liver, the bile acid concentration in the peripheral circulation increases only slightly, if at all. In contrast, where there is a direct communication between the portal and peripheral circulations, the concentration of bile acids in peripheral blood increases markedly.

Dynamic bile acid test

This protocol is specifically designed to demonstrate the existence of a portosystemic shunt. A blood sample is collected after an overnight fast. The patient is then fed – a normal meal if possible, but sick animals may have to be coaxed to eat. The second sample is collected about 90 minutes later. If no shunt is present there will be little or no change between the two samples. The presence of a shunt is characterized by a marked increase in bile acid concentration post-feeding – if the fasted value is normal, an increase of greater than 25 μmol/l identifies a probable shunt, but if the fasting value is already high the increase is usually greater than 50 μmol/l.

A screening protocol has been developed for Irish wolfhound puppies aged 6 weeks or more, which involves the post-prandial sample only. Samples are collected 90–120 minutes after feeding. A result of less than 30 μmol/l is normal, over 50 μmol/l identifies a probable shunt, and puppies testing between 30 and 50 μmol/l are required to be retested using the dynamic test. The main pitfalls are ensuring that every puppy in the group has eaten, and that the individual puppies are reliably identified. However, this protocol has not been fully validated in other breeds.

Cholesterol

Normal plasma concentration under about 7–8 mmol/l in dogs, 5–6 mmol/l in cats and 2–3 mmol/l in herbivores.

Cholesterol is both absorbed from the gut (carnivorous diet) and synthesized in the body. It is a component of cell membranes where it lies between the fatty acid 'arms' of the lipid molecules and increases the rigidity of the membrane structure. Excess cholesterol is excreted in the bile, partly as bile acids and bile salts, partly as unchanged cholesterol (which may be reabsorbed). Interestingly, the bile salts are themselves necessary for the absorption of dietary or recycled cholesterol from the gut. In man, hypercholesterolaemia is associated with arteriosclerosis and ischaemic heart disease, but no such association has been found in domestic animals.

Increase (hypercholesterolaemia)

Clinically speaking, cholesterol is only of diagnostic importance in small animals. In herbivores levels are usually very low and increases are not specifically associated with particular conditions. A number of causes of hypercholesterolaemia are recognized in small animals.

(1)   Recent fatty meal. It is essential that a truly *fasting* sample be collected for a cholesterol result to be of diagnostic significance. However, dietary alterations in plasma cholesterol concentration are not particularly large, at most 2–3 mmol/l.

(2)   Liver or biliary disease. As the hepato-biliary system is involved in the excretion of cholesterol, patients with liver failure will often have elevated plasma cholesterol concentrations.

(3)   Nephrotic syndrome, partly due to its effect on plasma proteins.

(4)   Diabetes mellitus. The increased fat metabolism seen in diabetic patients leads to increased cholesterol in most cases, particularly as these patients also often suffer from fatty infiltration of the liver and consequent reduced liver function.

(5)   Cushing's disease. Elevated plasma cholesterol concentrations are commonly seen in cases of Cushing's disease, partly due to a hormonal disturbance of lipid metabolism and partly due to the steroid hepatopathy which often accompanies this condition.

(6)   Hypothyroidism. While dietary effects are unlikely to produce a plasma cholesterol of more than 10 mmol/l at the outside, and liver/kidney/diabetes/Cushing's problems seldom increase it above 15 mmol/l, hypothyroidism can cause hypercholesterolaemia up to as much as 30 mmol/l and concentrations of this order are more or less pathognomonic for this condition. However, milder cases can be difficult to differentiate from Cushing's disease (haematology can be very helpful in this), and up to 30% of genuinely hypothyroid patients have normal plasma cholesterol concentrations.

Decrease

Paradoxically, severe liver dysfunction is sometimes associated with abnormally low plasma cholesterol concentrations. Unusually low concentrations have also been reported in cases of hyperthyroidism, but this is not considered to be a diagnostically useful finding.

Triglycerides, glycerol and free fatty acids (FFAs)

Normal plasma triglyceride concentration is around 1 mmol/l in dogs, 0.4 mmol/l in horses. Free glycerol is normally below 100 µmol/l.

In fat depots fat is stored as triglycerides, which consist of three fatty acid residues esterified to a glycerol unit. Normal fat mobilization is stimulated by adrenaline and involves lipases and esterases acting *within the fat depot* to split the fatty acids off. FFAs and glycerol are released into the plasma. The normally low plasma triglyceride concentration is therefore unaffected by lipolysis. Increased plasma triglyceride levels occur in a number of conditions, and should be suspected when a white milky suspension (lipaemia) is seen in the plasma. If the lipaemia is due to triglycerides as such, the milkiness will remain in suspension. However, if it is due to chylomicrons in the plasma, the milkiness will gradually rise to the top (like cream on milk).

Note, however, that standard laboratory 'triglyceride' methods do not actually measure triglycerides, they measure *total glycerol* after pre-treatment of the sample with lipase and esterase. A high free glycerol concentration will therefore also register on the assay and may be misinterpreted as triglycerides unless a parallel assay for free glycerol is run (minus the lipase/esterase) and this value subtracted from the total glycerol. The remainder is genuinely triglyceride.

Conditions associated with high plasma triglyceride concentrations (or possibly high glycerol concentrations, many publications do not make this distinction) include the following:

(1)   Diabetes mellitus.
(2)   Hypothyroidism.
(3)   Nephrotic syndrome.
(4)   Renal failure.
(5)   Acute necrotizing pancreatitis.
(6)   Equine hyperlipidaemia. This is a peculiarly equine disease which is due to prolonged dietary carbohydrate deficiency, either because of very poor winter grazing after a fat summer, or anorexia secondary to other disease (e.g. colic). It has some similarity to acetonaemia of cattle, but instead of a build-up of the products of lipolysis (ketones) occurring, the actual fat depot mobilization appears to get out of hand. Affected animals usually stop eating completely while fat mobilization runs riot, and the finding of a plasma total glycerol concentration of over 2 mmol/l and plasma total lipids of over 5 g/l is virtually diagnostic. Plasma bilirubin is often also elevated. The triglycerides can be seen as a milky opacity in the plasma, and this 'lemon curd' appearance in an equine sample should be an immediate cause for alarm. The condition is often fatal if untreated, though prognosis is much better if the patient can be persuaded to continue eating. The most effective treatment is heparin: 5000 iu dissolved in about 10 ml saline, injected i/v twice daily. This reverses the hyperlipidaemia by potentiating the enzyme lipoprotein lipase. Treatment should be continued until plasma total glycerol concentration has fallen below 1 mmol/l. Administration of glucose by stomach tube is also beneficial, and some authors recommend glucose and galactose given on alternate days. Note that strenuous exercise will cause an elevation in plasma total glycerol concentration due not to triglycerides but to free glycerol, and therefore this finding is not clinically significant in horses which have just finished a race or an endurance event.

Fat absorption test

This test can be useful to demonstrate malabsorption in small animals. It has advantages over vitamin measurements in that it looks directly at the absorptive process rather than for deficiencies which may (or may not) be secondary to poor absorption. Note, however, that as described it does not distinguish between intestinal malabsorption and exocrine pancreatic insufficiency. A variant has been suggested in which the test is repeated with the addition of pancreatic enzymes to the maize oil (when EPI cases will give a normal result and intestinal malabsorption cases will remain abnormal), but in practice it is easier simply to confirm or deny pancreatic insufficiency using the immunoreactive trypsin (IRT) test (see p. 144) – if IRT activity is normal, an abnormal fat absorption result must be due to an intestinal problem.

(1)   The patient must be fasted overnight (at least 8 hours).
(2)   Collect fasting sample (at least 1 ml serum or heparinized plasma).
(3)   Administer maize cooking oil (sometimes called 'corn oil' – *not* sunflower oil) by mouth at a dose of 3 ml/kg, up to a maximum of 90 ml.
(4)   Wait about 90–120 minutes.
(5)   Collect second sample as above.

Centrifuge the samples and observe the colour of the plasma. If the second sample is obviously lipaemic compared to the first, the patient is not malabsorbing, and no further analysis is necessary. If the colour difference is not obvious (or obscured by slight haemolysis), total glycerol is measured on each sample.

In a normal dog or cat, the fasting result will be around 0.6–0.8 mmol/l; after maize oil administration this will rise to around 1.2–1.5 mmol/l. When malabsorption is present, both results tend to be around 0.4–0.5 mmol/l.

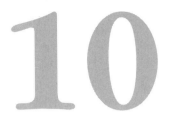

Clinical Enzymology – Plasma Enzymes in Diagnosis

Although all cells contain the same DNA, not every gene is expressed in every cell. Instead, those proteins proper to the cell's function are synthesized while other genes are suppressed, so that each cell type (e.g. hepatocyte or muscle fibre) contains its own 'fingerprint' of enzymes. Low levels of all of these enzymes normally appear in the plasma, reflecting the balance between the release of enzymes during normal cell turnover, and their catabolism or excretion.

Enzyme units and measurement

The total amount of all enzymes by weight in the plasma is less than 1 g/l. Results are not, however, expressed as concentrations but as *activities* – basically a measure of how fast the enzyme in the sample can convert substrate to product under the standardized assay conditions. However, few reaction products can be measured directly and a coupled series of several reactions is usually used with the final one producing an optically measurable change – NADH → NAD$^+$ is often used as this is easily followed at 340 nm. This means that enzyme measurement is much more method-dependent than other analytes. The *international unit (IU)* of enzyme activity is defined as 'the amount of enzyme which, under given assay conditions, will catalyse the conversion of 1 mmol of substrate per minute'. However, the sting is in the phrase 'under given assay conditions' – these conditions may vary quite considerably between laboratories, and choice of substrate, starter, co-factors, buffers, secondary reactions and in particular temperature will all affect the numerical result. Reaction temperature is now commonly standardized at 37°C, but results relating to 25°C or even 30°C may still be encountered. The numerical values quoted in this chapter are for commonly used methods at 37°C, but they are included mainly to give some impression of the orders of magnitude involved. When interpreting 'real' results, the reference values supplied by the laboratory which carried out the analysis should always be consulted.

Older texts sometimes quote outdated method-specific units such as King–Armstrong units or Wroblewski units. These can be very difficult to interpret as there is no simple numerical conversion factor. Some attempt has been made to introduce a new SI enzyme activity unit, the *catal*, but so far this has not come into general clinical use.

'Normal values'

In addition to the problems outlined concerning units and method variations, the distribution of plasma enzyme values in normal animals makes it difficult to put clear limits on the 'normal range'. Unlike most biochemical constituents, which form a fairly neat normal distribution curve (see Introduction, Fig. A.1), many enzymes, particularly in horses, show a very markedly skewed distribution with a sizeable number of apparently normal individuals demonstrating quite high values (Fig. 10.1). This leads to a very wide 'grey area' in enzyme interpretation, with creatine kinase (CK), aspartate aminotransferase (AST) and alanine aminotransferase (ALP) in horses being the worst offenders. Because of this grey area, it is very unwise to act solely on the basis of a single elevated enzyme activity unless this is *very* high, and corroboration should be sought either in the clinical findings or in other laboratory or radiological tests.

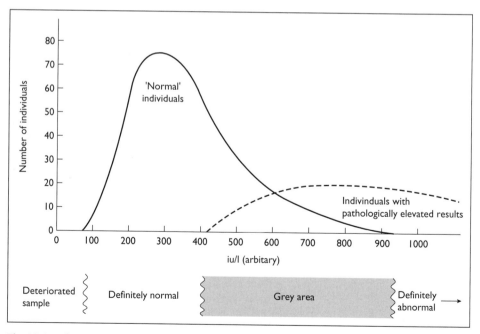

Fig. 10.1   Schematic representation of the distribution of results for a figurative plasma enzyme assay, showing how the skewed distribution of 'normal' results leads to a very wide 'grey' area.

Increase

An increase in plasma levels of an enzyme occurs mainly due to damage, rupture or necrosis of the cells of the organ or tissue which contains that enzyme. To a lesser extent cellular proliferation may also lead to plasma enzyme increases. The actual levels reached depend on the rate and extent of cell damage, balanced against the rate of catabolism or excretion. This means that relatively high levels will be reached transiently when even a small degree of damage occurs acutely, but during a chronic disease more extensive (and potentially more serious) damage may lead to little or no increase in plasma enzyme levels. In the latter case these enzymes with short plasma half-lives will show the smallest increases while those with longer half-lives will provide more useful information.

Impairment of enzyme excretion

This can occasionally lead to increased plasma enzyme levels in the absence of primary tissue damage which can itself be of diagnostic importance as in the huge increase in alkaline phosphatase which accompanies bile duct occlusion, or it may be an incidental finding as in the slightly raised amylase or lipase levels which are sometimes seen in renal failure.

Non-specific increases in enzyme activity

These should be borne in mind and include the following:

(1) Age. Neonates have fairly high levels of many enzymes, and young animals before the closure of the epiphyseal growth plates have higher plasma alkaline phosphatase levels than adults.

(2) Enzyme induction. Some drugs may stimulate the production of some enzymes – in particular note that *barbiturates* may increase alkaline phosphatase activities. The high γ-glutamyl transferase levels typical of alcoholism in man may be as much due to enzyme induction as to alcohol-induced liver damage.

(3) Haemolysis. Haemolysed samples are unsuitable for enzyme estimation as enzymes released from the red cells are liable to interfere with the assay.

Decrease

A decrease in plasma enzyme levels is much less frequently used for clinical interpretation, and the most that can be said for many low enzyme findings is simply that the sample has been badly stored (most enzymes are fairly labile, especially without refrigeration). However, there are a few specific cases where low plasma enzyme levels will indicate that the relevant organ is hypoplastic, atrophied or destroyed; hence the normal evidence of cell turnover is absent. The commonest example of this is immunoreactive trypsin (IRT) in exocrine pancreatic deficiency.

Localization of damage

Very few enzymes are specific for only one cell type. Many enzymes are actually present in nearly all cells, at different levels, and most enzymes have two or three different tissues in which they are particularly abundant. Specificity can be improved in two ways:

(1)   Isoenzyme determination. Where an enzyme is particularly prominent in more than one tissue it is often the case that each tissue has its own particular isoenzyme. If these isoenzymes can be separated this can be of major diagnostic importance; however, techniques tend to be tricky, and methods are often not readily available and designed in any case for human use. Selective inhibition of a particular isoenzyme and re-assay of the remainder is usually the simplest method, but electrophoretic separation can often yield more detailed information, especially when three or more isoenzymes are involved.

(2)   Estimation of more than one enzyme. Relative concentrations of enzymes are seldom exactly the same in two tissues and the damaged tissue can often be pinpointed by estimation of several enzymes. This approach can and should be widened to include other laboratory and radiological tests so that a composite picture of the individual pathology can be built up.

Note that there are some marked species variations in tissue enzyme distribution which must be taken into account when selecting the appropriate tests — for example, alanine aminotransferase (ALT) is predominantly liver-specific in dogs and cats, and virtually muscle-specific in horses.

Individual enzyme interpretation

Creatine kinase (CK or CPK)

CK is involved in high energy metabolism. Be careful to distinguish this from creatinine (see Fig. 7.3) as in clinical biochemistry terms the two analytes are quite unconnected. CK is present as a dimer and two subunit types are found — M and B. Thus three isoenzyme forms are possible — MM, MB and BB.

CK-MM is the *skeletal muscle* form and responsible for the very dramatic increases seen in generalized muscle lesions such as rhabdomyolysis, or iliac thrombosis in the cat. Total CK activity can increase from a normal of about 100 iu/l (a little higher in horses) to 500 000 iu/l in severe cases. Note, however, that a couple of days of lying on a major muscle mass will itself cause CK to increase to as much as 3000 iu/l in a recumbent large animal, so be wary of diagnosing a primary muscle lesion in cases which have been down for a while before the sample was taken. Surgery, muscular exertion and intramuscular

Case 10.1

A 10-year old part-thoroughbred mare was observed walking very stiffly after competing in a one-day event. What diagnosis is suggested by these blood results?

Total protein	71 g/l	
Albumin	32 g/l	
Globulin	39 g/l	
Sodium	144 mmol/l	
Potassium	4.2 mmol/l	
Calcium	3.24 mmol/l	
Urea	4.4 mmol/l	
CK	84 600 iu/l	high
AST	9640 iu/l	high

Comment

The muscle enzymes (CK and AST) are much higher than might be caused by an ordinary muscle injury and are consistent with rhabdomyolysis. Other results are normal, though that does not preclude an electrolyte disturbance being the initiating cause of the problem.

injections will all produce slightly to moderately increased plasma CK-MM activities.

CK-MB is the *cardiac muscle* form. It is used specifically in man in the diagnosis of actue myocardial infarction. However, this condition is extremely rare in animals and the more chronic cardiomyopathy-type conditions tend to cause few detectable enzyme changes due to the short half-life of this enzyme.

CK-BB is the *brain* form. If it can be assayed specifically it is useful in the diagnosis of conditions such as cerebrocortical necrosis, an actue CNS disease of young ruminants due to thiamine deficiency. However, few laboratories offer this test.

A slightly raised total CK activity is typical of hypothyroidism as CK catabolism is apparently promoted by thyroxine. In general, total CK measurement reflects the MM isoenzyme which is most abundant. MB and BB increases can usually only be appreciated by isoenzyme estimation as otherwise they will be swamped by the MM. Note that CK is a small enzyme with a very short half-life and even the most spectacular increases seen in rhabdomyolysis will be back to normal in 24–48 hours so long as ongoing damage has stopped. It is also quite labile, especially at room temperature or above, and samples should ideally be assayed on the day of collection. Freezing to $-20°C$ will preserve it; however, postal samples are not really reliable unless very large increases are expected.

Lactate dehydrogenase (LDH or LD)

The heart isoenzyme is also known as hydroxybutyrate dehydrogenase, HBDH or HBD.

LDH catalyses the reversible interconversion of lactate and pyruvate, and is one of the largest protein molecules in the body. It is a tetramer (four subunits per molecule) and the subunits come in two forms, H and L. Thus five isoenzymes exist (HHHH, HHHL, HHLL, HLLL and LLLL), referred to as LDH_{1-5} in descending order of electrophoretic mobility. LDH_1 (HBDH) is associated with *cardiac muscle*, *kidney* and *erythrocytes*, LDH_5 with *liver*. Other isoenzymes are associated with *skeletal muscle* and *lung*. Because of its wide distribution, increases in total LDH activity can be very difficult to interpret in veterinary medicine and electrophoretic isoenzyme separation is really essential if the source is to be pinpointed. However, due to its large size and long half-life LDH activity remains raised for some time after the initial damage and so can sometimes be useful in retrospective diagnosis; for example when a case of rhabdomyolysis is seen several days after the actual tying-up episode CK will be back to normal, but in conjunction with clinical signs LDH can be used to confirm what is (or has been) going on. Normal total plasma LDH activity is around 200–300 iu/l in most species; this can increase to several thousand iu/l in some conditions.

Aspartate aminotransferase (AST, formerly GOT)

For the function of this transaminase, see Fig. 7.1. No specific AST isoenzymes are recognized. It is quite widely distributed in the body; in particular it is found in *skeletal muscle*, *cardiac muscle*, *liver* and *erythrocytes*. It is used in all species to investigate muscle damage, where its half-life is intermediate between CK and LDH, and in large animals to investigate liver disease. It is not particularly specific for this purpose, especially in the horse (see below), and has largely been superseded by GDH and sometimes SDH.

Normal plasma AST activity is under 100 iu/l in all species except the horse. The horse is unusual in that activities of 200–400 iu/l are quite normal and some apparently healthy horses have been found to have activities in excess of 1000 iu/l – probably due to some subclinical muscle enzyme release (the same is true to a certain extent of CK). Accordingly, liver disease should *never* be diagnosed solely on the basis of an elevated plasma AST in a horse.

Alanine aminotransferase (ALT, formerly GPT)

This is also a transaminase with a similar function to AST, and again has no specific isoenzymes. In dogs and cats it is predominantly specific for *hepatocellular damage* – normal plasma activities of under 100 iu/l can increase to around 5000 iu/l in very acute conditions (acute hepatitis, steroid hepatopathy), but activities of more than 150–200 iu/l are clinically significant. Note, however, that it does also increase in severe muscle damage (rhabdomyolysis in greyhounds, iliac thrombosis in cats), and a raised ALT in a patient with such a condition need not indicate a concurrent liver disorder. Mild to moderate increases in ALT are also frequently seen in hyperthyroid cats. In large animals

ALT is in effect a muscle enzyme and in practice is not considered to be of diagnostic significance in these species.

Sorbitol dehydrogenase (SDH)

This is in effect an 'ALT substitute' of particular use in the horse. It is virtually specific for *acute hepatocellular damage* in this species, and has a very short (24–48 hour) half-life in the absence of continuing damage. Plasma levels above 5 iu/l would be considered clinically significant. Note that SDH is a very labile enzyme and should be assayed within a few hours of sample collection. It does not take kindly to being posted.

Glutamate dehydrogenase (GDH, GLDH or GMD)

This is used as an 'ALT substitute' in large animals and is specific for liver damage, particularly hepatic necrosis. It is much less labile than SDH, and therefore the test of choice in the horse if samples have to be posted. Normal plasma activity is under about 20–25 iu/l, and it can increase to over 100 iu/l in acute liver damage.

Gamma glutamyl transferase (γGT or GGT)

γGT occurs mainly in the *liver* and *kidney*, but in clinical terms its use is confined to liver conditions. In large animals it seems to be particularly associated with longer-term liver damage than SDH or GDH – often it is normal when they are raised, then when they are declining γGT begins to increase. In small animals it is raised roughly in parallel with ALT but is seldom requested clinically. In man it is said to be particularly associated with hepatic cirrhosis, metastatic carcinomata and hepatic infiltrations, but it is doubtful if such specific interpretations should be read into it in veterinary species. The half-life of γGT is particularly long – horses with ragwort poisoning have been observed still to have elevated plasma levels for a considerable time after clinical recovery. Normal values in horses and ruminants are below about 60 iu/l, and somewhat less than that in other species. In the cat, γGT is normally virtually undetectable.

Alkaline phosphatase (ALP)

This is one of the most widely distributed enzymes in the body. It really consists of a group of several isoenzymes which hydrolyse phosphates at an alkaline pH – these are found in particular in *bone* (osteoblasts), *liver* and *intestinal wall*. The range of normal levels is quite wide, anything up to 300 iu/l in most species, 100–500 iu/l in horses. The higher levels are found in young animals with high oesteoblastic activity; after closure of the epiphyseal growth plates rather lower levels are seen, mostly of liver origin. ALP is also the enzyme which is most seriously affected by differences in method of measurement, particularly

Case 10.2

A 13-year-old cob gelding in a riding school had been noticed to be dull and uninterested in food for several days. When the veterinary surgeon arrived the horse was observed head-pressing in the corner of the loosebox. On examination he was visually unresponsive, blowing at the nostrils and sweating slightly. Rectal temperature was 38.5°C and faecal consistency appeared normal. What do the biochemistry results below suggest and what is the most likely cause of the condition?

Total protein	76 g/l	
Albumin	33 g/l	
Globulin	43 g/l	
Urea	3.1 mmol/l	
Bilirubin	74 µmol/	raised
Bile acids	782 µmol/l	high
AST	1360 iu/l	high
GDH	129 iu/l	high
γGT	857 iu/l	high

Comment

The results suggest either hepatotoxicity or hepatitis, probably the former. The most commonly encountered hepatotoxin in the horse is ragwort (*Senecio jacobea*), which can cause extremely severe liver damage. Although this horse was stabled, this does not exclude the diagnosis, as ragwort is just as toxic dried in hay as fresh (if not more so), and considerably less unpalatable.

Examination of the hay revealed several ragwort plants, and blood tests on the other horses at the stables revealed three other (asymptomatic) individuals with high liver enzymes (but normal bile acid concentrations). The sick horse died, but the offending hay was destroyed and replaced by ragwort-free hay, and the other horses remained well.

buffer used (see p. 321). 'Normal' values will therefore vary widely between laboratories, and it is essential to ascertain the levels considered normal in the laboratory you are using.

Generalized bone diseases

Conditions such as rickets, osteomalacia, hyperparathyroidism, oesteogenic osteosarcoma, bone metastasis of non-skeletal carcinoma and cranio-mandibular osteoarthropathy can produce moderate to marked elevations in plasma ALP activity. Localized lesions such as (healing) fractures sometimes do not produce large enough changes to be visible against the background of the very wide normal range. Bone origin ALP elevations are quite easy to distinguish from hepato-biliary conditions by the lack of any elevation in liver parenchymal enzymes (AST, ALT, SDH, GDH or γGT depending on species) and the absence of jaundice; however, Cushing's disease may produce a very similar picture. Radiographic abnormalities or Ca/PO$_4$ abnormalities are also often present in generalized bone disease.

Liver damage

This will cause moderate increases in plasma ALP activity in all species. This tends to parallel the increase in activity of the other liver enzymes listed above. Raised ALP also accompanies the raised ALT in some hyperthyroid cats.

Cushing's disease

In the dog Cushing's disease is often associated with high plasma ALP activities, partly due to the frequent presence of a steroid hepatopathy in these animals, but also due to the production of a specific ALP isoenzyme by the adrenal cortex. A specific assay for this isoenzyme is available. However, it is not a sensitive or specific enough test to be used as a substitute for dynamic cortisol testing (see p. 150). Cats do not produce steroid-induced ALP.

Biliary tract disease

Biliary tract disease, especially obstruction, causes massive increases in plasma ALP activity – 50 000 iu/l may be reached. This was thought to be due to a failure to excrete the normal bone enzyme, but later studies indicate that during biliary stasis the cells of the bile duct canaliculi produce increased amounts of a specific biliary isoenzyme which is regurgitated into the plasma. In practice, biliary tract disease can be distinguished by marked elevations in ALP without (at first) any change in hepatic parenchymal enzymes in many cases. Unlike cases of bone disease, these patients will be jaundiced. As the condition progresses, 'damming back' of bile into the liver will cause actual liver damage and other liver enzyme activities will increase. Due to this biliary tract connection, ALP may be thought of to some extent as an index of hepato-biliary *function*, while all other enzymes simply measure cellular *damage*.

Non-specific increases in plasma ALP activity

These are seen in some cases of severe generalized skin disease in dogs, after barbiturate anaesthesia, and in many types of neoplasia.

Isoenzyme estimation

This could be extremely useful in aiding interpretation of elevated ALP activities. However, apart from IAP and SIAP, no practically useful methods of isoenzyme separation have been developed for veterinary use.

Intestinal alkaline phosphatase (IAP)

This may be measured by differential inhibition. Markedly increased plasma activities are particularly associated with parasite-induced damage to the intestinal wall in horses and can be very useful in the differential diagnosis of protein-losing enteropathy in this species.

Steroid-induced alkaline phosphatase (SIAP)

This is the isoenzyme associated with Cushing's disease; it may also be specifically assayed.

α-Amylase (AMS)

Amylase is concerned with the breakdown of dietary starch and glycogen to maltose. It is mainly present in the pancreas and salivary glands and is, unusually for a protein molecule, excreted by the kidney. Its main clinical use is in the diagnosis of *acute necrotizing pancreatitis*. This is essentially a canine (and human) disease associated with high fat diet, obesity (and alcoholism), in which the proteolytic enzymes leak from the cells and begin to auto-digest the organ. Symptoms of acute abdominal pain and vomiting may be mistaken for a small intestinal foreign body, and since surgery on a case of pancreatitis does not improve survival prospects, amlyase (and lipase) should always be checked if there is any uncertainty. The upper limit of normal is about 3000 iu/l and acute pancreatitis is associated with activities in the 5000–15 000 iu/l range, decreasing as recovery progresses. Note that amylase is not reliable for investigating pancreatitis in the cat.

Slight to moderate non-specific increases may be seen in other acute abdominal disorders (including intestinal obstruction) and in renal failure. These are not of diagnostic importance.

Lipase

Lipase is concerned with the breakdown of dietary fat and is also present in the pancreas. It is used in conjunction with amylase to investigate acute necrotizing pancreatitis and seems generally to be more specific for this condition, being less affected by non-specific changes. As a larger molecule it appears to remain increased for longer after the initial disease episode but in the early stage it does not increase as quickly as amylase and so assay of both enzymes is recommended. Normal values in dogs are under about 300 iu/l and in the acute stages of pancreatitis levels over 500 iu/l are usually found. As with amylase, smaller non-specific increases can be seen in other conditions such as renal failure. Again, this enzyme is not reliable for investigating pancreatitis in the cat.

Immunoreactive trypsin (IRT or TLI)

This is the one enzyme which is not measured by activity (it is inactive). Trypsin is a proteolytic enzyme secreted by the pancreas, and active trypsin does not leak out of the pancreatic cells under normal circumstances –

Case 10.3

An overweight bull terrier dog was presented as an emergency having been discovered in the morning extremely unwell and apparently in pain. There were pools of vomit on the floor of the kennel, but no evidence of diarrhoea. On examination rectal temperature was 40.3°C and the abdomen was extremely tense and painful to palpation. No foreign body could be demonstrated either by palpation or conscious radiography, so fluid and broad-spectrum antibiotic therapy was begun and laboratory results awaited. What do these suggest, and is surgery indicated? Are any complications evident?

Total protein	91 g/l	raised
Albumin	39 g/l	raised
Globulin	52 g/l	raised
Sodium	158 mmol/l	
Potassium	5.6 mmol/l	raised
Calcium	1.85 mmol/l	low
Urea	9.2 mmol/l	raised
Creatinine	88 μmol/l	
ALT	157 iu/l	raised
ALP	422 iu/l	raised
Amylase	13 400 iu/l	high
Lipase	1183 iu/l	high

Comment

Surgery is contraindicated. The results indicate acute necrotizing pancreatitis, which can present in a very similar way to an intestinal foreign body, but which can only be exacerbated by laparotomy. The dog is very dehydrated, though the electrolytes are relatively unaffected. The slight liver damage is almost inevitable considering the proximity of the liver to the pancreas. The main complication evident is the hypocalcaemia, which in fact started to become clinically apparent while the dog was on fluids.

when it does it causes acute necrotizing pancreatitis. However, something is present in normal plasma which will react with anti-trypsin antibodies in a radioimmunoassay while having no proteolytic activity – 'immunoreactive trypsin', probably in fact trypsinogen. In human medicine IRT is used as another index of acute pancreatitis in the same way as total amylase and lipase. In canine medicine the finding of a *decreased* plasma IRT is used (like pancreatic isoamylase in man) to assess *exocrine pancreatic insufficiency* and it appears to be quite specific and of good diagnostic value for this purpose. See also faecal trypsin, p. 173.

In addition, IRT has been recommended for investigation of acute pancreatitis in the cat – in this case looking for elevated results. However, even at best there is still considerable overlap between normal and affected cats, and some authors report it to be of no benefit at all. In addition, the specialized assay is available at only a few centres and results can take several days to appear. Ultrasonography may be a more practical approach to diagnosis of pancreatic disease in the cat.

Pepsinogen

Pepsinogen is present in the wall of the stomach or abomasum and is not activated to pepsin until after secretion. It is a gastric proteolytic enzyme. In cases of generalized damage to gastric mucosa, pepsinogen will leak back into plasma and plasma activities will increase. In practice the one clinical disease which this enzyme is used to assess is *type 2 ostertagiasis*, where the emergence of winter inhibited L_4 ostertagia larvae from the crypts causes massive damage to abomasal mucosa. Before about 1976 this condition was extremely common, but since the advent of larvicidal anthelmintics the incidence has declined dramatically and nowadays pepsinogen assay is seldom required. The enzyme is estimated after *in vitro* activation to pepsin and the assay involves an extended digestion step; therefore rapid results will not be forthcoming. Normal values in cattle are up to about 1000–1500 iu/l, while cases of type 2 ostertagiasis usually show marked increases into several thousand. Pepsinogen appears to have no value in assessing gastric ulcers, etc., in small animals.

Acid phosphatase (ACP)

This is a group of isoenzymes which hydrolyse phosphates at an acidic pH – these are found in prostate, liver, erythrocytes, platelets and bone. The single clinical use of acid phosphatase estimation is in the assessment of prostatic conditions and for this purpose the prostatic isoenzyme is specifically measured utilizing the fact that it is inhibited by tartrate. The difference in activity of the sample pre- and post-tartrate addition is the prostatic or 'tartrate labile' acid phosphatase. Normal values in dogs are under about 30 iu/l and really massive rises occur in cases of *prostatic carcinoma*, particularly when it has metastasized (but beware of tumours too undifferentiated to produce enzymes at all). Smaller increases are often seen in cases of *prostatitis* but simple prostatic hyperplasia is not generally associated with any change in plasma acid phosphatase activity. Note that palpation of the prostate *per rectum* may itself cause a slight increase in plasma acid phosphatase which can persist for up to a week; also note that acid phosphatase is a very labile enzyme and samples must be delivered to the laboratory without delay. Postal samples are unsuitable.

Urinary enzyme analysis

None of the above plasma enzymes appears to be of any use in detecting kidney damage – not even γGT which is known to be present in renal tissue in large amounts. However, renal damage is accompanied by high *urine* activities of certain enzymes, and these may be detectable before plasma urea and creatinine begin to rise. γGT is the main enzyme involved, but N-acetyl glucosaminidase has also been measured. Urine enzyme measurement is seldom employed clinically in veterinary practice.

Glutathione peroxidase (GSH-Px)

This is in quite a different category from all the other enzymes. It is present within the erythrocyte cell membrane and each enzyme molecule contains four atoms of selenium. It is measured not on plasma but on whole lysed blood and in this case the enzyme is being investigated *in its normal situation*, like a biopsy. The actual whole blood concentration is not the final answer, however, as the figure of interest is the GSH-Px activity in *packed red cells* (i.e. any effect of variations in PCV must be eliminated). This is done by dividing the whole blood GSH-Px activity by the PCV (expressed as a decimal fraction) in the same way as the MCHC is calculated from whole blood haemoglobin concentration and PCV (see p. 8). Normal values are about 30–40 iu/ml RBCs in cattle and about 70–80 iu/ml RBCs in sheep. Lower levels correlate with selenium deficiency. The enzyme is of no value in the investigation of selenium toxicity.

Endocrine tests are becoming increasingly routine in general practice, thanks to advances in analytical techniques which mean that radioisotopes are no longer essential for most common tests, and results are often available within 24 hours. However, the warnings about ensuring that test methodology is appropriate for the species in question still apply. Enzyme-linked immunosorbent assay (ELISA) or concentration immunoassay technology (CITE) should not be used for tests such as cortisol or thyroxine in non-human species – the only valid alternative to radioimmunoassay is chemiluminescence. In addition, the assay must be validated for the individual species in question. This means that in practice it is usually easy to get common analytes (like cortisol or thyroxine) measured in dogs and cats, but less common requests, including requests for these tests in other species, are still mainly the provenance of the specialist endocrinology laboratory.

Methods do vary as to the sample requirement; for example, some chemiluminescence methods cannot be performed on samples in anticoagulant, so it is essential to check your particular laboratory's preferences before embarking on the tests.

The adrenal cortex

The main hormone of diagnostic value is cortisol, which is secreted by the adrenal cortex in response to adrenocorticotrophic hormone (ACTH) produced by the pituitary gland. Overproduction of cortisol (Cushing's disease) can be due either to a cortisol-producing tumour of the adrenal cortex itself (about 20% of canine cases) or to an ACTH-producing tumour of the pituitary gland (80% of canine cases). Idiopathic Cushing's disease is rare in the cat and is again usually pituitary in origin. In the horse, Cushing's is a disease of elderly animals (usually ponies) and is invariably pituitary in origin. Underproduction of cortisol (Addison's disease) is almost entirely confined to the dog, and is believed to be a result of autoimmune destruction of the adrenal cortex.

Hyperadrenocorticism, Cushing's disease

This is a chronic condition which seldom becomes critical before a diagnosis can be reached. The emphasis is on building up a picture which is sufficiently convincing of Cushing's disease before embarking on treatment, and this is sometimes a drawn-out process involving three or four investigatory steps. This is often no bad thing, as the time taken to carry out each test in order and then assess the significance of the result can allow the clinical condition to become more obvious and so aid in the decision-making.

The first step is the demonstration of a convincing case for Cushing's as a *possibility*, based on the combined pattern of clinical and routine biochemistry and haematology results (see p. 229). This is one of the most classic pattern-recognition processes. It is not unusual to encounter Cushing's cases lacking one or even two of the cardinal findings on the routine analysis, and the skill lies in deciding when there is a sufficiently Cushingoid pattern to justify further investigation and when to dismiss the idea. The Cushing's pattern is less easy to recognize in the cat than in the dog, as the ALP does not tend to increase and the haematology changes are less marked. However, most cases of idiopathic Cushing's in cats present with insulin-resistant diabetes mellitus, which in itself must be considered grounds for investigating for possible Cushing's.

In dogs, diabetes mellitus itself can mimic the Cushing's pattern in the bio-chemistry results quite effectively, and so this pattern is of relatively little use in diabetic patients. Again, any diabetes mellitus which has been demonstrated to be insulin resistant should be considered as a possible Cushing's, while a diabetes which is insulin-responsive is very unlikely to be consistent with Cushing's.

One might think that all that would be necessary to confirm or deny the diagnosis would be to measure a single cortisol level, but this is not the case. Only a small minority of Cushing's cases have elevated cortisol levels on a single random sample, and most (especially the pituitary cases, which are about 80% of the total) give a normal result. Thus dynamic cortisol testing (that is stimulation or suppression with exogenously administered hormones) is necessary to confirm or deny the diagnosis.

ACTH stimulation test

This is the most practical approach in a first opinion situation once the decision has been taken to proceed with a Cushing's investigation. It is quicker and cheaper than the dexamethasone screening test, it is much less likely to give a false positive result (which can be dangerous), and if the result is clear-cut it can save the need for any further testing. In addition, it is never a wasted test. Because it is the ACTH stimulation test which is used to monitor Cushing's cases on treatment (dexamethasone response is unhelpful for that purpose), it is essential to carry out a pre-treatment test in any case, to act as a baseline for follow-up investigations.

ACTH stimulation test protocol

It is preferable to begin this test in the morning, as close as is practical to 9 a.m. This is designed to standardize for the diurnal rhythms of cortisol secretion which cause blood levels to vary quite considerably during the day. However, it has to be said that there is little regular diurnal rhythm detectable in most Cushing's cases in any event.

(1) Collect baseline blood sample.
(2) Inject one vial (250 µg) of tetracosactide (Synacthen: Alliance Pharmaceuticals) intravenously. Half a vial is sufficient for a dog of 5 kg or less, or for a cat.
(3) Wait *90 minutes* (some protocols suggest 2 hours, but recent studies suggest that the peak in cortisol is closer to 90 minutes).
(4) Collect second blood sample.

An alternative protocol has been suggested for cats in which three samples are collected: baseline, 1 hour and 3 hours. Interpretation is similar to the two-sample protocol, the 3-hour sample is included because of a suggestion that some cats show a delayed response.

Interpretation. (See Fig. 11.1.) In the normal dog the baseline result is usually around 100–300 nmol/l, rising to less than 500 nmol/l post-ACTH. An increase to over 1000 nmol/l is a conclusively positive result, consistent with pituitary-dependent Cushing's. Between 500 and 1000 nmol/l post-ACTH the probability of Cushing's increases – 500–600 nmol/l is still unlikely and requires further investigation to confirm; 600–700 nmol/l is possible but depends very much on the clinical context; 700–800 nmol/l is quite likely, but again one would consider it in relation to other findings; anything over 800 nmol/l can reasonably be considered diagnostic *in an unstressed patient, in the presence of typical clinical and routine biochemistry and haematology results.*

Adrenal Cushing's is often associated with a different pattern of ACTH response. The baseline result may be elevated above 400 nmol/l, while there is much less of an increase post-ACTH. Unless the values are quite high, however, it is usually preferable to confirm these cases by the dexamethasone screening or suppression test. Abdominal ultrasound can also provide useful diagnostic information in this context.

A small proportion of Cushing's cases (usually adrenal tumours) do in fact show a normal ACTH response; thus in a very suspicious clinical situation a negative result from an ACTH stimulation test should not be regarded as the last word on the subject, and a dexamethasone screening test is advisable.

If the cortisol results appear depressed in a suspected Cushing's case, consider whether the Synacthen actually went into the vein (intramuscular injection sometimes works, but it is difficult to ensure that the injection doesn't go into a fascial plane where it is ineffective), or whether it is possible that the animal might, in fact, be on some corticosteroid therapy – it happens!

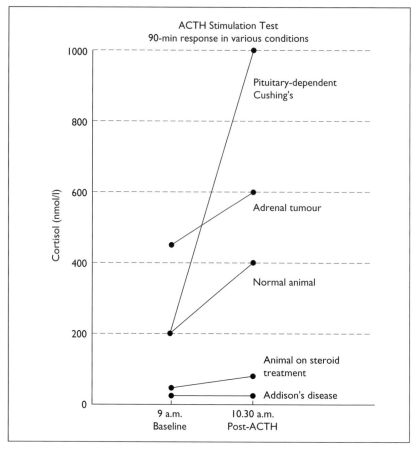

Fig. 11.1   Interpretation of various patterns of ACTH response.

The ACTH stimulation test in cases on treatment.   A well-controlled Cushing's case will usually have both values less than 100 nmol/l, and an apparently Addisonian result (<20 nmol/l in both samples) is not necessarily a cause for alarm unless the animal is clinically unwell. Post-ACTH values of 100–200 nmol/l may be acceptable so long as the animal is clinically well, though it is worth keeping an eye on these cases as the Cushing's may be heading for a comeback. Post-ACTH values of over 200 nmol/l are generally an indication that it may become necessary to get a bit braver with the mitotane in the foreseeable future (depending on clinical condition). It is also worth noting that animals which appear to be well controlled according to the ACTH response and not apparently Addisonian according to plasma sodium and potassium results can show a noticeable malaise, particularly in the day or two following mitotane administration. This is in fact due to low glucocorticoid levels, and a low dose of prednisolone can improve matters appreciably. The recent introduction of trilostane (Vetoryl: Arnolds, a reversible 3β-hydroxysteroid dehydrogenase inhibitor) as an alternative to mitotane may make the management of Cushing's disease a little less fraught.

When working up a suspected Cushing's case, the aim at this stage is to assess *all* the results available to date – clinical findings, routine biochemistry and haematology and ACTH response – and decide whether the overall evidence is sufficient to justify proceeding with treatment (or alternatively so poor as to justify abandoning the idea entirely), or whether further evidence is necessary.

The dexamethasone screening test (low dose)

If further investigation is still necessary, this is the next shot in the armoury. In a normal animal even a very low dose of dexamethasone will depress cortisol secretion very effectively and keep it depressed for over 8 hours. In Cushing's disease the cortisol either doesn't suppress at all (usually adrenal tumours) or bounces back in less than 8 hours (pituitary-dependent cases).

Low-dose dexamethasone screening test protocol

(1)   Once again, begin the test first thing in the morning (about 9 a.m.) by collecting the baseline sample.
(2)   Inject soluble dexamethasone intravenously at a dose rate of 0.01 mg/kg.
(3)   Three hours later (about 12 noon) collect the second sample.
(4)   Five hours after that (8 hours from the injection, about 5 p.m.) collect the third sample.

Note that this is a very low dose of dexamethasone, and it is fairly easily overcome by endogenous ACTH secretion if the patient is stressed. Therefore, decide in advance on the best way to conduct the test to avoid stress throughout the day – some dogs relax happily in a hospital kennel, while others are better returning home and coming back for each sample. In a very excitable patient it may be best to omit the 3-hour sample completely in the interests of getting a true reading at the 8-hour stage.

Interpretation. In a normal unstressed dog a baseline cortisol of about 100–300 nmol/l will fall by at least half (often to less than 40 nmol/l) by the 3-hour mark, and will definitely have fallen below 40 nmol/l by the 8-hour sample. An 8-hour result of greater than 40 nmol/l is considered to be consistent with Cushing's. However, bear in mind that stress during testing can cause a false positive result, and be very wary of a definite diagnosis from an 8-hour value of 40–70 nmol/l in an excitable patient, particularly where the rest of the evidence for Cushing's is not very convincing. A 3-hour result of less than half the baseline value is considered to point to a pituitary-dependent case, while a value higher than this raises the possibility of an adrenal tumour. However, as with the ACTH stimulation test, the pituitary/adrenal differentiation with this protocol is not necessarily clear-cut.

Once again, examine all the available clinical and laboratory evidence and decide if the case is strong enough to justify initiating treatment for Cushing's disease. If there is still room for doubt by this stage, it is generally best to put the question on hold and re-assess in a few months. It is sometimes simply too early in the course of the disease to be sure, and these cases will take no great harm from a delay, whereas it can be very dangerous to treat a non-Cushingoid patient with mitotane.

The dexamethasone suppression test (high dose)

Many would argue that once a diagnosis of Cushing's has been established beyond reasonable doubt there is little need to proceed further to differentiate pituitary from adrenal cases, if the intention is to treat medically whatever the cause. Others prefer to know exactly where they stand, or even be in a position to consider surgery of an adrenal tumour in suitable cases. The high-dose dexamethasone suppression test is designed to differentiate more specifically between the causes.

High-dose dexamethasone suppression test protocol

This is identical to that of the low-dose screening test described above, but the dose of dexamethasone is ten times higher, 0.1 mg/kg. This exploits the fact that the higher dose will feed back and suppress ACTH secretion from a pituitary lesion at least to some extent, but will have little or no effect on secretion from an adrenal lesion.

Interpretation.   In an adrenal tumour neither the 3-hour nor the 8-hour result will fall below half the baseline value – in fact, most cases show little or no change. In contrast, a pituitary case will show one or other (or perhaps both) results falling to less than 50% of the baseline. However, note that *it is not possible to distinguish definitely between a pituitary-dependent Cushing's and a normal dog by this method.* Therefore this protocol should only be used after Cushing's as such has been demonstrated beyond reasonable doubt by other means.

Combined ACTH/dexamethasone tests

Several protocols have been described which combine these two tests, with the aim of getting all the way to a final diagnosis in one investigation; however, these are not recommended. Generally there is no great hurry to diagnose a Cushing's case, and more time and money can be wasted by trying to cut corners than might be saved. Protocols where the dexamethasone is given first should be avoided at all costs, as the ACTH part of the test is impossible to interpret under these conditions – *never* do an ACTH stimulation test on a patient which has been given steroids. Protocols which begin with a standard ACTH stimulation test have the merit of allowing that part to be interpreted without interference, but often the second part of the test proves to be of little use. It is more satisfactory all round simply to do the ACTH stimulation test and assess the results of that before deciding where to go next.

'Steroid-induced alkaline phosphatase'

Prolonged exposure to high levels of corticosteroids induces the canine liver to produce an isoenzyme of ALP which is different from the usual isoenzymes found in the serum (see pp. 143–4). A method exists to detect this particular isoenzyme, and it has been suggested that it might be helpful in investigating possible Cushing's cases. However, the test is not especially sensitive or specific, and it does not reduce the necessity for dynamic cortisol testing. Experience demonstrates that once a reasonable suspicion of Cushing's disease exists based on clinical and routine laboratory results, it is better to get right on and perform the dynamic testing, and that carrying out further inconclusive screening tests at this stage is unhelpful.

Urinary cortisol/creatinine ratio

This test was used many years ago to investigate Cushing's, but fell into disuse after the dynamic blood testing protocols were developed. There has recently been a revival of interest in the method, again as a screen to determine whether continued investigation of possible Cushing's disease is worthwhile. It takes advantage of the fact that a urine sample represents something of a mean of the situation during the time when that aliquot of urine was being secreted, which in this case can be more useful than a single spot blood cortisol result. The ratio of cortisol to creatinine is then introduced to compensate (partially) for the error introduced by variations in the degree of concentration of the urine at the time of sampling.

The disadvantage of this test is again that it is merely a guide, and it does not do away with the need to confirm the diagnosis by dynamic blood tests before treatment can be begun. Once again, it is preferable simply to proceed to the dynamic testing once the clinical suspicion has been established. It is important to stress that this test is *less* specific than the dynamic blood tests, and it should not be used as a decision-maker in cases where these tests are inconclusive.

ACTH measurement

This test is technically difficult, and it is offered by comparatively specialized endocrinology laboratories. It provides a further means of differentiating between pituitary and adrenal Cushing's cases – in the former, levels are abnormally high, while in the latter they are abnormally low. However, special transport of frozen samples to the laboratory has to be arranged, which makes the test somewhat impractical for routine use.

Cushing's disease in the horse

Equine Cushing's disease is a pituitary condition, and is quite common in elderly ponies. The primary abnormality is believed to be an under-secretion of dopamine, which leads to hypertrophy of the pars intermedia of the hypothalamus, which then progresses to the characteristic adenoma. The easiest and most straightforward means of diagnosing equine Cushing's is the demonstration of a significant hyperglycaemia. Most cases progress eventually to diabetes mellitus, and Cushing's is practically the only cause of diabetes mellitus in the horse. Therefore, in the absence of recent exercise, stress, excitement or a concentrate feed, hyperglycaemia is essentially pathognomonic for the condition. The main problem lies with cases of acute laminitis (which can be part of the presentation of equine Cushing's disease), where it can be difficult to be sure that a raised glucose is not caused by the pain of the sore feet. In these cases it is best to wait until the acute pain has subsided and the patient is more comfortable before repeating the test.

Where hyperglycaemia is absent or mild it can also be helpful to measure insulin (see p. 166).

Dynamic cortisol tests

Various dynamic cortisol methods have been used to investigate the non-diabetic equine Cushing's case. A test which uses thyrotrophin-releasing hormone (TRH: Protirelin) to stimulate cortisol secretion has been described, but in practice this is difficult to interpret because it is not unusual for normal horses to produce results similar to the 'Cushing's' category in certain circumstances. In addition, the quantity of TRH required to carry out the test in a horse can be extremely expensive. An ACTH stimulation test can be performed more or less in the same way as in the dog (using about ten times the amount of tetracosactide (Synacthen)). Interpretation is similar to the dog, but the test is not nearly so well characterized, results are frequently not clear-cut, and it is not recommended. A combined dexamethasone/TRH test has also been described, but once again that has the cost drawbacks associated with TRH, and (as with dogs) protocols which combine stimulating and suppressing hormones in a single test can be problematical.

The most satisfactory technique is probably the overnight (19-hour) dexamethasone suppression test.

Overnight dexamethasone suppression test protocol

This test is usually begun mid-afternoon, for convenience of sample timing.

(1)   Collect baseline blood sample.

(2)   Inject soluble dexamethasone at a dose rate of 20 mg for a 500 kg horse (0.04 mg/kg), either intravenously or intramuscularly.

(3)   Wait 19 hours.

(4)   Collect second blood sample.

Interpretation.   In the normal horse, as in the dog, the baseline result is usually around 100–300 nmol/l, and this will fall to below 40 nmol/l by the second sample. A 19-hour result greater than 40 nmol/l is considered to be consistent with Cushing's, though again one has to take care to ensure that the patient is unstressed during the period of the test.

However, when a suspected equine Cushing's case is proving difficult to confirm, there is often a good argument for simply waiting a bit longer. An animal which gives inconclusive results one month may well produce a very clear-cut diagnosis a few months later, and as the disease is very slowly progressive little may be lost by the delay.

Iatrogenic Cushing's syndrome

This term describes the clinical appearance of Cushing's-disease-like signs as a result of administration of exogenous corticosteroids. It is almost unavoidable when treating autoimmune disease with immunosuppressive doses of steroids, but can also be seen with lower doses, especially when prolonged administration is involved. Routine laboratory results will demonstrate a steroid pattern, and both baseline and post-ACTH cortisol levels will be depressed – the latter especially in long-term administration. However, the same pattern of results will be seen in any patient on corticosteroid treatment, and these laboratory findings are in no way specific for or diagnostic of 'iatrogenic Cushing's'. In fact this is a purely clinical diagnosis. If a patient on corticosteroid treatment looks or behaves 'Cushingoid', then the inference is pretty obvious. The only other thing to do is to withdraw the corticosteroids (with care!) and observe whether the signs resolve. Running routine profiles or ACTH stimulation tests in an attempt to prove 'iatrogenic Cushing's' is a waste of time. In fact, this clinical appearance is sometimes an unavoidable sequel to essential corticosteroid therapy, and if the clinical consequences of withdrawing the treatment are less desirable than a bit of polydipsia and hair loss, then one simply has to go for the lesser of two evils.

Hypoadrenocorticism, Addison's disease

Many dogs with Addison's disease present in an Addisonian crisis, and the diagnosis is obvious from the routine biochemistry and haematology results (see pp. 84 & 228). In these circumstances it is not really necessary to confirm this by hormone measurements; it is more important to initiate treatment. Where the presentation is less acute or there is genuine doubt about the diagnosis, hormone investigations are required.

Although the main clinical signs of Addison's disease are due to hypo-aldosteronism rather than low glucocorticoid levels, in practice it is cortisol which is measured for diagnostic purposes. A single random cortisol is conclusive in ruling out Addison's if the result is obviously normal, say over about 150 nmol/l. A very low result (generally undetectable, less than 20 nmol/l) from a sample taken before any corticosteroids have been given is very suggestive indeed of Addison's, if not entirely conclusive. It is certainly possible for a normal dog to have a very low random cortisol, but if the animal is under stress (as most cases showing signs suggestive of possible Addison's are), this is very unlikely. However, exogenous corticosteroid administration depresses cortisol secretion very efficiently (by feeding back to depress ACTH secretion), and so a sample collected after steroids have been given is likely to give a false diagnosis and should not be used.

For the most reliable confirmation of the diagnosis, an ACTH stimulation test is preferable – if cortisol is still undetectable after ACTH stimulation, there is really no argument. However, again it is essential to carry out this test *before* any corticosteroids are administered to the patient; thus if a dog has been given steroids 'just in case' the problem arises as to how long the treatment must then be discontinued before a valid ACTH response can be measured. It is therefore worth considering performing an ACTH stimulation test whenever Addison's disease is suspected, before beginning corticosteroid treatment. If the results of routine biochemistry and haematology tests then prove to be conclusive either way the blood samples can be discarded without bothering to measure the cortisol, but if the routine results are inconclusive then the samples are available for testing without delay. This way, corticosteroid treatment can be started with a clear conscience as soon as the post-ACTH sample has been collected. For this reason ACTH should always be stocked in a small animal practice, as it is unsafe to delay treating a dog which might be in an Addisonian crisis until a supply can be obtained from the pharmacy. If a delay is unavoidable, ensure that fluid therapy is begun as soon as the initial samples for routine analysis have been collected, so that the dehydration and electrolyte abnormalities are corrected.

ACTH stimulation test protocol for Addison's investigation

(1) Collect baseline blood sample for routine biochemistry and haematology and cortisol estimation.
(2) It is now permissible to begin intravenous fluid or other therapy *except* for corticosteroid administration.
(3) Inject one vial (250 µg) tetracosactide (Synacthen: Alliance Pharmaceuticals) intravenously. Half a vial is sufficient for a dog of 5 kg or less.
(4) Wait at least 45 minutes (note that this timing is inappropriate for the investigation of Cushing's disease, see above).
(5) Collect second blood sample for cortisol estimation.
(6) Corticosteroid treatment may now be given.

Interpretation. In the normal dog baseline cortisol is usually around 100–300 nmol/l, rising to around 300–500 nmol/l post-ACTH administration. Most dogs with acute Addison's disease have undetectable (<20 nmol/l) cortisol in both samples; however, any case where both figures are below 100 nmol/l, especially where there is a *fall* post-ACTH, is probably Addisonian, especially where there is other corroborating evidence of the condition. As an aside, it is worth noting that dogs under acute stress sometimes demonstrate an exaggerated ACTH response which might under other circumstances be considered consistent with Cushing's disease. Thus if a stressed, dehydrated dog proves to have an extremely high post-ACTH cortisol concentration the only safe conclusion is that it is not suffering from Addison's disease, and instant diagnoses of Cushing's disease are probably unwarranted!

'Iatrogenic Addison's'

This can occur in two situations – a Cushing's case on treatment which has over-reacted to the mitotane dose, and an animal which has been on corticosteroid treatment which has then been withdrawn too suddenly. While a *normal* ACTH response in either of these situations will tend to rule out Addison's, it must be remembered that in both these situations the therapy will in any case tend to depress cortisol levels whether or not the patient actually becomes clinically Addisonian. Thus diagnosis should be on clinical grounds backed up by routine biochemistry investigation (especially sodium and potassium), and cortisol measurements are not necessarily helpful.

The thyroid gland

The two hormones secreted by this gland are thyroxine (T_4) and tri-iodo-thyronine (T_3). Secretion is controlled by thyroid stimulating hormone (TSH) and thyrotrophin releasing hormone (TRH), both secreted by the pituitary gland. T_3 is the more physiologically active hormone; however, it is T_4 (in different forms) which is the usual routine diagnostic measurement, because abnormalities show up more readily in this hormone. Total T_4 is exactly what the term implies, while free T_4 is a measurement of the small fraction of this total which is free in the plasma as opposed to being protein-bound.

Hyperthyroidism

This is extremely common in elderly cats, with most cases being due to benign adenoma of the thyroid gland which often is or becomes bilateral. Carcinomas of the thyroid are uncommon. Nevertheless, even after a bilateral thyroidectomy some cases show a recurrence of signs, apparently due to proliferation of extra-thyroid tissue. This condition was generally unrecognized until the mid to late 1980s, and there is some debate as to whether cases were being misdiagnosed as chronic renal failure before that time, or whether the condition is genuinely new. While most hyperthyroid cats are over the age of 10 years, the condition occurs sporadically in younger cats, with a few cases having been recorded as young as 5 years old. Below this age, hyperthyroidism can be essentially discounted.

The condition is much less common in the dog, but again it is a condition of older animals, and affected dogs are usually obviously unwell. Suspicions of hyperthyroidism in young, hyperactive dogs are invariably unfounded. Thyroid carcinomas (malignant) are the more common cause of canine hyperthyroidism, though adenomas similar to the feline condition have also been recorded.

Confirmation of hyperthyroidism, especially in the cat, is generally very simple, with a single elevated total T_4 measurement being diagnostic. In the old cat, anything above 50 nmol/l is considered to be conclusive, with values between 40 and 50 nmol/l regarded as highly suspicious, especially in conjunction with a typical hyperthyroid pattern on routine biochemistry results (see p. 234). Note, however, that T_4 levels of up to 70 nmol/l have been recorded in normal *young* cats, and that age is an important criterion when interpreting results from this test. Free T_4 can also be used as a diagnostic test for hyperthyroidism, and where the result is clearly abnormal (over about 20 pmol/l) it is just as valid. However, results around the cut-off point are less easy to interpret than with total T_4; therefore the latter is generally regarded as the test of choice.

T_4 levels below 40 nmol/l in clinically suspicious cats present a particular problem. One approach is simply to wait for a couple of months and re-investigate. However, sometimes a trial 2–3 week course of carbimazole (Neo-Mercazole: Roche) is worth considering in such cases. There are no reports of this having caused any harm, and if a dramatic clinical improvement is obtained that itself can be a very useful diagnostic pointer.

Alternatively, the *T_3 suppression test* may be employed. The rationale is similar to the dexamethasone suppression tests for Cushing's disease. In the euthyroid animal, exogenous thyroid hormone will suppress secretion of endogenous hormones by negative feedback to the pituitary, while in the hyperthyroid animal hormone secretion continues regardless. Tri-iodothyronine (Tertroxin: Goldshield) is employed because there is no back-conversion *in vivo* of T_3 to T_4, and T_3 does not interfere with T_4 measurement.

T_3 suppression test protocol

(1)   Collect baseline sample.
(2)   Dispense tri-iodothyronine (Tertroxin), 175 µg. This is sufficient for seven doses of 25 µg.
(3)   Owner administers 25 µg Tertroxin three times daily (8-hourly intervals) orally, starting the morning after the baseline sample was collected, and finishing with the seventh dose on the morning of the third day.
(4)   Two to four hours after the seventh dose of Tertroxin, collect the second blood sample.

Interpretation.   Conventionally, total T_4 is measured on both samples, though it is the second sample which gives the critical result – less than 20 nmol/l indicates a normal (euthyroid) cat, while greater than 25 nmol/l is diagnostic of hyperthyroidism. One would also expect to see a decrease in T_4 concentration in the euthyroid cat, but interpretations based on percentage or absolute decreases are not necessarily reliable. Measurement of T_3 in addition to T_4 is only a means of checking that the owner has actually dosed the cat as directed, and is not strictly necessary.

In the dog, while again a high T_4 concentration is diagnostic in conjunction with the right clinical signs, normal total (or free) T_4 levels are not especially unusual in hyperthyroid cases. This is one situation where measurement of T_3 is sometimes used to improve diagnostic accuracy. However, since the vast majority of cases have palpable lumps in the neck, histopathology of a biopsy sample is often the best approach at this stage.

Hypothyroidism

This is primarily a condition of the dog, and it is rare in other species. Most fat, lazy cats are simply fat, lazy cats, and although owners of unwilling or lethargic horses often suggest hypothyroidism as a possible cause, few such allegations stand up to investigation. Iodine deficiency causing goitre and hypothyroidism has been recorded in horses, but it is uncommon under modern management conditions where proprietary horse feeds with properly formulated mineral content are employed. Even in dogs, overeating and lack of exercise are commoner causes of obesity than are thyroid problems.

The commonest age for presentation of hypothyroidism in the dog is around 4 years, and there are definite breed predispositions. As with so many of the conditions presenting in this age of dog, an autoimmune aetiology is postulated. Once again it is a question of weighing up the clinical signs and the routine biochemistry and haematology results before deciding whether pursuit of a possible diagnosis of hypothyroidism is justified, and then trying to build up the whole picture to the point where you feel you have satisfactorily confirmed (or excluded) the diagnosis.

Choice of initial screening test for suspected hypothyroidism may vary according to test availability, and it is essential to be guided by the laboratory you are using. In addition, bear in mind that non-thyroidal illness will also cause thyroid hormones to be depressed, so test strategies concentrating exclusively on thyroid measurements are only justified if you are confident that other medical conditions are not at issue. If the differential diagnosis list is not limited to hypothyroidism, a wider profile approach is indicated (see p. 217). Concentrating on the thyroid, the preferred initial screening test is free T_4 in conjunction with cholesterol. Failing that, total T_4, again plus cholesterol, may be used. The critical question is the availability of an assay method properly validated for the dog, and sensitive at low concentrations, and while free T_4 is preferred if available, a properly validated total T_4 method is preferable to a free

T_4 method which is not validated for dogs. The main problem is what is known as the 'sick euthyroid syndrome', where an animal suffering from a non-thyroidal illness demonstrates a depressed T_4 result as a consequence of that illness. Total T_4 is affected to a much greater extent than free T_4, and total T_4 results in the 8–25 nmol/l range can be very difficult to interpret one way or another, which covers an annoyingly high proportion of cases. Free T_4 is also affected but to a lesser extent, with the 'grey area' covering about 5–10 pmol/l. The cholesterol is included as an aid to decision-making in the inconclusive range.

Interpretation. Hypothyroid dogs seem to fall into two categories – the extremely obvious, which give grossly abnormal results for virtually any test you choose, and the difficult ones, which remain stubbornly in the grey area of any screening test and require dynamic testing before any decision can be made. Free T_4 results below about 5 pmol/l and total T_4 results below about 8 nmol/l are a very strong indication indeed of hypothyroidism, as is a cholesterol concentration greater than about 15 mmol/l *in the absence of diabetes mellitus or Cushing's disease.* Free T_4 results over about 10 pmol/l and total T_4 results over about 25 nmol/l suggest that the dog is almost certainly euthyroid, especially if the cholesterol is normal, but note that about 30% of hypothyroid dogs have normal or only slightly elevated cholesterol concentrations, so a normal cholesterol result never excludes hypothyroidism.

However, rather than applying rigid rules, a pragmatic approach taking into account clinical presentation (including results of skin biopsies, if available) together with biochemistry tests, is most fruitful. Once more, weigh up *all* the available information, and decide whether the situation is clear-cut enough to justify declaring a diagnosis and instituting treatment (or alternatively to justify excluding the diagnosis completely), or whether further investigation is warranted. Dynamic testing (TSH or TRH stimulation tests) is considered the most definitive approach, but other methods are available and may be helpful in certain circumstances.

TSH stimulation test

This is the preferred test if TSH is obtainable, which at the time of writing it has not been (or not legally, anyway) for a number of years. However, it may be that it will become available again, and so the protocol is included more in hope than expectation. If you are offered TSH for injection from any source other than a pharmacy or a legitimate pharmaceutical wholesaler, it is prudent to ask some very searching questions before accepting it.

TSH stimulation test protocol

(1) Collect baseline sample for T_4 measurement.
(2) Inject thyroid stimulating hormone (TSH) intravenously at a dose of 0.1 iu/kg. (This must be a pharmaceutical-grade preparation.)

(3)   Wait 6 hours.
(4)   Collect second sample.

Interpretation.   In the normal dog, the T_4 will increase to at least 50% over baseline and reach a value of at least 35 nmol/l. Less than this is indicative of hypothyroidism. However, be cautious in cases where the baseline value is itself high – in this situation a further increase of 50% may be expecting too much, and the high baseline itself suggests the patient is normal.

TRH stimulation test

This is capable of producing results almost as good as those of the TSH stimulation test *if* a sufficiently high dose of TRH is used, and it has the inestimable advantage of not breaking the law, as a pharmaceutical-grade preparation of TRH with a product licence for human use (Protirelin) is available from pharmacists. As the dose rate is quite high, be sure to weigh the dog before ordering the TRH, otherwise there is a danger of finding yourself short on the day.

TRH stimulation test protocol

(1)   Collect baseline sample for T_4 measurement.
(2)   Inject TRH intravenously at a dose of 0.02 mg/kg. This must be done slowly over a period of 2 minutes, so an intravenous cannula is necessary.
(3)   Wait 4 hours.
(4)   Collect second sample.

Interpretation.   In the normal dog, the T_4 will increase to at least 20% over baseline and reach a value of at least 30 nmol/l. Less than this is indicative of hypothyroidism. However, the same caution as above applies if the baseline value is itself high – though this is unlikely if preliminary investigations have shown reasonable cause for suspicion of hypothyroidism.

Measurement of endogenous TSH

This is the test of choice for the diagnosis of hypothyroidism in man. It has been known for many years that canine patients are much less accommodating, and that TSH levels correlate poorly with clinical hypothyroidism in dogs. More recently, the lack of availability of injectable TSH and the indifferent performance of the (lower dose) TRH stimulation test has led to a revival of interest in the test, and attempts have been made to improve its performance by calculating a ratio of either total T_4 or free T_4 to TSH. However, even employing the ratio, results have been disappointing. A very high TSH result is indeed a good pointer to hypothyroidism, but a normal or slightly elevated result is of little help – unfortunately the very high levels tend to occur in precisely those cases which are already clear-cut on the T_4 or free T_4 assay. Once again, the easy cases which have 'read the book' behave as predicted, but the 'definite maybe' ones are often no further advanced. The test does not reduce the need for dynamic T_4 testing, and even as a screening test its performance is, if anything, somewhat poorer than the (free) T_4/cholesterol approach.

Free T_4 by equilibrium dialysis

This is a specialized method of measuring free T_4 which is generally the province of the specialist endocrinology laboratory. It is more sensitive and specific than the simple radioimmunoassay or chemiluminescence methods, and may approach the TRH stimulation test in diagnostic usefulness. It may be particularly helpful in large dogs, where the cost of the TRH for injection can become almost prohibitive at the recommended dose.

Thyroglobulin autoantibodies

Canine hypothyroidism is almost invariably of autoimmune aetiology, and it might be expected that a test for the appropriate antibodies would provide a definite answer. However, the usefulness of this approach depends very much on the age of the patient. While the majority of hypothyroid dogs under the age of 4 years are indeed positive for thyroglobulin autoantibodies, over the age of 6 years this situation is reversed – probably due to decay of humoral antibody with time. A positive result is an extremely strong pointer to hypothyroidism, but as 'false' negatives can occur at any age, a negative result is of little value in excluding the condition.

Anti-T_4 antibodies

Occasionally anti-T_4 antibodies occur in the plasma of patients with auto-immune thyroid disease to such an extent as to interfere substantially with the test methodology – which of course uses anti-T_4 antibody as a reagent to detect the T_4. This produces a falsely high T_4 or free T_4 reading, which in fact bears no relation to the true concentration in the blood sample. Thus if an anomalously high T_4 or free T_4 result is obtained in a dog being investigated for hypothyroidism, it is useful to assay the sample for endogenous anti-T_4 antibodies. A high level both confirms that the original result was an artefact and supports a diagnosis of autoimmune thyroid disease.

Therapeutic monitoring

The test of choice for monitoring dogs on thyroxine treatment is total T_4. Samples should be taken about 6 hours after the last tablet has been given to ensure that you are not measuring hormone which has just been absorbed from the gut. Ideally, you are looking for a result of between 30 and 50 nmol/l;

however, this has to be viewed in conjunction with the clinical response – if a dog is very well clinically then levels which are a bit outside this range may be regarded as acceptable.

A hyperthyroid cat which has been started on carbimazole therapy should demonstrate a marked decrease in total T_4 by 2–4 weeks after beginning treatment. It is a good idea to check that this has occurred. However, it must never be forgotten that carbimazole is not necessarily a 'cure' for hyperthyroidism, and that the drug is principally used to achieve a euthyroid status *in order to facilitate surgery*. Some cats will indeed stay well on drug treatment alone for 2 years or more, but sooner or later the effect is usually lost and you will be back at square one. Therefore, unless the cat is so old that it seems likely to die of something else in less than a couple of years, a normal T_4 some weeks after beginning carbimazole therapy should be regarded as the green light to schedule surgery, not as an indication to continue indefinitely on maintenance therapy.

The endocrine pancreas

Insulin is the only pancreatic hormone commonly measured in general practice. Indications are in the investigation of diabetes mellitus, for the diagnosis of insulinomas, and in the investigation of equine Cushing's disease.

Hyperinsulinism

This can be caused by overdosage of insulin in a diabetic patient (not usually a great diagnostic challenge!), accidental administration of insulin to a non-diabetic animal (rare), or an insulin-producing tumour of the β-cells of the islets of Langherans (insulinoma). In practice the usual question is whether a hypoglycaemia which has been observed in a collapsing animal is or is not due to an insulinoma (see p. 120). For this purpose measurement of insulin alone is insufficient, it is necessary to calculate an insulin/glucose ratio using glucose and insulin results obtained from the same sample. This is because many insulinoma cases have circulating insulin levels similar to those seen in normal animals; the point is that these insulin levels are *not* normal in association with hypoglycaemia.

Samples for insulin/glucose ratio measurement should normally be collected after at least a 12 hour fast; however, if the clinical signs are so severe that such a fast is impractical, the absolute minimum period is 4 hours. Collect simultaneous serum (for insulin) and fluoride plasma (for glucose) samples – a glucose result from a side-room reflectance meter is inadequate for this purpose, and both samples should be submitted to the laboratory.

Insulin/glucose ratio is calculated as

$$\frac{\text{Insulin (mU/l)} \times 100}{(\text{Glucose (mmol/l)} \times 18) - 30}$$

and expressed as a percentage. However, if the plasma glucose concentration is below 1.7 mmol/l, this formula gives an invalid (negative) result. In that situation, any measurable insulin at all, above the limit of sensitivity of the assay, is generally indicative of an insulinoma.

Interpretation.   Ratios of under 30% are normal. Anything above that may well be an insulinoma, but results between 30% and 60% should be viewed as equivocal, especially if the pre-fasting requirement may not have been rigorously followed.

Diabetes mellitus

Insulin measurement is helpful in distinguishing between type I ('insulin-dependent') and type II ('non-insulin-dependent') diabetes mellitus. In the former, insulin is generally so low as to be undetectable, even in the presence of gross hyperglycaemia. In the latter, insulin levels are in the lower part of the normal range (around 8–20 mU/l). Where actual insulin resistance is present, measured insulin concentrations may be quite normal (20–40 mU/l).

Equine Cushing's disease/diabetes mellitus

The upward pressure on glucose concentration exerted by chronically excessive cortisol secretion is countered by increased insulin secretion (see Fig. 8.1, p. 112), and it is only when that itself proves inadequate that actual diabetes develops. Thus in Cushing's disease in any species there is a tendency to increased serum insulin concentration even if frank diabetes is not yet evident. In the horse, where diagnosis of the pre-diabetic Cushing's case is often less than straightforward, insulin measurement can be a useful extra indicator. Again a fasting sample is required, which in this case means no concentrate feed for at least 15 hours before sampling. An insulin level of greater than about 20 mU/l is very suggestive of Cushing's under these circumstances, and levels up to 80–90 mU/l may be encountered.

Sex hormones

Measurement of sex hormones is generally only of benefit in a few specific situations, and it is wise to be absolutely certain of what you are measuring and why before embarking on the tests. In particular, random requests for any or all of the sex hormones in suspected 'sex hormone alopecia' are invariably unrewarding. An investigative protocol for this condition has been described in which five sex hormones are analysed pre and post ACTH injection, but this is an expensive undertaking, and experience in evaluating the significance of the results in individual cases is very limited.

Oestradiol

This is the main biologically active oestrogen, and the one usually measured in clinical situations. The two situations where this measurement is helpful are suspected Sertoli cell tumour in the male dog and suspected residual ovarian tissue in a supposedly spayed bitch or cat.

The Sertoli cell of the testis secretes oestradiol, and abnormally high levels (over about 200 pmol/l) are seen in most cases of Sertoli cell tumour where feminization is evident.

Receptal stimulation test

This test was originally described as a means of proving that a bitch is unspayed for Kennel Club purposes, but it is also useful in situations where an allegedly spayed bitch is showing signs of possible oestrus, and it also appears to be valid in the cat. The difficulty with a single random oestradiol measurement in this situation is that while a high level is positive proof that ovarian tissue is present, a low level does not conclusively rule it out. However, if ovarian tissue is pre-stimulated by buserelin (a synthetic FSH/LH analogue, Receptal: Intervet), it will produce measurable oestradiol in circulation within 60–90 minutes after i/v injection. The dose rate given in the original publication is '0.32 µg, based on a body weight of 12 to 15 kg', and this may be scaled up or down as appropriate. A more recent publication suggests that hCG (human chorionic gonado-trophin, Chorulon: Intervet, also an FSH/LH preparation) may be substituted for buserelin, at a dose rate of 20 iu/kg. A single blood sample is collected 60–90 minutes after injection, and an oestradiol measurement of greater than 20 pmol/l is indicative of the presence of ovarian tissue. Entire bitches generally show levels greater than 50 pmol/l.

Progesterone

The only routine indication for progesterone measurement is when it is necessary to demonstrate the presence of a functional corpus luteum.

'Ovucheck Premate' test

This is a semiquantitative ELISA kit test (marketed by Guildhay) for proges-terone in the serum of bitches, which is useful for detecting the time of ovu-lation and so helps achieve the optimum timing of mating. It is more sensitive to the 'right moment' than vaginal cytology, particularly in less experienced hands. The kit produces a colour change which can be read by eye, and it can be used in the practice side-room if necessary.

Testosterone

This test is primarily useful in determining whether a male is castrate or cryptorchid. Once again, however, a single random sample is inappropriate, as a low level does not conclusively rule out the presence of testicular tissue, and a stimulation test is necessary. The procedure (in all species) is to inject human chorionic gonadotrophin (hCG) intravenously at a dose rate of 20 iu/kg, and sample 90 minutes later. In castrated males the testosterone level will remain very low (less than about 0.5 nmol/l), while males with one or more retained testes generally show much higher levels, certainly over 1 nmol/l and usually considerably higher than this. Post-hCG testosterone in a (normal) entire adult male is around 30–50 nmol/l in all species. However, note that the human nose is a very sensitive detector of testosterone in the cat and laboratory tests are often unnecessary: if it smells like a tom-cat there *must* be testicular tissue present – though the opposite is not necessarily the case in the young adult (under 2–3 years of age).

Elevated testosterone levels are also found in mares with granulosa cell tumours of the ovary.

Oestrone sulphate

The equine testis is unique in being able to convert testosterone to oestrone sulphate. Unlike testosterone, there is little diurnal variation in plasma oestrone sulphate concentration, which allows this measurement to be used as a single random-sample (no gonadotrophin stimulation required) test for cryptorchidism. However, it is only useful in *horses* over 3 years old, and not in any other species (including donkeys). Anything over about 0.1 µg/l is suggestive of the presence of testicular tissue.

Non-blood Body Fluids

Urine

General

Urine biochemistry, unlike plasma biochemistry, is very seldom concerned with accurate *quantitative* measurements. This is because the important information regarding normal urine constituents is the rate of excretion by the kidney, not the concentration in the urine, which is entirely dependent on the amount of water excreted at the same time. In fact, since many urine constituents show a pronounced diurnal rhythm in their excretion rates, the really useful measurement is the amount of a substance excreted in 24 hours. This necessitates carrying out a 24-hour urine collection, which is not particularly difficult with human patients, but is so impractical with animals that not only is it seldom attempted clinically but the baseline normal values are not readily available. A compromise can be made by expressing the concentration of a substance in a spot urine sample as a ratio of the concentration of creatinine, a substance with an excretion rate which is fairly constant. However, once again diurnal and other variations pose a problem. The concept of 'clearance ratios' is discussed on p. 96.

For these reasons clinical urine analysis is usually concerned *qualitatively* with the appearance of substances in the urine which are not normally present, and accurate measurements of concentrations are not necessary.

Specific gravity (SG)

This is a general measurement of the concentration of the sample, expressed as a ratio of the weight of the sample to the weight of the equivalent volume of distilled water. Normal values are about 1.020 to 1.050. Lower values are quite common during diuresis and in most conditions the important fact is not the SG of one random sample but whether or not this rises during water deprivation – that is, whether or not the kidney can concentrate the urine. Extremely low values (under 1.005) are virtually diagnostic of diabetes insipidus.

In diabetes mellitus, urine SG is high due to the glucose concentration in spite of the fact that other constituents are very dilute due to the osmotic diuresis. Note that the SG patch on the Bayer/Ames dipstix gives completely erroneous results for non-human urine and must not be used. Refractometry is the method of choice, see p. 304.

Dipstix tests

Urine test strips are available in a number of permutations of the following tests: nitrite, pH, protein, blood, glucose, ketones, bilirubin and urobilinogen. The multiple patch strips are most useful in the consulting room while one- or two-patch strips are convenient for home use by owners if required.

(1) *Nitrite.* This is produced in urine from natural nitrates by nitrite-forming bacteria. A positive result on a *fresh* sample indicates bacterial contamination, i.e. urinary tract infection, and the next step is to culture the urine sediment. A negative result does not prove the absence of bacterial infection.

(2) *pH.* This is normally acid in carnivores and alkaline in herbivores. In cases of urinary tract infection pH often becomes more alkaline, but stale urine also becomes alkaline with time. Disturbances of acid/base balance (acidosis or alkalosis) will also be reflected in the urine pH. Therapeutic manipulation of urine pH is often useful when treating urolithiasis.

(3) *Protein.* Normal urine occasionally has a trace of protein, but any more than this is clinically significant. There are two possible causes:

   (a) Urinary tract infection such as cystitis or prostatitis. This is much the commoner cause of proteinuria. In the majority of cases blood will also be present in the urine, especially where the infection is severe or of acute onset. Urine pH will often be alkaline and a positive nitrite reaction may also be seen. Plasma albumin concentration is usually normal.

   (b) Protein-losing nephropathy such as glomerulonephritis, where the plasma proteins (especially albumin) leak out through the glomerular basement membrane. This should be suspected where a maximum urine protein reading is not accompanied by any blood. These patients will be hypoalbuminaemic (see p. 78).

(4) *Blood.* This can appear in the urine in two forms – as red blood cells (haematuria) or as free haemoglobin (haemoglobinuria). Small amounts of either can be differentiated on the test strip – red blood cells create a stippled pattern on the test patch while haemoglobin produces a uniform wash of colour. Strongly positive reactions cannot be differentiated in this way and it is then necessary to examine the urine sediment for the presence (or absence) of erythrocytes.

   Red blood cells almost always originate from the lower urinary tract, e.g. as in cystitis. Loss of blood from the kidney is very rare and, when it occurs, is usually the result of trauma. In contrast, free haemoglobin does originate at the kidney. It appears in the urine when there is a large amount of haemoglobin free in the plasma, i.e. in acute haemolytic disease. (Both haematuria and haemoglobinuria will also produce a positive protein reaction.)

(5) *Glucose.* The presence of glucose in the urine simply means that the plasma glucose concentration has exceeded the renal glucose threshold at some time during the hours before the sample was collected (see p. 112). While it is true that a very strongly positive urine glucose reading is virtually diagnostic of diabetes mellitus in most cases, remember that the correlation between plasma and urine glucose concentrations is poor, and that other causes of hyperglycaemia should always be considered especially where the urine glucose reading is less than the maximum. The possibility of glycosuria without hyperglycaemia due to an abnormally low renal glucose threshold (e.g. Fanconi syndrome), though unusual, should also be borne in mind. For these reasons it is essential to measure plasma glucose before making a firm diagnosis of diabetes mellitus. It is also most important to monitor plasma or blood glucose during stabilization of a diabetic, as otherwise it is extremely difficult to attain optimum control.

(6) *Ketones.* Normally, plasma levels of ketones are very low. However, when an animal becomes ketotic (see p. 124) the 'ketone bodies', acetone, acetoacetic acid and β-hydroxybutyrate, are readily excreted in the urine and in fact become more concentrated in urine than in plasma. Urine testing is therefore one of the easiest ways to demonstrate ketosis. Ketosis in a diabetic is a bad sign as it indicates that virtually no glucose is getting into the cells, which is the reason for the inclusion of a ketone patch on urine strips for home monitoring of diabetics.

(7) *Bilirubin.* Positive urine bilirubin reactions at the trace, + and even ++ level are extremely common in normal, unjaundiced dogs (particularly when the sample is not absolutely fresh), and so only the highest (+++) reading can really be said to be clinically significant. It might be expected that, as unconjugated bilirubin is albumin-bound, only conjugated bilirubin would appear in the urine. In practice, however, haemolytic patients often do show strongly positive urine bilirubin reactions, and so the presence of bilirubin in the urine is not really a realiable method of distinguishing between conjugated and unconjugated bilirubin. Due to the frequency of 'false positive' bilirubin readings and the lack of specificity for conjugated bilirubin, urine bilirubin readings are not, on their own, a very reliable clinical tool, and investigation of plasma bilirubin should be the first priority.

(8) *Urobilinogen.* This is used in human medicine as a diagnostic aid for investigating liver disease. The test is of no value in veterinary medicine, and false positives and atypical colour changes on the strip are common. Note that a positive urobilinogen reading is often a sign that the test strips are *out of date!*

Protein/creatinine ratio

This measurement provides a more quantitative guide to whether sufficient protein is being lost in the urine to be consistent with a protein-losing nephropathy. It is derived by the formula

$$\text{Protein/creatinine ratio (g/mmol)} = \frac{\text{Urine protein concentration (g/l)}}{\text{Urine creatinine concentration (mmol/l)}}$$

Note the units, especially the creatinine units. Note also that reference values given in publications using gravimetric units (mainly US publications) will be different, as the unit used (which is often not stated) is g/g (see p. xv). Many authors quote about 0.1 g/mmol as the upper limit of 'normal', but relatively small increases are frequently caused by lower urinary tract disease (e.g. cystitis), and anything below 0.3 g/mmol is of relatively little diagnostic significance.

Protein losing nephropathy is associated with hypoalbuminaemia and urine protein/creatinine ratios of greater than 0.3–0.5 g/mmol – some cases, especially patients with renal amyloidosis, demonstrate very high ratios, sometimes as high as 3–4 g/mmol. The test is also used as a screen for hereditary nephritis in the Bull Terrier, a glomerular condition associated with marked proteinuria and progressive renal failure. The cut-off value chosen is 0.3 g/mmol, and dogs should be tested twice, samples being collected at least one month apart. It is difficult to predict that an apparently normal dog will not develop proteinuria subsequent to testing, but the finding of two normal results in a dog over two years old is regarded as reassuring.

Protein/creatinine ratio is not especially helpful in assessing other renal conditions, at least at a first opinion presentation, due to interference from protein originating elsewhere in the urinogenital tract. In addition, chronic interstitial nephritis, the commonest cause of renal failure in the dog and cat, is not usually associated with appreciable proteinuria.

Urine sediment examination

This is a simple technique to perform on fresh urine (see p. 304) and a number of different things can be recognized. Its greatest use is probably in the recognition of the cells (red blood cells, white blood cells and epithelial cells) typical of urinary tract infections of different types and severity. Recognition of crystal morphology can be useful in conjunction with calculus analysis in cases of urolithiasis. Identification of tumour cells is however the province of the specialist cytology or histopathology laboratory.

Faeces

Biochemical analysis of faeces is of relatively small importance in diagnostic work, but two or three tests are, or have been, of use in specific situations.

Occult blood

Where haemorrhage into the gastrointestinal tract is suspected, it is important to be able to demonstrate the presence of blood or altered blood in the faeces. Frank blood is, of course, easy to recognize when bleeding is into the lower part of the intestine, but blood in the stomach or small intestine will be digested and appear in the faeces only as a black colour (melaena), or not even that in mild cases. A number of impregnated paper type tests are available to detect this. Ensure that the test used is applicable to animals (i.e. not specific for human haemoglobin only), and beware of false positives due to haemoglobin in meat contained in the diet (a meat-free diet should be fed for 3 days before testing), or to ingested blood resulting from the patient licking a bleeding wound or swallowing blood from a bleeding nose or mouth.

Trypsin

When trypsin production by the pancreas is normal the enzyme is quite easy to detect in the faeces. The usual method used is the X-ray film digestion test, and the ability of the faeces to clear the film at dilutions of 1:80/1:160 or above indicates that a normal amount of trypsin is present. This generally rules out exocrine pancreatic insufficiency. However, note that many faecal samples of dogs with normal exocrine pancreatic function still fail to digest the film, especially when diarrhoea is present, and so the absence of digestion is not definitely diagnostic. In the past the procedure was to repeat the test at weekly intervals and to presume a positive diagnosis after three samples showed no evidence of trypsin. Now, however, it is usually more convenient to proceed to plasma enzyme testing (IRT) after one faecal sample has proved negative (see p. 144).

Undigested food elements

Striated muscle fibres, starch granules and fat globules can all be visualized microscopically on an iodine-stained wet preparation of faeces. The finding of significant amounts of any or all of these in canine faeces is a good indicator of exocrine pancreatic insufficiency, particularly when the X-ray film digestion test is also abnormal. However, note that striated muscle fibres are normal in cat faeces.

Peritoneal and pleural fluids

Whenever ascitic or thoracic fluid is detected, a sample of the fluid should be drained off for identification. Note that these fluids should always be collected into *plain* sterile tubes (sterile universal bottles are ideal). Such fluids are in no danger of clotting in the way that a blood sample will clot, and no anticoagulant is necessary. EDTA does *not* preserve cells; it is used for haematology samples because it is the anticoagulant which will *least damage* the cells, and if it is present in a fluid sample it will simply make some of the essential tests (especially protein estimation) impossible to carry out. It also kills bacteria making the sample useless for bacteriological culture.

Some nine different types of fluid may be encountered in the abdominal cavity, each of which has its own characteristic composition. One of the most informative pieces of information is simply the gross appearance of the fluid, and it should be standard practice to make a note of this when the sample is collected. In addition, any variation in the appearance of the fluid during collection should be noted – for example, a fluid may be clear when first aspirated, but blood may appear subsequently. This is usually due to nicking a blood vessel during sampling, whereas a sample which runs uniformly bloodstained throughout collection is more likely to be representative of the true appearance of the fluid.

True transudate

This fluid forms as a result of severe hypoproteinaemia – the resulting low osmotic pressure is insufficient to retain plasma water in circulation and it accumulates in the peritoneal and pleural cavities. Oedema may also be present – in general large animals tend to form oedema while small animals (especially dogs) become ascitic.

Physical appearance. Clear, colourless and non-viscous; may look just like tap water. There is no change on centrifugation and little or no frothing when shaken.
Total protein. Less than 5 g/l, with negligible albumin.
Total white cell count. Less than 1×10^9/l.
Cytology. Often no cells at all, or a very few mesothelial cells.

There is often fluid present in both the chest and the abdomen. Plasma albumin (and usually total protein) will be low, and as the two likely causes are nephrotic syndrome or protein-losing enteropathy, there is likely to be either marked proteinuria (urine protein/creatinine ratio greater than 0.3 g/mmol) or obvious diarrhoea.

Modified transudate

This fluid forms as a result of impaired circulation.

Physical appearance. Clear, perhaps slightly viscous, and either colourless or very slightly yellow-tinged. There may be small fibrin clots and occasionally it may be slightly milky. There is no change on centrifugation, but the fluid will froth when shaken.
Total protein. Around 20–40 g/l, about half of which will be albumin.
Total white cell count. Less than 1×10^9/l.
Cytology. A few mesothelial cells, possibly a very few erythrocytes also, and the occasional neutrophil or lymphocyte.

The two likely causes of a modified transudate are congestive heart failure and liver disease. When the cause is cardiac, fluid tends to accumulate in both the chest and the abdomen, and there may also be oedema. Very occasionally, acute congestive heart failure produces a bloodstained modified transudate due to leakage of erythrocytes from a congested spleen. Plasma urea and creatinine concentrations may show a pre-renal pattern, and albumin is usually normal. When the cause is hepatic, fluid tends to accumulate only in the abdomen, as impaired local circulation is the main precipitating factor. Plasma albumin may be low, and there will be other evidence of liver dysfunction, principally high serum bile acid concentration.

Pyothorax/septic peritonitis

This fluid (sometimes termed 'pseudochyle' due to its turbid appearance) is essentially pus, due to bacterial infection of the pleural or peritoneal cavity. However, note that like all accumulations of pus, it is quite frequently sterile on bacteriological culture due to the large numbers of neutrophils present.

Physical appearance. Opaque, turbid, usually creamy or beige-coloured, occasionally somewhat bloodstained, and often slightly viscous. On centrifugation there is usually a large amount of beige sediment and a more translucent supernatant. The fluid may have an unpleasant septic smell.
Total protein. Around 60–100 g/l, but it may be impossible to measure accurately due to the turbid nature of the sample.
Total white cell count. Over 20×10^9/l, often considerably higher.
Cytology. Almost all cells are degenerating neutrophils.

Haematology usually demonstrates a marked neutrophilia, and the patient may be pyrexic.

Neoplastic effusion

This fluid forms because the vascular bed associated with an abdominal or thoracic neoplasm is allowing leakage into the body cavity.

Physical appearance. Bloodstained pink or orange, or the fluid may resemble frank blood (though if a PCV is performed on the sample it is usually less than 0.05). Sometimes it is slightly milky or turbid. It is important to distinguish a genuinely bloodstained fluid from blood introduced at sampling; however, this can usually be appreciated when the sample is collected. Over 80% of visibly bloodstained fluids are neoplastic effusions (the rest being very bloody pyothorax/septic ascites, due to trauma, or very occasionally to acute congestive heart failure). On centrifugation there will be an appreciable erythrocyte button, but the supernatant usually remains pink as the cells will be partially haemolysed.
Total protein. Around 20–40 g/l, about half of which will be albumin.

Total white cell count. Less than 5×10^9/l, except for thymic lymphosarcomas, when it may be around $30–50 \times 10^9$/l.

Cytology. With one exception, neoplastic effusions in the chest or abdomen do not contain characteristic tumour cells. Instead the cytology shows erythrocytes, but is otherwise quite similar to a modified transudate. The exception is the thymic lymphosarcoma of the cat, in which large numbers of lymphocytes, often appreciably atypical, may be seen along with the erythrocytes.

There is likely to be clinical and/or radiological evidence of tumour activity in the abdominal or thoracic cavity, and in the case of abdominal neoplasia the pattern of blood results described on p. 225 may also be seen. A cat with a thymic lymphosarcoma is likely to be FeLV positive.

Blood

Although this is distinguished from the bloodstained effusions, the cause of frank blood in a body cavity is also often neoplastic, in that a blood-filled neoplasm (e.g. a haemangiosarcoma) has ruptured. Alternatively, the cause may be traumatic (e.g. road accident or gunshot wound) or post-surgical bleeding.

Physical appearance. Looks like blood! On centrifugation there is a *large* erythrocyte button and the supernatant will look like plasma which may be slightly haemolysed. The PCV of the sample will be around 0.20–0.50. (Although fluid is reabsorbed from the body cavities faster than erythrocytes, there is usually some clot formation which reduces the PCV of the aspirated sample.)

Total protein. This cannot be measured on the sample as such, but protein concentrations of the supernatant will be similar to those of plasma.

Total white cell count. Perhaps around 10×10^9/l – similar to that of whole blood.

Cytology. This will look just like a blood film, and if the haemorrhage was very recent there will usually be platelets present.

Unless the haemorrhage was *extremely* recent the patient will be anaemic, and depending on the source of the haemorrhage there may be evidence of damage to organs such as the liver.

Urine

There are two explanations for collecting urine from an abdominal tap – one is a ruptured bladder; the other is inadvertently putting the needle into a full bladder when attempting to sample ascitic fluid, thus performing an accidental cystocentesis.

Physical appearance. Clear non-viscous fluid, usually slightly yellow. No change on centrifugation, and if shaken it will not froth.

Total protein. Very low, less than 1 g/l.

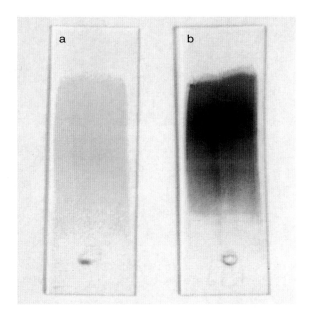

Plate 1 Well made blood films.
(a) Unstained; (b) stained.

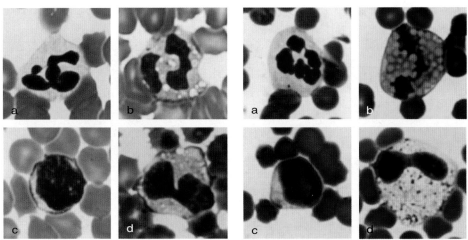

Plate 2 Dog blood: some normal white cells.
(a) Neutrophil; (b) eosinophil; (c) lymphocyte;
(d) monocyte.

Plate 3 Horse blood: some normal white cells,
(a) Neutrophil; (b) eosinophil; (c) lymphocyte;
(d) basophil.

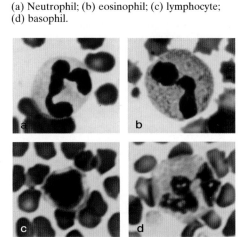

Plate 4 Cat blood: some normal white cells.
(a) Neutrophil; (b) eosinophil; (c) lymphocyte;
(d) basophil.

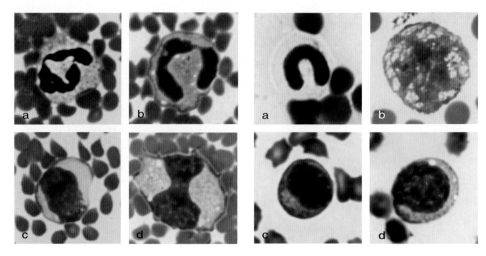

Plate 5 Goat blood: some normal white cells.
(a) Neutrophil; (b) eosinophil; (c) large
lymphocyte; (d) monocyte.

Plate 6 Dog: some abnormal white cells.
(a) Band neutrophil; (b) basket cell (degenerate);
(c) reactive (antibody-producing) lymphocyte;
(d) prolymphocyte (large, vacuolated cytoplasm,
necleolus).

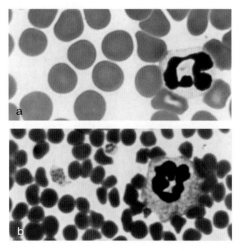

Plate 7 Normal red cells. (a) Canine; (b) caprine,
each with a neutrophil for size comparison.
(b) also shows very prominent platelets.

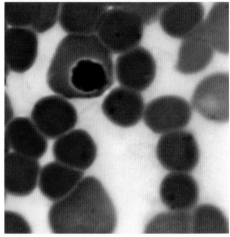

Plate 8 Regenerative anaemia (dog). Note
polychromatophilic macrocytes and nucleated
red cell.

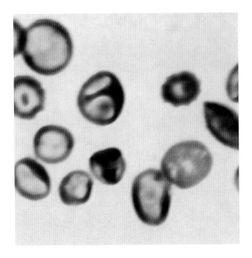

Plate 9 Chronic haemorrhagic anaemia (dog). red cells are regenerative (polychromatophilic) but also very hypochromic with leptocoytes and microcytes.

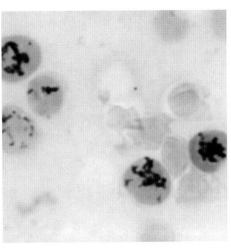

Plate 10 New methylene blue vital stain for reticuloctye counting. Reticuloctyes show up with dark blue inclusions.

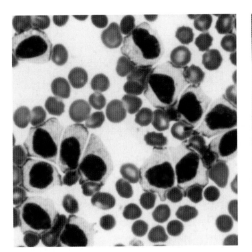

Plate 11 Leukaemia (dog), low power view. Enormous numbers of atypical neoplastic lymphocytes dominate the film.

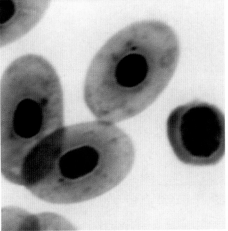

Plate 12 Reptile (tortoise) blood – both erythrocytes and platelets (right) are nucleated.

Total white cell count. Less than 1×10^9/l.

Cytology. Often no cells at all, or a very few mesothelial or epithelial cells.

Note that these characteristics are very similar to those of a true transudate – on these standard tests the only appreciable difference is the colour of the sample, and even that might not be immediately obvious. The sample *may* smell of urine, but again this is easily overlooked. It is vitally important not to mis-identify urine (however it got there) as a transudate; therefore any ascitic fluid with a very low total protein concentration which is not *absolutely* colourless should have creatinine measured as routine. Usually this is unambiguous (the highest possible ECF creatinine concentration is about 2000 μmol/l, while even very dilute urine starts about 3 mmol/l (3000 μmol/l). However, if there is any doubt (and doubt is more likely if urea is measured instead of creatinine, as very high ECF concentrations and very low urine concentrations might overlap), plasma urea and creatinine should be measured. If the fluid is a transudate (ECF), fluid concentrations will be essentially identical to plasma concentra-tions (and if the concentration is high, then a renal problem must be present), while if the fluid is urine, concentrations will be appreciably higher than plasma concentrations.

If urine is found on a peritoneal tap, it is essential to re-examine the patient for evidence of an intact bladder. If an intact bladder is definitely present, then the sample must have come from an inadvertent cystocentesis, and a further attempt to sample the ascitic fluid is necessary. Otherwise, proceed as for a presumed ruptured bladder.

Chyle

This may appear in either the chest or the abdomen, but almost never both together.

Physical appearance. White, opaque, non-viscous or only slightly viscous – occasionally there may be slight blood-staining; this is more likely with thoracic samples due to the difficulty of entirely excluding blood when performing a thoracocentesis. There is no change with centrifugation, other than any erythrocytes present forming a button leaving the supernatant less blood-stained.

Total protein. It is impossible to measure this accurately due to the colour of the sample – if attempted it may seem very high, but this is likely to be an artefact.

Total white cell count. Around 5–20 $\times$ 10^9/l.

Cytology. Almost all the cells are normal lymphocytes.

The main opportunity for misidentification here is between a chylothorax and a mediastinal lymphosarcoma, though the cytology (normal lymphocytes in chyle, atypical ones in a lymphosarcoma) and the presence of less blood in a chyle sample should help to differentiate. On occasion, a slightly chylous modified transudate may also cause some difficulty. If in doubt, a crude but effective 'chyle test' can be helpful.

Chyle test

Mix sample with ether in 1:1 proportions (this should be done carefully in a fume cupboard or other well ventilated place). If the turbidity in the sample clears, the sample is chyle (this almost never happens). If the resulting mixture is one homogeneous layer, the sample is not chyle. If the mixed sample forms two distinct layers, take a few drops of the upper layer, place them on a microscope slide, and allow the fluid to evaporate. If a white, waxy deposit forms on the slide, the fluid is chyle; if it does not, it isn't.

Bile

Neat bile escaping into the abdomen from a ruptured bile duct is rare. It is characterized by being opaque, non-viscous and almost black in colour – a greenish-yellow tinge can be seen at the side of the meniscus. If bilirubin is measured it will be extraordinarily high; however, it is necessary to dilute the sample considerably before attempting to assay it. Ascitic fluid which is simply bright yellow is not bile, it is usually a modified transudate from a jaundiced patient.

Feline infectious peritonitis (FIP) effusion

This may appear in the chest or the abdomen (more usually the latter), or occasionally both. It is quite distinctive, but its appearance does not always match the descriptions given in some publications. Most commonly, it looks exactly like a plasma sample – same colour, same consistency – it is not often bright yellow, and it often does not clot.

Physical appearance. Translucent, moderately viscous, straw-coloured or yellow – looks like plasma. May contain fibrin clots. No change on centrifugation.
Total protein. High, usually over 60 g/l, with a relatively low albumin concentration, often below 10 g/l.
Total white cell count. Less than 3×10^9/l.
Cytology. Mixed population of mesothelial and inflammatory cells.

Diagnosis of FIP is discussed in more detail on p. 192. The finding of the characteristic effusion is an important part of the diagnostic decision, and in the right circumstances (i.e. the young pedigree cat) it may be considered virtually pathognomonic. However, it is important to take all relevant information into consideration, and in particular to bear in mind that a very similar fluid may be found in cats suffering from lymphocytic cholangitis.

Cerebro-spinal fluid

The CSF is essentially an ultrafiltrate of plasma. It is normally crystal-clear, colourless and non-viscous. Both biochemical and cytological examination can be helpful in the investigation of CNS disorders. The cytology can be quite labile, and it is advantageous to be able to examine the fluid, at least to a first approximation, in the practice side-room. However, a sample in a plain tube transported as quickly as possible to the laboratory will still provide useful information. The addition of 10% (v/v) of the patient's own serum to the sample has recently been advocated to improve cellular preservation, but if this is done, note that any sample so treated will be useless for anything *other* than cytology, and so a separate untreated aliquot must be preserved for the other tests. Some publications have suggested the addition of a drop of formalin to the fluid for the same purpose, but this does more harm than good. A small sample of fluid in a fluoride tube *in addition* to the plain tube is also helpful for glucose estimation. However, if sample volume is limited, it is better to send what is available in a single plain tube than to mess around with several aliquots and different additives.

Total white cell count. A total white cell count may be performed on undiluted CSF in a standard haemocytometer slide. Normal CSF has less than 8/µl, and frequently no cells at all are seen. Where there has been blood contamination of the sample the white cell count is meaningless – formulae to allow for this contamination by comparing red and white cell numbers in CSF and blood are pure wishful thinking.

Cytology. This may be investigated on a dried smear, but gentle centrifugation may be necessary to concentrate the cells if the count is below 200/µl. Cells seen are generally neutrophils, lymphocytes or macrophages.

Colour. Normal CSF is crystal clear. A yellow colour (xanthochromic) is a consequence of red blood cells being broken down, while turbid CSF occurs in a number of conditions. If the sample is turbid it may be necessary to centrifuge it to appreciate xanthochromia. (Jaundiced patients may also have yellow CSF.)

Total protein. Normal CSF protein concentration is very low, under 0.25 g/l. Levels as low as this cannot be accurately measured by methods designed for plasma protein measurement (including the refractometer), and specialist laboratory methods (such as Coomassie brilliant blue or trichloroacetic acid) are employed. However, the protein block on a urine dipstick may be used for an approximate assessment, as it is also sensitive at very low concentrations.

Glucose. Glucose is usually similar in concentration to plasma glucose, or slightly lower.

Enzymes. CK, AST and LDH have all been measured and may be of diagnostic use. Enzymes do not normally cross the blood–brain barrier and so elevated CSF levels suggest tissue damage in the CNS.

Inflammatory conditions

Total cell count and protein are invariably significantly increased. In bacterial infections neutrophils are the predominant cell, CSF glucose concentration is extremely low and the fluid is usually turbid. In viral infections mononuclear cells predominate, glucose is normal and CSF AST may be elevated. Toxoplasmosis and cryptococcosis are both usually associated with xanthochromic CSF.

Neoplastic conditions

Total protein is nearly always elevated while the cell count is usually normal (so-called 'albuminocytological dissociation') – tumour cells only rarely escape into the CSF. Occasionally the fluid is slightly turbid or xanthochromic.

Degenerative conditions

CSF is usually normal in this type of abnormality.

Traumatic damage

Sub-arachnoid haemorrhage is associated with increased protein and moderately increased cell count (mostly neutrophils), and particularly with markedly xanthochromic CSF. However, if the haemorrhage is very recent (less than 48 hours old), actual blood may be evident. This is difficult to distinguish from blood contamination at sampling, except that in the latter case the sample usually runs progressively clearer during collection.

Hydrocephalus

Associated with increased CSF CK and LDH activities.

13

Feline Virus Testing

The immunology of virus disease is an enormous subject outwith the scope of this book; however, two or three of the common feline virus tests have found their way into the routine testing repertoire and have thus become part of standard profiling in many practices.

Feline leukaemia virus (FeLV)

In contrast to most virus testing, routine FeLV tests do not detect antibody to the virus, but detect a part of the virus itself, known as the p27 antigen. This is enormously helpful when investigating cats which have been vaccinated against FeLV, as vaccination does not interfere with the test.

After a cat acquires the infection there is an intervening period of about 8 weeks before a positive result can be expected to any routine test. Some cats do mount an effective immune response and eliminate the virus over the following weeks; therefore whenever a positive result is obtained in a healthy individual (no matter how reliable the test), it is always wise to retest in about 3 months. Cats which are still positive at this stage are usually permanently infected. Nevertheless, the incubation period for FeLV is both long and variable. While many cats succumb to the disease in the months following infection, and the majority are dead within 2 years, there are recorded cases of cats being persistently FeLV positive but clinically healthy for as much as 8 or 9 years before going down with classic signs of FeLV-related disease.

While the vast majority of FeLV-infected cats show up positive to at least one (usually all) of the tests available, it is known that a few cats remain stubbornly negative to every blood test known to science, probably because the virus is confined to the haemopoietic tissue. The exact incidence of this 'latent infection' is obviously difficult to ascertain, but thankfully it appears to be uncommon. Infection can usually be proved by immunofluorescence assay (IFA) examination of bone marrow or spleen impression smears.

ELISA tests for FeLV

These come in two forms, the read-by-eye CITE tests designed for practice side-room use, and plate ELISA methods which require a photometric plate reader used by professional laboratories. The performance of both types of test is similar, though as one might expect the plate reader used by the laboratory technician tends to be more standardized than reading by eye.

There has been a great deal of confusion surrounding the reliability of these tests and some entirely preposterous statements have been made, particularly regarding the reliability of a negative result. It is therefore worth taking the time to try to understand what is meant by sensitivity and specificity, and what effect these performance indicators have on the reliability of negative or positive results, respectively. At the end of the day it can be seen that the correct approach is one of simple common sense; nevertheless, certain essentially fallacious arguments have gained such wide acceptance that it is helpful to understand what is being said even if only to be able to refute it with confidence.

Sensitivity is a measure of reliability of negative results: 100% sensitivity means that no infected animals test negative; therefore a negative result is always indicative of freedom from infection.

Specificity is a measure of reliability of positive results: 100% specificity means that no uninfected animals test positive; therefore a positive result always identifies an infected individual.

In the real world, however, test performance tends to be something of a trade-off between these two attributes. Improvements in sensitivity tend to result in more false positives occurring, and attempts to eliminate false positives tend to lead to more infected animals being missed. A well-thought-out test will generally have somewhat better sensitivity than specificity, because it is preferable to have to check some unexpected positives than to be constantly in doubt about the validity of a negative result. However, it is rare to find any test with either sensitivity or specificity of 100%, never mind both.

In general, commercial kits tend to have sensitivity/specificity figures of around 97–99%, which is not bad, but at the same time not necessarily as good as it might sound. Bear in mind that a specificity of 98% means that one in fifty uninfected animals will give a false positive result, while a sensitivity of 98% means that one in fifty genuinely infected animals will be missed. It is always a good idea to translate any percentages quoted into this format, as it allows a much clearer idea of reliability (98% may be a splendid result in an exam, but it is not necessarily all that stunning in terms of test sensitivity or specificity). Anything below about 95% (that is, one in twenty animals giving the wrong result) is probably not worth having, as the amount of doubt generated means that you are probably better off not doing the test at all.

A great deal has been written and said (much of it nonsense) about how the reliability of a result 'depends on the prevalence of infection in the population', and goes on to 'prove' that 'a negative result is therefore highly reliable, even if the sensitivity of the test is not so good'. This, however, is a complete contradiction in terms, a bit like 'proving' that black is white. The fallacy in the arguments is that they are based on the assumption that all the animals being tested are clinically healthy and have no known history of exposure to FeLV, i.e. they are exclusively considering the mass screening of well cats either for breeding purposes or pre-vaccination. In this situation, so the story goes, only (say) about 1% of cats tested will be infected. If only one in fifty of that 1% then appears as a false negative (98% sensitivity), only 0.02% of total tests performed (one in 5000) will be a false negative. Or to put it another way, nearly 99.98% of all the negative results you get will be correct. Say that fast enough, and it almost sounds like 100%. Even if the sensitivity of the test drops as low as 90% (that is one in ten infected animals being missed, a very bad performance), by this calculation 99.89% of all negative results obtained will still be correct, therefore 'a negative result is still highly reliable, even if the sensitivity of the test is not so good'. It is worth pointing out at this stage that even if the test has a sensitivity of *zero*, i.e. it always reports a negative result for every sample regardless, in this scenario 99% of the results will still be right (Fig. 13.1)! In fact, all this piece of striking illogic is saying is that if you get a negative result in a healthy cat with no specific history of FeLV exposure, it is probably right – or even more crudely, when almost all the cats you test are negative, almost all your negative results will be right, even if you are only guessing. Quite so.

The same argument can be (and is) used to suggest that all positive results are highly unreliable and should never be accepted at face value. Under the same conditions, with test *specificity* at 98%, 1.98% of total tests performed will be false positives, and no less than 66.7% of all the positive results you get will be incorrect. If the specificity of the tests drops to only 90%, then a staggering 91.7% of all the positive results will be wrong. This is because the very few genuinely infected cats are vastly outnumbered by all the false positives piling up in the uninfected majority. However, once more all this bandying of figures is saying is that if you get a positive result in a healthy cat with no specific history of FeLV exposure, there is a pretty good chance that it is a false positive.

This is perhaps easier to follow from Fig. 13.2. This illustrates graphically how the percentage of positive or negative results which are correct varies according to the likelihood of the patient being infected. If you consider the screening situation, where healthy cats with no known history of exposure to FeLV are being tested, then the probability that a cat is infected is indeed equal to the incidence of infection in the general population from which the cat comes – possibly only 1% or even lower. Thus (again at 98% sensitivity) two-thirds of all positive results will be false, but virtually all of the negative results will be right. Even at the 95% sensitivity level the line is still almost indistinguishable from the 100% mark up to about 10–15% prevalence, and even at the worst, it is difficult to imagine a 'population' (in the geographical sense) with much more than a 10% infection rate. Thus by this logic, even where FeLV is rife, a negative result is still almost 100% reliable, and it is impossible to imagine

New! Cutting-edge technology!
Statistically proven!

THE

NEG-TEST™

Over 99.5% of all negative results
guaranteed correct!*

NEVER produces a false positive!

Simple and inexpensive!

Method: Simply take the Neg-Test™ ballpoint pen provided, find the cat's clinical record,
   and write the words "FeLV negative". That's it. No need to take a blood sample, no
   messy reagents, no fiddly timing, no laboratory skill required.

Change to the Neg-Test™
in your practice today!

* Statistics only valid when the prevalence of infection in the population being tested is less than 0.5%

Fig. 13.1   Reliability of a test with 0% sensitivity when testing clinically well animals in an
area of low prevalence.

a situation where this is not so, even if the test is known to miss as many as one
in 20 infected cats. This is the logic which has been used for many years to
bolster the assertion that negative FeLV ELISA results are essentially infallible.

However, this logic breaks down completely the moment you move away
from screening entire healthy populations to testing sick cats for diagnostic
purposes – exactly the way the test is used in most practices. When dealing

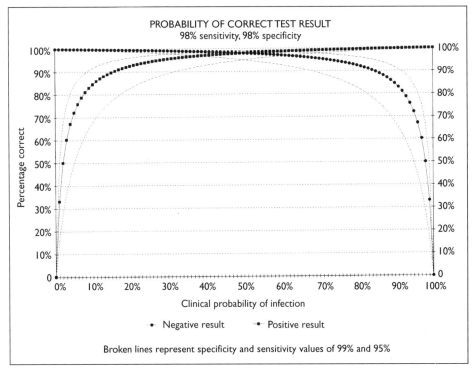

PROBABILITY OF CORRECT TEST RESULT
98% sensitivity, 98% specificity

Clinical probability of infection

• Negative result   •— Positive result

Broken lines represent specificity and sensitivity values of 99% and 95%

Fig. 13.2   Variation in reliability of a test result with sensitivity, specificity and the clinical probability of infection (or incidence of infection in the 'population' being tested).

with a sick cat it is essential to remember that so far as the x-axis represents the incidence of infection in a population, that population has to be *representative of the cat in question*. In the case of a cat with known exposure to FeLV which presents with signs suggestive of FeLV-related disease, the population to be considered consists, of course, of cats with known exposure to FeLV presenting with signs suggestive of FeLV-related disease. In other words, the x-axis represents the probability (clinical and as regards known exposure) that the cat in question is infected. Looked at in this way, it can be seen that the right-hand area of the graph is just as important as the left-hand one, and is the area to bear in mind when the clinical probability of infection is high. Here, of course, the opposite situation applies. *Positive* results are close to 100% reliable, while *negative* results have a fair chance of being wrong.

Thus, in fact, the figure merely demonstrates statistically what clinicians generally know instinctively. It is not simply wishful thinking to declare that you will believe the result if it is what you expected and doubt it if it is not. When dealing with a test which is not entirely 100% reliable either way, it is indeed the unexpected result which is likely to be the error. False positives occur in uninfected animals, and most uninfected animals are well; false negative results occur in infected animals, and most infected animals are sick. Therefore, rather than demanding that all positives be checked no matter how clinically likely the result is, and insisting that all negatives *must* be right irrespective of whether the cat has gross lymphocytic leukaemia and a known FeLV-positive mother (and the test is known to miss about one in ten infected cats), it is much more rational to follow common sense and check any result you find clinically surprising. Certainly, if sensitivity or specificity (as appropriate) are better than 98%, even the relatively unexpected result should be taken seriously. Nevertheless (and this is true for any test with less than 100% sensitivity and/or specificity), it should be viewed as part of the general pattern-recognition process rather than as a diagnosis set in stone.

The IFA test for FeLV

To be able to state the sensitivity and specificity of a test such as the ELISA, it is necessary to have some sort of 'gold standard' test which is regarded as giving the correct answer to run the comparison. In the USA and continental Europe the indirect immunofluorescence assay (IFA) is used for this purpose, as studies have shown a very close agreement between this test and virus isolation. It is also the test of choice in these countries for checking doubtful results obtained from in-practice ELISA/CITE kit tests. The test is also used for routine diagnostic purposes as it is actually somewhat cheaper and quicker than running a plate ELISA. It is, however, impossible to adapt for in-practice use as it requires both specialist laboratory equipment and considerable technical experience.

The IFA test is carried out on patient blood smears. The fluorescent-labelled anti-p27 antibody adheres to any viral p27 protein in the neutrophils and platelets, and positive samples show a very clear pattern of fluorescence when viewed under a fluorescent microscope. Ideally, a blood smear made from newly collected blood with no anticoagulant is used, which is yet another reason for acquiring and maintaining skill in making good blood smears. However, the test can be carried out on smears made in the laboratory from blood in anticoagulant, and in spite of assertions that this can interfere with the result, this does not appear to be a significant problem at the practical level – certainly much less so than the false positive and false negative rates of the ELISA method. (If you are concerned by this point, EDTA has been said to cause false positives and heparin to cause false negatives – but the easy way round it is simply to submit well-made, fresh smears instead.)

The IFA method has another useful attribute. In newly exposed cats, in the period before the infection becomes established, it can be seen that less than 100% of the cells on the blood film are fluorescing. If such cats are checked regularly over the following weeks one of two things happens. In cats which are mounting an effective immune response and eliminating the virus, the proportion of cells fluorescing gradually drops off until the result is negative, while in cats which are destined to become persistently infected, the proportion of fluorescing cells increases until the result becomes 100% positive. Therefore with this test it is possible to distinguish the transient from the persistent infection. Any result with greater than 90% of cells fluorescing may be regarded as indicating persistent infection, while cats with a lower proportion of fluorescing cells should be retested in about 3 months to verify whether they have progressed to this state or have eliminated the infection.

Virus isolation

This test is also generally very reliable, but it is a highly specialized procedure requiring cell culture facilities and is only available through centres specializing in research into FeLV. It also takes 1–2 weeks to get a result by this method. Nevertheless, it has been the recommended method in the UK for checking doubtful results from ELISA/CITE kits.

A positive result by virus isolation is a true 'gold standard' – if the virus can be grown from the sample, that cat is infected beyond any doubt. The position with negative results is slightly less clear-cut. While again the method is reported to agree very well with IFA results, there is anecdotal evidence that the virus can be difficult to recover from certain samples and that occasional false negative results can occur. Once again, the common-sense approach to Fig. 13.2 should be adopted. A cat with clinical signs suggestive of FeLV-related disease and which is positive for p27 antigen (especially by the IFA method) is probably infected, and this probability should not be discounted simply because one serum sample from the cat failed to grow virus in tissue culture.

Pre-vaccination testing for FeLV

Testing any cat for FeLV solely because it has been presented for vaccination is a *bad idea*, no matter what it may say on the vaccine box. In particular, testing it by ELISA or CITE is a *bad idea*, again no matter what it may say on the box.

(1)   Vaccination of an FeLV-infected cat is not harmful. There is no evidence that it is of any benefit either, but it will not adversely affect the cat in any way.

(2)   If a clinically healthy cat is found to be FeLV positive, there is absolutely nothing you can do about it. There is no known way of preventing the cat from eventually developing FeLV-related illness, or of prolonging the period before this happens. All that a positive result can achieve is to cause the owners unnecessary distress, perhaps years before their pet becomes ill.

(3)   FeLV is not foot-and-mouth disease, and there is no national test-and-remove scheme in operation. Owners who request a vaccination for their cats should not find that they have unwittingly entered their pets in an *ad hoc* local eradication programme.

(4)   No vaccine can be guaranteed to be 100% protective to all individuals, and the efficacy of the FeLV vaccines in this respect is lower than (for example) parvovirus or canine distemper vaccines. To imply that a

negative test result before vaccination guarantees that the cat will never become infected is misleading.

(5)   When using the ELISA/CITE method to screen clinically healthy cats, at least half the positive results you get will be false positives, probably more (see Fig. 13.2 above).

A number of questions tend to come up in the context of pre-vaccination testing.

Vaccinating an infected cat is a waste of the client's money, so isn't it better to check first?

The amount of money 'wasted' in vaccinating the very small percentage of healthy cats which are infected with FeLV pales into insignificance beside the enormous cost of testing the more than 99% of cats which are uninfected. It is unreasonable to expect the majority to take on this extra expense in order to save the minority a bit of money. Indeed, once the cost of the test is considered, and the cost of checking the unexpected result if an ELISA method has been used, the owner of the FeLV positive cat will usually end up paying just as much money as if the vaccination had simply been given in the first place. In addition, the combined price of the test-and-vaccine package can be enough to completely deter some clients from having their pets vaccinated against FeLV, which is counterproductive. One also has to consider the amount of distress caused by a positive result. If this proves to be a false positive or a cat which happens to have been tested while it was in the process of eliminating the infection then all that is for nothing, and the owner may well be aggrieved at having to pay for the testing and follow-up. Even if it is a true positive there is nothing which can be done to help the cat, and most owners would probably prefer simply to pay for the vaccine and continue in blissful ignorance until the cat actually becomes ill.

But if we don't test, we'll never know how effective the vaccine really is

It is the responsibility of the vaccine manufacturers to conduct (and pay for) clinical efficacy trials.

Am I not protecting myself by advising that the test is done?

No. Possibly even the reverse. There are a number of reasons for a cat which has tested FeLV negative subsequently succumbing to the disease after vaccination:

(1)   False negative result. Uncommon, but only because healthy FeLV-positive cats are fairly uncommon. A recent study has shown that in-practice FeLV tests miss between one in 3 and one in 12 infected animals.

(2)   Cat tested less than 8 weeks after becoming infected. It takes about 8 weeks before an infected cat will give a positive result.

(3) Latent infection. A small proportion of infected cats do not give a positive result on any test, probably because the virus is confined to the bone marrow.

(4) Vaccine breakdown. No vaccine can be guaranteed to provide 100% protection in all individuals; some will simply fail to mount an immune response.

However, it could be argued that by advising the test, you are in some way implying that once a negative result has been demonstrated protection from infection can be guaranteed. The best way to protect yourself is simply to explain to clients that the vaccine offered is the best that is available and is efficacious in most cases, but that nothing can be 100% guaranteed. This in fact applies to all vaccinations, not just FeLV.

I give the client the choice and leave it up to them

This is unfair. It is the responsibility of the veterinary surgeon to advise what tests are necessary. If a test is clinically advisable, you should recommend it. If it is not, then 'leaving it up to the client' can come unpleasantly close to moral blackmail. The problem is that even the mention of the test can be enough to set many pet owners worrying about what the result might be, worry which can only be set at rest by doing the test, no matter how improbable it is that their cat is infected. In some cases owners who have heard that a test is involved may even decide against presenting their pets for vaccination out of an almost irrational fear of the result.

But what about the risk of infection to other cats?

Bear in mind that it was not normal practice to test healthy pet cats routinely for FeLV before the vaccines were available. There is arguably even less reason to do so now, when the 'other cats' at hypothetical risk also have the option of being vaccinated.

The fact is that the best way to eliminate FeLV infection from the feline population is to vaccinate as many cats as possible, no questions asked. Pre-vaccination testing puts up quite unnecessary barriers to this goal, some financial, some psychological, and offers no benefit to either the cats or their owners.

Pre-mating testing for FeLV

This is a requirement of most pedigree studs, and one which needs to be adhered to even if the cats in question are vaccinated. It is still possible for a vaccinated cat to acquire FeLV infection, and it is foolhardy to allow any outsider into a known FeLV-free cattery without testing.

Some studs insist on 24-hour testing, that is a negative test from a sample taken less than 24 hours before entry into the cattery, but this is something of an over-reaction. A negative result cannot *entirely* guarantee that a cat is uninfected; apart from anything else there is the 8-week period after acquiring the infection to consider. Therefore insistence on 24-hour testing, which often necessitates the use of in-practice ELISA/CITE kits, is probably unnecessary, and a negative result within the past week by a more reliable method such as the IFA may, in fact, be a more satisfactory solution.

Pre-homing testing for FeLV

The incidence of FeLV is highest among stray and feral cats, and there is enough trouble in the world without adopting it. The cat rescue centre is one situation where a policy of test-and-remove has some merit. A homeless FeLV-positive cat is arguably best put to sleep (or at least moved to an isolation colony) before it infects anyone else, and it is unfair to put a cat like that up for adoption when there are always more needy cats than there are homes available. However, for best effect the test should be carried out on admission to the rescue centre, before the cat is allowed to mix with the other residents and definitely before it has been picked out by a potential new owner. Once the owner has bonded with the cat it is really too late to test, and cats newly acquired from rescue centres are arguably best vaccinated without asking too many questions.

Feline immunodeficiency virus (FIV)

Routine FIV tests look for antibody to the virus, not the virus itself. Nevertheless, a positive result does correlate with actual infection, as it appears that cats do not mount an effective immune response to this virus and once acquired it is not eliminated. The pathology of the virus is similar to that of HIV in that it destroys the immune system and affected cats succumb to conditions which would be comparatively trivial in an uninfected animal.

However, the latent or incubation period for FIV can be even longer than that of FeLV, and there are many reports of confirmed antibody-positive cats living normal lives for 10 years or more with no indication of impaired immune competence. As this is an infection which is more often acquired in adult life (entire toms with a fighting record are the top incidence group, as the main route of spread is by biting), it is not especially unusual for an FIV-positive cat to live an apparently normal lifespan and eventually die of one of the common diseases of old age. Therefore owners should be discouraged from thinking of FIV as a sort of analogue of human AIDS, and dire prognoses should only be given on clinical grounds, not simply on the basis of a positive test result.

The sorts of specialist lymphocyte function tests which are used to monitor immune function in HIV-positive individuals are not generally available for cats. The most obvious pointer to FIV-related disease in routine haematology is a marked and persistent neutropenia, though it should always be borne in mind that there are other causes of neutropenia (endotoxin exposure and other viruses such as feline infectious enteritis (FIE), for example), and that some cats with clear clinical evidence of impaired immune competence do not have abnormally low neutrophil counts.

ELISA tests for FIV

Again these tests are available in two forms, the plate ELISA for use in the professional laboratory and the read-by-eye CITE kit for in-practice use. Performance of the two types of ELISA is again similar, with the plate reader producing more standardized results.

Exactly the same arguments regarding specificity and sensitivity, and the reliability of positive or negative results in different circumstances that are presented for FeLV, apply to FIV, though they have been much less talked about in this context. However, in practice false positive results seem to be unusual, and the suspicion at least of a false negative occurs comparatively frequently. Follow-up testing of suspect negatives by a more sensitive method such as IFA or Western blotting will certainly demonstrate at least some of these cats to be genuinely positive, but there remains a suspicion that some FIV-infected cats simply do not produce detectable antibody. Estimates of the incidence of these infected negatives range up to 10% of infected cats or even more, but it is difficult to be sure just how well this relates to the field situation.

The IFA test for FIV

Like the FeLV IFA, the comparable method for FIV is used as a 'gold standard' to check doubtful results from ELISA/CITE methods, but it is also quick enough and cheap enough to be used for routine diagnostic screening. However, the requirement for a fluorescent microscope and a high degree of technical skill means that it cannot be adapted for practice side-room use. Because it is detecting antibody rather than antigen, this test works on slightly different principles from the FeLV IFA. Pre-prepared slides coated with feline kidney cells infected with FIV are used. Patient serum is then applied, and the presence of antibody binding to the cells is demonstrated by fluorescent marker. Because this method uses whole virus rather than the two or three antigens employed by the ELISA methods it is more sensitive than the ELISA, and results correlate extremely well with 'research' methods such as Western blotting. Nevertheless, if a cat is producing no antibody to the virus, then no antibody test will be able to pick it up.

Pre-breeding testing for FIV

Any circumstance where cats which are strangers to each other are introduced is a potential FIV hazard, especially if entire toms are involved. Feline mating in itself often involves some biting, and it is entirely possible that FIV may be sexually transmitted in a similar way to HIV. It is therefore simple common sense to insist on a negative FIV test as well as FeLV as a prerequisite for admission to a pedigree stud, and stud toms and resident queens themselves ought to be tested at regular intervals. Once again it is preferable to test by the more sensitive IFA rather than relying on an in-practice CITE kit, as minimizing false negatives is more important than having a result *right now*. Breeders should be warned that a negative result for either virus cannot entirely guarantee freedom from infection; nevertheless, it is better to take what precautions one can rather than leave the door wide open by omitting to test.

Pre-homing testing for FIV

This is more of a grey area than for FeLV. Some FIV-positive cats live normal lives for many years, and when a cat is neutered and living in harmony in its own home, transmission to other cats seems to be fairly uncommon. Therefore it is not entirely unreasonable to expect a potential new owner to be prepared to take on such a cat. Nevertheless, it is preferable that the potential owner *knows* what he or she is taking on. In addition, given the potentially explosive feline sociodynamics in some rescue catteries, it is unwise to introduce new individuals without testing for FIV first. Thus routine testing before admission to such a cattery can be considered good practice. However, bear in mind that in kittens born to FIV-positive mothers, maternally derived antibody may be a problem – and not all such kittens are in fact infected with the virus. Any kitten testing FIV positive should be retested at 6 months of age.

Pre-vaccination testing for FIV

There is no vaccine available for FIV. However, many in-practice CITE kits present FeLV and FIV tests as a single package, and as a result some practices do both tests at once as a pre-FeLV vaccination screen. This is completely pointless, and a positive result can achieve nothing but to alarm the owner.

Feline infectious peritonitis (FIP)

Unlike FeLV tests, 'routine' FIP tests detect antibody to the virus rather than the virus itself. And unlike FIV infection, cats exposed to FIP infection can and frequently do produce protective antibody. Thus a positive test result to this virus merely indicates exposure, and does not prove either that the cat has clinical FIP or that it will develop clinical FIP in the future. Even more disconcerting, the time-course of antibody levels in clinical FIP somewhat resembles a bell curve. Many infected cats do die while antibody levels are still high, but in the later stages of disease measurable antibody can actually decrease, possibly because it is becoming bound up in immune complexes, and it is not uncommon for moribund FIP cases to produce a negative result at this stage. It is therefore unwise to regard the FIP test in the same way as (with appropriate caveats) the other two can be regarded, i.e. as producing a meaningful positive or negative result. Testing for FIP antibody should therefore be confined to situations where there is already reasonable cause for suspicion that a diagnosis of clinical FIP is on the cards, and it should not be included in routine screening profiles.

To understand the interpretation of FIP antibody tests it is necessary to understand the epizootiology of the condition and its most common means of transmission. The main reservoir of FIP virus is in multi-cat breeding households, i.e. pedigree cat breeders, and infection rates among non-pedigrees are very much lower than among pedigrees. Although it is something of a taboo subject, the fact is that the majority of pedigree breeding households have enzootic FIP in the premises. In these households most cats have antibody, some higher levels, some lower, but this is protective antibody and the adult residents seldom develop clinical FIP. However, up to about 5% of kittens emerging from such a household will present with clinical FIP in adolescence or young adulthood – the earliest age of presentation is about 4 months, the peak age is around 10 months, and cases are rare over the age of 2 years. The effect of this disease pattern is to cause many breeders to be unaware that they have a problem. Many deaths from FIP occurring in 1-year-old cats are not reported back to the breeder, and even if they are there is an understandable tendency to declare that the infection must have been picked up after the kitten was sold.

After the age of about 2 or 3 years clinical FIP is much less common, and the incidence seems to go on declining with age. Middle-aged cats with FIP are just as likely to be non-pedigree as pedigree, and it seems likely that these cases represent unprotected cats who have had the misfortune to encounter the virus in the field as adults and failed to mount an effective immune response. However, great caution should be exercised when diagnosing FIP in cats over the age of 3 years. The classic low albumin/high globulin plasma protein pattern associated with FIP is quite easily mimicked by inflammation of other kinds, in particular by gingivitis/stomatitis. This is comparatively unusual in young cats, which makes these protein results a good pointer to possible FIP at that age. However, in middle-aged and older cats gingivitis is common, and a knee-jerk reaction associating raised globulins with FIP infection can be very dangerous in this situation, especially if the cat happens to have some antibody present. Electrophoresis can provide some extra help in differentiating between FIP-related hyperglobulinaemia and non-specific chronic inflammatory reactions in older cats (see p. 76).

There have been suggestions of a second, lower peak of FIP incidence in the elderly cat, but it appears that this is not the case – clinical FIP is rare in old cats. However, the low albumin/high globulin plasma protein pattern is extremely common at this age as a result of stomatitis, and some of these cats will, of course, prove to have FIP antibody due to a long-standing immunity, so it is easy to be misled. Again a diagnosis of dry FIP should be made with extreme caution, and based on more than simply plasma protein and FIP antibody results.

'Enteric coronavirus'

A second coronavirus affecting cats has been postulated, the so-called 'enteric coronavirus'. This was held to explain the presence of FIP (coronavirus) antibody in households where there was no apparent history of clinical FIP, and was associated with a comparatively mild, non-lethal enteric condition. However, mounting evidence points to the two viruses being essentially one and the same thing, with some differences in virulence and individual susceptibility to disease, the latter being the more important factor. Households where the enteric form of FIP is present have a tendency to acquire cases of effusive FIP sooner or later, and the two conditions are so closely interlinked that whether one labels the virus or the antibody as 'FIP' or 'feline coronavirus' seems largely academic.

FIP tests

A number of different methods have been employed, but once again IFA techniques seem to be the most favoured. It is important to ensure that the result reported is either an antibody titre or something (like an optical density ratio) which can be related to an antibody titre, simple positive/negative results are inadequate.

Side-room FIP kits

A CITE kit for FIP does exist, but it is not recommended and should be avoided. Misreading of the result is common because the test is based on a descending reaction rather than the ascending reaction of the FeLV and FIV kits; even if properly read the simplistic positive/negative readout is inadequate, and results appear to correlate poorly with laboratory reference methods.

Interpretation of FIP results

Diagnosis of FIP is another of the classic pattern recognition situations, and in fact the FIP antibody level is arguably one of the less important factors in the decision-making process. It must always be borne in mind that healthy cats can have antibody to FIP – therefore so can cats with cat 'flu or any other minor ailment – and that some cats terminally ill with FIP have no detectable antibody in either blood or ascitic fluid. Nevertheless, having said that, it is still the case that the classic clinical FIP cat will usually have a high antibody titre (1:640 or above, often greater than 1:10 240), while the unaffected cat will usually be antibody negative, so the test does form a useful *part* of the diagnostic investigation.

An approach to diagnosis based on a 'rule of three' has been found to be useful. Three aspects of the case are examined: clinical signs, including the composition of any ascitic fluid; routine biochemistry and haematology results; and antibody level. Scoring is as follows:

(1)   Score 1 for classic 'wet FIP' signs, with a typical FIP composition to the ascitic fluid (globulin over about 60 g/l, albumin under about 10 g/l, see p. 178). In the absence of this classic pattern, score $\frac{1}{2}$ for a clinical picture somewhat suggestive of dry FIP, e.g. uveitis.

(2)   Score 1 for a classic FIP picture on biochemistry and haematology (see p. 235), especially globulin over about 70 g/l and albumin under about 20 g/l, but be careful to discount the effects of stomatitis when assessing this finding in older cats. Score $\frac{1}{2}$ for a pattern which is a bit suggestive but not really classic, e.g. raised globulins which are still less than 70 g/l.

(3)   Score 1 for a high antibody level of 1:640 or greater; score $\frac{1}{2}$ for a moderate antibody level of 1:40 to 1:320.

(4)   Add an extra $\frac{1}{2}$ point if the patient is a pedigree cat less than 2 years old which is actually ill.

If a cat scores two or more points, a diagnosis of FIP is reasonable. One point or less, and the diagnosis can reasonably be discounted. One-and-a-half points is inconclusive, and the best thing to do is to continue with symptomatic treatment and hope for the emergence of further evidence one way or the other. However, in practical terms the finding of classic wet-FIP ascitic fluid in a young pedigree cat is pretty much pathognomonic for the condition, and further testing is a bit academic.

'Virus shedders'

The source of trouble in enzootically infected households is thought to be adult cats which, while clinically well themselves, shed virulent virus which then infects susceptible kittens. Cats with higher antibody levels are statistically more likely to be virus shedders, but the relationship is not strong enough to allow accurate prediction in respect of an individual animal.

Testing for FIP virus

Since a positive antibody test for FIP cannot be specific for clinical FIP, it has been suggested that tests which actually identify part of the virus particle itself might be more useful for diagnostic purposes. However, it appears that cats with FIP antibody also test positive for the virus whether or not they are sick and whether or not they are virus shedders. Thus testing for the virus as such does not really yield much extra diagnostic information.

Pre-mating testing for FIP

This is a minefield. The only way to ensure that FIP is not introduced into an FIP-free household is to insist that all visiting cats are shown to be antibody negative. However, this may be found to limit the available gene pool within the breed quite substantially! A breeder considering adopting a policy of accepting only FIP-negative cats should be advised that all resident cats must be tested first, even if no recent cases of FIP associated with the stud are known. There is no point in shutting the stable door after that particular horse has bolted. They should also be advised that (although very few will admit to it in public) most breeders *do* have FIP in their catteries, and a positive result is not the equivalent of leprosy or the Black Death.

Owners of queens requesting an FIP test before visiting a stud should be advised in the first instance to ascertain whether the stud household is, in fact, known to be free from FIP. Amazingly enough, some breeders do demand certificates of freedom from FIP from visiting queens without having tested their own cats at all. If the status of the stud is unknown, then insisting that incoming cats be tested is pointless. If the stud is genuinely FIP-free then the request is, of course, justified. However, once again the owner of the cat to be tested should be advised about how common FIP antibody is in pedigree cats, and reassured that the only thing a positive result means is that the cat will not be able to visit that particular stud. It does *not* mean that the cat herself is going to develop clinical FIP, and there will be plenty of other studs which will be in no position to make any stipulations about FIP certificates before entry.

Eradication of FIP from an affected household is a difficult process, and probably impossible in the short to medium term. However, there is some evidence that the most dangerous period regarding infection may be around weaning, as protection from maternal antibody wanes, and that kittens which are never allowed to mix with the household in general and whose dams are not themselves virus shedders seldom seroconvert. Therefore it has been suggested that isolation of the queen and her litter from late pregnancy, with the kittens never mixing with other cats before sale, may be effective in minimizing the chance of the kittens contracting the disease. This may indeed be valuable as regards kittens going to pet homes, but kittens to be introduced to the same or another breeding colony must still be at risk. Nevertheless, the morbidity from FIP is low, most kittens emerging from enzootically infected FIP households do not develop the disease, and it is arguable that contracting FIP is just one of the hazards of being a pedigree kitten, a bit like being hit by a car. However, that is not much help when advising a breeder how much (or how little!) to tell prospective buyers.

Pre-homing testing for FIP

This is worth considering when buying a pedigree kitten, and is essential when introducing new stock into a known FIP-negative breeding cattery. However, as so many pedigree breeding households are enzootically infected with FIP, repeated disappointments are commonplace. The best prospect of acquiring an antibody-negative pedigree kitten may be to look for breeders who keep litters segregated from the other cats in the household, as described in the previous paragraph. The incidence of FIP in non-pedigree cats is relatively small, and testing kittens before rehoming is not usually considered necessary.

III
Systematic Investigation

14

Investigation on an Individual Organ Basis

Damage and/or dysfunction associated with certain organs or tissues (principally the kidneys, liver, pancreas and musculo-skeletal system) can affect quite a wide variety of biochemical constituents and aspects of metabolism. It is therefore helpful to have a checklist of the various analytes which might be relevant to these organs to assist with further investigation.

The kidneys

Renal damage

Actual damage to kidney tissue is impossible to detect from a blood sample as there are no typical increases in plasma activity of any specific enzymes. However, urinary enzyme analysis (especially γGT) can be helpful in identifying acute nephrotoxicity.

Renal dysfunction

Primary tests (most appropriate for initial diagnosis)

(1) *Urea.* Not entirely renal-specific, also increases with pre-renal effects.
(2) *Creatinine.* More renal-specific, little influence by pre-renal effects.
However, these analytes do not usually increase until more than about 60% of nephrons are dysfunctional, so they are not much of an early warning system.
(3) *Phosphate fractional excretion (clearance ratio)* is a crude guide to glomerular filtration rate which can be useful in earlier cases and as a prognostic guide.

Secondary tests (useful to assess severity and prognosis)

(1) *Phosphate.* High where secondary hyperparathyroidism is present.
(2) *PCV.* Non-regenerative anaemia may be present in chronic cases, and is often severe in young, growing animals.

(3)   *Potassium.* High in acute renal failure, but may be low in chronic cases, especially end-stage when accompanied by vomiting.

(4)   *Total carbon dioxide.* Low when acidosis is present.

Incidental findings

(1)   *Ammonia (and uric acid).* These analytes increase in parallel with urea.

(2)   *Calcium.* Usually low where secondary hyperparathyroidism is present. However, bear in mind that hypercalcaemia can *cause* renal dysfunction.

(3)   *ALP.* May be raised where secondary hyperparathyroidism is present.

(4)   *Amylase (and lipase).* One or both are sometimes raised due to interference with excretion.

(5)   *Total protein (and albumin).* May be raised if dehydration is present.

(6)   *Magnesium.* May be raised.

Protein-losing nephropathy

Primary tests

(1)   *Albumin.* Inevitably low, will be very low if actual nephrotic syndrome (oedema/ascites) is present.

(2)   *Urine protein/creatinine ratio.* Inevitably high if renal loss is the cause of the hypoalbuminaemia.

Secondary tests

(1)   *Urea.*   } Both analytes *may* be elevated, but often not by much, and in
(2)   *Creatinine.* } some cases both may be normal.

Incidental findings

(1)   *Calcium.* Inevitably low when significant hypoalbuminaemia is present.

The liver

It is often very easy to conclude from the biochemistry findings that a liver problem is present. It may also be possible to characterize this problem to some extent, especially as regards chronicity and which aspects of hepatic metabolism are affected. Nevertheless, it can often be extremely difficult to translate these findings into an aetiological diagnosis, and although it may be possible to make an intelligent guess, definitive aetiological diagnosis is usually only possible by means of a liver biopsy.

Liver damage

A number of different enzymes are released into the plasma when the liver is damaged; their usefulness varies from species to species.

(1)   *ALT.* Acute/medium-term damage, dogs and cats.

(2)   *SDH.* Acute damage, horses (and ruminants).

(3)   *GDH.* Acute damage, horses and ruminants.

(4)   *AST.* Acute/medium-term damage, most species (but not very liver-specific).

(5)   *γGT.* More chronic damage, large animals (little use in small animals).

(6)   *ALP.* Moderate rises in acute/medium-term damage in all species, but not very liver-specific. Very marked increases accompany biliary obstruction.

(7)   *LDH.* Very non-specific, little diagnostic usefulness.

Liver dysfunction

This is not necessarily accompanied by the enzyme changes typical of liver damage, as dysfunction may occur without actual cellular disruption, and more chronic cases of liver failure may have little hepatic tissue left to release enzymes into the circulation.

The liver has many different functions, and it is unusual for all of them to be affected equally. Often one or more functions may be severely deficient while others may be virtually unaffected, depending on the actual pathology involved and the chronicity of the condition.

(1)   *Albumin.* Low when synthetic ability is impaired. However, half-life is quite long; therefore hypoalbuminaemia is only seen in long-standing conditions.

(2)   *Prothrombin time.* Low when synthetic ability is impaired. Half-life is shorter than albumin; nevertheless, again hypoprothrombinaemia is a feature of chronic conditions.

(3)   *Urea.* May be low if urea cycle is impaired, but this is not invariably the case.

(4)   *Ammonia.* Inevitably high if urea cycle is impaired.

(5)   *Bilirubin.* High if anion transport is impaired. May go very high very quickly in acute conditions. (See 'jaundice', below.)

(6)   *Bile acids (single test).* High if anion transport is impaired. Increases earlier than bilirubin in chronic conditions.

(7)   *Bile acids (dynamic test).* Excessive increase seen post-prandially when a portosystemic shunt is present.

(8)   *Cholesterol (non-specific finding).* Sometimes elevated, but may be depressed in severe chronic liver dysfunction.

(9)   *ALP.* Very high (over 10 000 iu/l) if biliary obstruction is present.

Jaundice (hyperbilirubinaemia)

Separation of bilirubin into conjugated/unconjugated (direct/indirect) fractions is usually a complete waste of time. However, the basic cause of the jaundice – haemolytic (sometimes referred to as 'pre-hepatic'), hepatic, or bile duct obstruction (sometimes referred to as 'post-hepatic') – is usually fairly easy to determine by other means.

Haemolytic disease

The patient will inevitably be anaemic! The anaemia is usually regenerative and not hypochromic. Plasma bilirubin is usually only slightly/moderately elevated, and very marked glow-in-the-dark jaundice probably has some other explanation. Liver enzymes will be normal (except in copper poisoning).

Hepatic disease

Hepatic parenchymal enzymes (ALT, SDH, GDH, depending on the species) and ALP (γGT in large animals) will be elevated in parallel. In small animals ALT activity is often extremely high (1000–4000 iu/l) while ALP activity is only moderately elevated (1000–4000 iu/l). Occasionally in certain chronic liver conditions there may be no change in liver enzymes, but the hepatic aetiology is demonstrated by other signs of liver dysfunction (such as hypoalbuminaemia) and the absence of any evidence of either haemolysis or biliary tract obstruction. In hepatic lipidosis, especially in the anorectic cat, normal liver enzymes may be accompanied by surprisingly marked jaundice; mild/moderate hypoalbuminaemia is also evident in some cases.

Biliary tract obstruction

In an extra-hepatic obstruction the hepatic parenchymal enzymes will be normal or only slightly increased, while ALP activity is extremely high (10 000–50 000 iu/l). Where the obstruction is intra-hepatic the results will also reflect the hepatic disease, and the parenchymal enzymes may also be relatively high.

The pancreas

Pancreatic damage

Note that acute pancreatitis is not described in herbivores, and that in the cat none of the plasma enzymes commonly used in human or canine medicine is reliable for investigating the condition. The laboratory approach, in effect, only applies to the dog, and where pancreatitis is suspected in a cat then other diagnostic methods (such as ultrasound) should be adopted.

Primary tests

(1)   *Amylase.* Usually very high relatively early in the disease process.
(2)   *Lipase.* Increases more slowly but remains elevated for longer.

Secondary tests

(1)   *Calcium.* Some cases of pancreatitis are significantly hypocalcaemic.

Incidental findings

(1)   *ALT.*
(2)   *ALP.*   } All three will be increased if there is concurrent hepatitis.
(3)   *Bilirubin.*
The pancreas is so close to the liver that a degree of hepatitis is almost inevitable when severe pancreatitis is present. However, it is usually clear which is the primary condition by the relative severity of the changes.
(4)   *IRT.* This will also be high, but it offers no particular diagnostic benefit over amylase and lipase (and takes a great deal longer to measure).

Exocrine pancreatic dysfunction

Once again this applies almost exclusively to the dog. The condition is not described in herbivores, and it is *extremely* rare in the cat.

Primary tests

(1)   *IRT.* Will be low.
(2)   *Faecal trypsin and demonstration of undigested food elements.* Trypsin will be low or absent, and fat globules, starch granules and muscle fibres will be seen in the faeces. However, this investigation is best reserved as part of a faecal screen (including microbiology) for diarrhoeic dogs, and it should not be the sole basis for a diagnosis of exocrine pancreatic insufficiency. If the suspicion arises, IRT should always be assessed.

Secondary findings

(1)   *Albumin.* Low in severe, long-standing cases.
(2)   *Prothrombin time.* Prolonged in severe cases due to vitamin K deficiency (secondary to fat malabsorption).

Incidental findings

(1)   *Calcium.* Low if albumin is low.
(2)   *Urea.* May be low due to protein malabsorption.
(3)   *Cholesterol.* May be low.

Endocrine pancreatic dysfunction (diabetes mellitus)

Primary tests

(1)   *Glucose.* See p. 116 for detailed interpretation.
(2)   *Urine glucose.* Will be positive if plasma glucose has exceeded the renal glucose threshold in the period before collection.
(3)   *Fructosamine.* High if hyperglycaemia has persisted for more than a few days.

Secondary tests

(1)   *β-Hydroxybutyrate.* High if patient is ketotic.
(2)   *Urine ketones.* Positive if patient is ketotic.
(3)   *Cholesterol.* Almost invariably elevated in diabetes mellitus.
(4)   *ALT and ALP.* Elevated when hepatic lipidosis is present.

Incidental findings

(1)   *Neutrophilia.* Often present in association with the hepatic changes.

Endocrine pancreatic neoplasia (insulinoma)

Note that this condition is almost exclusively confined to the dog. Glucagonoma has also been described, but that is extremely rare in comparison to insulinoma.

Primary tests

(1)   *Glucose.* Low, usually below 3.0 mmol/l, but suspect if below 3.5 mmol/l in the presence of suspicious clinical signs.
(2)   *Insulin.* Must not be interpreted in isolation; it is essential to measure insulin/glucose ratio on a *fasted* sample (see p. 165).

Incidental findings

Surprisingly few – even amylase and lipase tend to be normal.

The small intestine

Intestinal damage

The only enzyme which increases in intestinal damage is the ubiquitous and non-specific ALP. In the horse a specific assay for the intestinal isoenzyme is available, but in other species the finding of a raised total ALP can only be associated with the intestine by elimination and guesswork.

Intestinal dysfunction (malabsorption)

Note that while animals with malabsorption frequently have abnormal faecal consistency, not every patient presenting with diarrhoea is a malabsorption case. For simple diarrhoea the appropriate initial investigation is faecal microbiology to identify pathogens or (more commonly) deranged bowel flora, and absorption tests should be reserved for chronically sick animals showing real signs of malabsorption (especially weight loss).

Primary tests

(1)   *Fat absorption (small animals)*. Abnormal where malabsorption is present for any reason.
(2)   *Glucose absorption (horses)*. 'Flat curve' when malabsorption is present.

Secondary tests

(1)   *Folic acid*. May be low due to chronic poor absorption.
(2)   *Vitamin B_{12}*. Also may be low due to chronic poor absorption.
(3)   *PCV*. Anaemia may occur secondary to folate and/or B_{12} deficiency.
(4)   *Prothrombin time*. May be prolonged due to malabsorption of vitamin K.

Incidental findings

(1)   *Albumin*. May be low.
(2)   *Calcium*. Will be low if albumin is low.
(3)   *Urea*. May be low.
(4)   *Cholesterol*. Often low.

The musculo-skeletal system

Bone damage

The primary enzyme affected by bone disease is (once again) ALP, which is present in high concentrations in osteoblasts. High plasma ALP is therefore associated with osteoblastic activity, that is the laying down of new bone, rather than bone destruction. Thus an elevation in this enzyme is normal in young animals while the growth plates are still open. Conditions involving substantial bone remodelling, such as osteoblastic osteosarcoma, osteitis, and even healing fractures, can be associated with particularly marked increases. Nevertheless, even where bone destruction is extensive (e.g. secondary hyperparathyroidism, metastatic carcinoma) the dynamic nature of the process may again lead to elevations in plasma ALP activity. However, bone lysis alone, without new bone formation, will not produce any change in ALP activity.

No routine method is available for differentiating the bone isoenzyme of

ALP, and diagnosis generally relies on the pattern recognition approach described in Chapter 15.

Muscle damage

The three enzymes commonly used to assess muscle damage demonstrate different time-courses with respect to the initial injury (Fig. 14.1). Really spectacular increases are confined to conditions where there is generalized, or at least very extensive, muscle damage, such as rhabdomyolysis (horses and dogs), muscular dystrophy (cattle) and iliac thrombosis (cats). However, lesser or more localized damage (injury, recumbency – especially in heavy individuals – and eosinophilic myositis) can also produce elevations in enzyme activity.

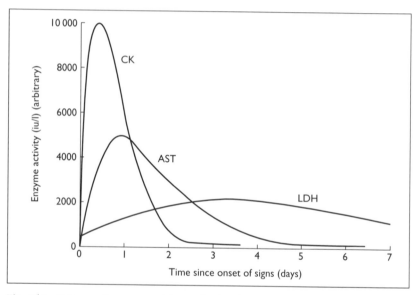

Fig. 14.1 Patterns of enzyme activity in the first few days following an uncomplicated episode of rhabdomyolysis.

(1) *CK*. This increases very quickly to very high levels, and in the absence of continuing injury can return to normal in less than 48 hours.
(2) *AST*. Very high levels reached 12–24 hours after initial injury, returning to normal in less than a week.
(3) *LDH*. High levels peak several days after initial injury; return to normal takes several weeks.

All these enzymes will remain elevated for longer periods if injury is recurrent or there is continuing damage.

Note that ALT, though it is usually seen as a 'liver' enzyme in small animals, will behave in a very similar way to AST in response to muscle damage in large animals, and will also increase quite appreciably in small animals with severe muscle damage. Therefore, if rhabdomyolysis or iliac thrombosis is obviously present, there is no need to postulate liver pathology as well, simply on the basis of an elevated ALT.

Muscle dysfunction

This is generally a consequence of mineral or electrolyte deficiency.

(1) *Potassium.* Hypokalaemia is associated with severe weakness. Common in elderly cats, also seen in farm animals; sometimes a cause of prolonged recumbency.

(2) *Calcium.* Hypocalcaemia is associated with trembling, hyperaesthesia and tetany, particularly in association with late pregnancy/lactation or compromise to parathyroid gland during thyroidectomy, but can be idiopathic in dogs.

(3) *Phosphate.* Hypophosphataemia is a relatively common cause of prolonged recumbency in cattle.

(4) *Magnesium.* Hypomagnesaemia is associated with violent tetany.

(5) *Selenium/vitamin E.* Deficiency is associated with chronic wasting, muscular dystrophy, 'white muscle disease' in cattle and sheep. Investigated by measuring erythrocyte glutathione peroxidase.

15 Diagnostic Profiling and Pattern Recognition

The concept of pattern recognition

A simplistic approach to interpretation of laboratory results sometimes seeks to identify one test with one condition or organ system, and run through a report on a one-to-one correspondence – urea is the kidney test, ALT is the liver test, and so on. It should be perfectly obvious by now, though, that matters just aren't that simple – and this is very fortunate.

If it were a simple matter of one test relating to one condition, then a panel of, say, six tests, would only be able to confirm or deny six conditions. However, if one considers the report in terms of pattern recognition, it becomes clear that the potential is much greater. Even if each of the six analytes is considered as having only three possible results (normal, high or low), this gives a total of 729 different combinations (3^6). For ten analytes, there would be 59 049 combinations (3^{10}), and if five possible results rather than three were allowed for (very low, low, normal, high and very high), this would increase to 9 765 625 combinations (5^{10}). Naturally this is not the number of different diagnoses which can actually be made – some combinations of results (low urea and high creatinine for example) will be impossible, some will be duplicates, while others will be uninformative. Nevertheless, this does illustrate the huge potential for information coding inherent in even a fairly restricted number of tests when considered as a pattern rather than as individual results.

Pattern recognition is a difficult thing to teach, but it is not difficult to learn. It is one of the things the human brain does best. Attempts to teach computers to recognize faces have been fraught with difficulty and largely unsuccessful, but even young babies readily recognize familiar faces without any formal instruction – even from strange angles or wearing silly hats. This is the reason why attempts to derive a computer program to interpret laboratory data have been generally unhelpful – approaching the problem in terms of algorithms, while it can be extremely constructive, does not entirely reproduce the way the human mind works.

Nevertheless, some consideration of the algorithmic approach is useful. Algorithms, or decision trees, are the art and science of knowing not only which questions to ask, but also the order in which to ask them. It is important to know that a pale animal is actually anaemic before looking for specific causes of anaemia, or that an ascitic animal is actually hypoalbuminaemic before looking at possible routes of protein loss. Whole pyramids of algorithms may be built to codify procedure in all sorts of situations, and some texts present extremely helpful sets of these. The approach is particularly useful in difficult cases, where a condition may not have been encountered before, or where an obvious pattern does not emerge. A structured, logical approach which considers all possible causes of each observed abnormality in turn and then pursues each one relentlessly until the problem is solved is really the basis of the scientific method.

However, this laborious process of deduction soon becomes unconscious, and with some experience the mind is able to skip the detail of the algorithms and go straight to the answer, or probable answer. This is the basis of pattern recognition – once the 'typical' presentation of a particular condition is encountered and recognized, subsequent cases are compared to this pattern. As more and more patterns are recognized, and more and more variations on the 'classic' pattern are encountered, interpretive skill increases – much like learning to recognize the faces of a wide range of acquaintances, no matter what hairstyle, or lighting, or angle of view may be involved.

Approach to test requesting

All algorithms begin, not with a laboratory abnormality, but with a clinical one – a presenting sign. There is always a reason for carrying out an investigation, even if it is as slim as an apparently groundless owner worry. More often, of course, there is a specific clinical complaint such as polydipsia or weight loss.

The next stage is, of course, a full history-taking and clinical examination, which are essential before considering further investigation of any kind – laboratory, radiological or whatever. The information from this purely clinical stage is the next part of the pattern to be revealed. It may well be that the diagnosis is obvious already – the ability to do this reliably is what is commonly referred to as having 'good clinical skills', which itself is usually pattern recognition in action. When sufficient cases of a particular condition have been encountered, it becomes easier to recognize the next one.

Nevertheless, it makes sense to confirm even a strong suspicion where confirmation is reasonably quick and easy – sometimes appearances can be remarkably deceptive. And of course there are always cases where even the most comprehensive examination still leaves several possibilities open, or occasionally a nasty sinking feeling that this one may not fit easily into any neat little box. But by this stage you should have a provisional diagnosis, or a manageable list of differential diagnoses, or at the very least enough of an idea of the likely nature of the problem to allow a rational choice of further investigation.

Assuming that laboratory investigation appears to be the next step, the next question is, which tests to do? Adopting the strict algorithmic approach, asking for confirmation or denial of a single specific question before moving on to the next one, can create a number of problems – it can lengthen the time to diagnosis by introducing repeated delays while the next test on the decision tree is requested and carried out; it can vastly increase the costs of the investigation by missing out on standard laboratory profile prices; it can lead to secondary, intercurrent problems being missed because the net has not been cast widely enough; and it can sometimes result in misdiagnosis when a secondary condition is identified rather than the main problem.

On the other hand, requesting every test in the laboratory's repertoire is not necessarily very constructive either. Not only can it increase costs unacceptably, it can result in the main findings being almost lost in the midst of a lot of relatively unimportant detail, and a lot of time wasted trying to figure out the reasons for minor abnormalities in tests which really weren't indicated in the first place.

This is where tailored profiling or panel requesting comes into its own. An attempt is made to consider the range of conditions which might be raised by the finding of a particular presenting sign, in other words, the directions of as many of the branches of the appropriate algorithm as possible. Analytes are then chosen on the basis of their relevance to the investigation of these conditions. This has the advantage of allowing all the routine information likely to be needed to follow the appropriate decision tree to be delivered in one request, thus speeding up the investigation and frequently reducing costs. It also allows easy exploration of alternative arms of the tree, thus reducing the chance of an incidental finding being mistaken for the main condition, and the chance of an important secondary abnormality being missed.

It is at this point that logical exploration of the algorithm metamorphoses into pattern recognition. Choice of the right analytes, including all that might be relevant (even if only to rule out a remote possibility) but excluding irrelevant tests that might simply muddy the issue, allows optimum recognition of the patterns which emerge, and the findings can be compared to the 'classic' patterns for several possibilities to enable the best match to be selected.

The panels or profiles which emerge from this approach are radically different from the panels offered by many laboratories before the 1990s. These tended to be designed on an organ or system-based grouping – thus there was the 'kidney profile', the 'liver profile', and so on. The difficulty there is that unless you know already whether the problem is in the kidneys or the liver or wherever, it doesn't really help decide which one to choose. However, by the time you come to fill in your lab request form you should at least have a good idea what the main clinical presenting sign is, and if test groupings are offered on that basis, life becomes considerably simpler.

When interpreting the results, the main maxim is, look at the *whole* picture, take into account *all* the relevant information available, including clinical and behavioural findings. On occasion the clinical pathology patterns exhibited by two or even three different conditions can be very similar, but when the clinical information is added to the decision tree it is perfectly clear which one is actually involved. Sometimes the pattern of the results alone may look quite extraordinarily typical of a particular condition, but anyone looking at the patient can immediately see that that diagnosis is, in fact, out of the question. This is why clinical pathologists will not comment on requests submitted without a clinical history (or with no indication of the age of the patient) – it is far too easy to look a complete idiot when the conjurer whisks away the screen covering over the other half of the picture. Laboratory results don't exist in a vacuum – always consider them in the context of the patient itself.

Tailored diagnostic panels

Core panels

These are groups of tests of very general relevance, which give a wide (though not necessarily very deep) overview of the patient's metabolism. They arguably represent the minimum that should be requested if you are going to the trouble of taking a diagnostic blood sample at all, and are extremely useful for patients with vague presenting signs such as lethargy or weight loss, and for patients with signs that don't fit easily into one of the later categories (such as respiratory presentations).

Basic core panel – small animals

A definitive diagnosis may not always be possible from the panel given in Table 15.1, but the list of conditions of which, if present, it is reasonable to expect some suggestive abnormality to be evident, is fairly extensive and includes those given in Table 15.2.

Table 15.1   Basic core panel for small animals

Biochemistry	Haematology[a]
Total protein	PCV
Albumin	Haemoglobin
Globulin (calculated result)	Red cell count
Urea	MCV
Creatinine	MCHC
ALT	Total and differential white cell count
ALP	Blood film examination
Plus bilirubin if sample is visibly yellow	
[a] This is commonly termed 'full' or 'general series' haematology.	

Table 15.2   Conditions of small animals identifiable from the core panel[a]

Abdominal neoplasia
Acute or chronic blood loss
AIHA/autoimmune thrombocytopenia
Allergic reactions/parasitism
Blood parasites
Bone marrow aplasia
Circulatory problems (including congestive heart failure, Addison's disease and
   simple dehydration)
Cushing's disease
FeLV
FIP
FIV
Hepatitis
Hyperthyroidism
Infection/inflammation
Leukaemia
Liver failure
Nephrotic syndrome
Paraproteinaemia
Polycythaemia
Protein-losing enteropathy
Pyometra
Renal failure
Systemic mastocytosis
Viral conditions (such as canine parvovirus and feline panleucopenia (FIE))

[a] This list is far from exhaustive.

Basic core panels – horses

The only difference between the panel for the performance horse (Table 15.3) and that for the non-athlete horse or pony (Table 15.4) is that the choice of enzymes in the former is slanted towards the muscles, while in the latter it is slanted towards the liver.

There is little to be gained from checking creatinine routinely in the horse, as renal dysfunction is relatively rare – if it is indeed present; the urea will be enough to ring the alarm bell to trigger further investigation. It is always important to make a point of checking the plasma of all sick horses for visible lipaemia, so that hyperlipidaemia can be recognized and treated as early as possible.

The list of conditions which might be identified from Tables 15.3 and 15.4 is shorter than the equivalent small animal list (Table 15.2), merely because horses tend to suffer from fewer conditions identifiable by clinical pathology investigation. It includes those given in Table 15.5.

Table 15.3 Basic core panel for the performance horse

Biochemistry	Haematology
Total protein	PCV
Albumin	Haemoglobin
Globulin (calculated result)	Red cell count
Urea	MCV
CK	MCHC
AST	Total and differential white cell count
γGT	Blood film examination
Plus creatinine if urea is elevated	
Plus total glycerol if sample appears lipaemic	

Table 15.4 Basic core panel for the non-athlete horse or pony

Biochemistry	Haematology
Total protein	PCV
Albumin	Haemoglobin
Globulin (calculated result)	Red cell count
Urea	MCV
AST	MCHC
GDH	Total and differential white cell count
γGT	Blood film examination
Plus creatinine if urea is elevated	
Plus total glycerol if sample appears lipaemic	

Table 15.5 Conditions of horses identifiable from the core panels[a]

Anaemia (true anaemia is comparatively uncommon in horses)
Dehydration
Infection/sepsis
Muscle damage/rhabdomyolysis
Parasitism/allergies
Protein-losing enteropathy
Ragwort poisoning and other hepatopathies
Renal dysfunction (also uncommon in horses)
Viral infections/post-viral syndrome

[a] This list is not exhaustive.

Basic core panel – ruminants

The panel given in Table 15.6 is an analogue of the diagnostic panels for small animal and equine use, and will give pointers to the same general range of conditions. However, as so many ruminant investigations tend to relate to metabolic problems, often on a herd/flock basis, more specific panels focusing on particular metabolic areas are commonly employed. Examples of these are included on p. 217.

Table 15.6   Basic core panel for ruminants

Biochemistry	Haematology
Total protein	PCV
Albumin	Haemoglobin
Globulin (calculated result)	Red cell count
Urea	MCV
Creatinine	MCHC
GDH	Total and differential white cell count
γGT	Blood film examination

Expanded panels

These are the panels specifically tailored to particular presenting signs. They are formulated by adding to the core panel those routine tests which, while not really indicated in the absence of these signs, must be included whenever the clinical picture is suggestive. The ruminant panels are geared mainly to nutritional problems.

Polydipsia/polyuria panel (dogs and cats)

Add to basic panel (Table 15.1): calcium, glucose, cholesterol.

The calcium is included to avoid missing cases of primary hyperparathyroidism or pseudohyperparathyroidism. This is a relatively rare finding; nevertheless, it is important to bear it in mind. Significant hypercalcaemia causes polydipsia, so there is little point in routinely checking for this if no polydipsia is reported, but if it is omitted in polydipsic animals there is a risk of missing the hypercalcaemia and making a mistaken diagnosis of primary chronic renal dysfunction.

The glucose is included because the presence of polydipsia immediately raises the question of possible diabetes mellitus, and it can also add some information to the Cushing's pattern. Cholesterol is included to allow maximum appreciation of a possible Cushing's pattern.

Acute abdomen/vomiting panel (dogs)

Add to basic panel (Table 15.1): sodium, potassium, amylase, lipase (plus calcium if these two enzymes are high). Chloride and total carbon dioxide might also be included.

The sodium and potassium are included partly because appreciation of any electrolyte disturbances is important in a vomiting animal when fluid therapy is likely to be instituted, and partly because some cases of Addison's disease present mainly as vomiting.

The amylase and lipase are included to identify cases of acute pancreatitis (note that this approach is not appropriate for the investigation of suspected exocrine pancreatic insufficiency, which does not present as an acute abdomen and for which amylase and lipase are not useful diagnostic tests). The calcium is included when indicated because a proportion of dogs with acute pancreatitis develop hypocalcaemia as a complication.

Note that this panel is not appropriate for cats – not only does pancreatitis not present as an acute abdomen in that species, none of the 'pancreatic enzymes' used in dogs or man is at all reliable in the cat. The best non-invasive technique for investigating suspected pancreatitis in the cat is ultrasound.

Fits/faints/collapse panel (dogs and cats)

Add to basic panel (Table 15.1): sodium, potassium, calcium, glucose.

The sodium and potassium are included because Addison's disease in the dog often presents as weakness/collapse, and because idiopathic hypokalaemia is a common cause of the same presentation in the cat. The calcium is included because idiopathic hypoparathyroidism is a relatively unusual cause of collapse/ fits in the dog and hypocalcaemia occurs in the cat both post-thyroidectomy and in antifreeze poisoning. The glucose is included to identify hypoglycaemic collapse/fits. Other causes of fits such as uraemia/hyperammonaemia may be identified or suspected from the tests included in the core panel.

This panel is frequently used in patients presenting with neurological signs/ epileptiform fits, and where the cause of the problem is primarily neurological then the investigation may draw a complete blank (except, perhaps from an obvious stress pattern). Nevertheless, it is a valuable part of the routine, as it can be extraordinarily embarrassing to start a patient on anticonvulsants and then discover that the true cause of the fits is an insulinoma or hypocalcaemia.

Skin panel (suspected endocrine alopecia in the dog)

Add to basic panel (Table 15.1): cholesterol, CK, AST.

The cholesterol is included both to aid in the assessment of possible hypothyroidism, and to allow maximum appreciation of a possible Cushing's pattern. CK and AST are also reported to be increased in a proportion of hypothyroid dogs.

Further relevant information can be obtained from the tests in the core panel, for example pyoderma and hypersensitivity reactions are likely to be appreciable from the white cell picture.

Sick horse panel

Add to basic panels (Tables 15.3 and 15.4): creatinine, glucose, total glycerol, and include all relevant enzymes – CK, AST, ALP, GDH, γGT.

When a horse is really ill (as opposed to mildly off colour or simply not jumping high enough), it is prudent to assay total glycerol as routine to guard against hyperlipidaemia being missed on visual inspection of the sample. Glucose is included to help identify possible cases of equine Cushing's disease.

Energy metabolism (ruminants)

Glucose, β-hydroxybutyrate, free fatty acids, GDH and γGT (with or without full haematology).

Glucose *may* be reduced in the face of inadequate energy intake, as ruminant control of plasma glucose is less tight than in monogastrics, but normal levels do not prove that energy provision is adequate, particularly if there has been any excitement associated with sample collection. Raised β-hydroxybutyrate is a definite indication of carbohydrate deficiency, but this analyte usually remains normal until only a couple of days (or even a few hours) before the onset of clinical acetonaemia.

Increased plasma FFAs suggest increased mobilization of fat depots, thus again implying energy deficiency. However, adrenaline also promotes lipolysis, and so excitement at sampling may again influence the results. Liver enzymes are included to give some indication of fatty change in the liver, which often accompanies energy deficiency.

Protein metabolism (ruminants)

Total protein, albumin (globulin calculated), urea, PCV (with or without remainder of full haematology).

PCV, haemoglobin (and possibly MCHC) and albumin are usually reduced in protein deficiency. Total protein is not invariably reduced, as the globulin fraction may actually increase. Urea is usually quite markedly decreased, but where poor quality protein rather than an absolute deficiency is the problem, urea may actually increase.

Mineral panel (ruminants)

Sodium, potassium, calcium, magnesium, phosphate, copper, GSH-Px, CK (with or without full haematology).

Sodium and potassium are of no value when screening for a chronic or low-grade production problem, but can be helpful in the downer cow – hypokalaemia is a factor in a proportion of cases.

The other analytes, while also being relevant to the diagnosis of the individual downer cow, can also be of some help in the investigation of more chronic production issues. Calcium is under quite tight homeostatic control, and 'low normal' concentrations are normal in newly calved cows and in hypoalbuminaemic animals, but sometimes a problem is appreciable before clinical signs are evident. Plasma magnesium concentration falls gradually in chronic deficiency states and so a problem may be uncovered well before clinical disease occurs, but in acute deficiencies such as 'grass staggers' the fall is usually very precipitous. The paradoxical effects of parathyroid hormone on plasma phosphate concentration make investigation of dietary adequacy by this means fairly tricky, but low levels should probably be considered significant.

Low plasma copper concentrations in clinically normal cattle may be considered important because copper supplementation often improves productivity in these situations. Much the same is true of selenium, which is investigated by measuring GSH-Px. CK not only gives some measure of muscle damage in an acutely collapsed animal, it is often raised when a mineral deficiency has given rise to a low-grade myopathy – selenium is probably the prime example.

Other panels may be devised for particular circumstances (such as musculoskeletal conditions or chronic enteric signs), and a similar approach may be used to devise suitable panels for other species.

Screening panels

A different approach is required when tests are carried out not for the investigation of a definite clinical problem, but as a prophylactic routine in particular circumstances, in animals with no clinical signs. One of the first things for the clinician to consider is under what circumstances this sort of investigation is really appropriate.

Ruminant metabolic profiles

The term 'metabolic profile' is a very specific one, referring to the biochemical and haematological investigation of a selected group of cattle (usually clinically normal) from a dairy herd. It is incorrect to use the term to describe a diagnostic or individual screening panel. In a metabolic profile, mean results rather than individual ones are considered in a thorough statistical analysis of the findings to provide information about the 'metabolic' status of the herd.

The Compton Metabolic Profile test was first introduced in 1970, and was designed to provide an insight into the clinical status and performance of dairy herds by comparing a range of biochemical and haematological measurements from selected groups of animals in the herd with standard reference values. Twenty-one cows is the chosen number – seven dry cows, seven average milkers and seven maximum yield animals – and the original list of tests carried out was PCV, haemoglobin, total protein, albumin (globulin calculated), sodium, potassium, calcium, phosphate, magnesium, copper, iron, urea and glucose. Free fatty acids, β-hydroxybutyrate and other tests were added at a later date.

This approach contains some oddities: PCV and haemoglobin are treated as statistically independent variables (although they are essentially two ways of measuring the same thing); sodium and potassium are not analytes which could be considered to be indicative of metabolic or subclinical disease; and plasma iron is not usually considered to be of any value without a corresponding figure for total iron binding capacity, which is not included. However, the main problem the concept is up against is homeostasis. Many of the analytes are variables which are under fairly tight hormonal and metabolic control, with the very specific aim of maintaining the ECF (and thus the plasma) concentrations within 'normal' limits even in the face of sub-optimum nutrition or excessive metabolic stress. Thus for certain conditions (energy metabolism is a good example) there may be nothing to see in the metabolic profile until the problem is becoming critical. Conversely, problems with protein metabolism are more easy to appreciate because the relevant analytes are not under such tight control.

Since the 1970s dairy farming has come under increasing economic pressure, and in this climate the metabolic profile concept has not proven itself to be a really cost-effective management tool. In herds with no identifiable clinical problem, where the aim might be to identify either a potential production increase or a potential cost-saving by fine-tuning the nutrition, experience demonstrates that approaching the matter directly by means of feed analysis is likely to be more fruitful. Exact nutritional requirements have been characterized for farm animals in every conceivable management regime and stage of production, and looking directly at what is going in eliminates the problems posed by homeostatic control of ECF composition. If a specific clinical or production problem is being investigated, the choice of groups of animals at random and a wide range of analytes makes for a very blunt tool. This type of presentation is more suited to the traditional approach to diagnosis, with history-taking and clinical examination being used to derive a rational group of differential diagnoses which is then used to select the most appropriate further investigations (see p. 215). In addition, it is often most constructive to select the most severely affected individuals for testing, on the grounds that they are the ones most likely to be demonstrating diagnostically useful abnormalities.

When this type of investigation is being contemplated, the vital importance of analytical precision and accuracy must be appreciated. Side-room analysers are entirely unsuitable for this sort of work, and ideally the samples should be referred to a laboratory with a particular interest in the subject so that statistical comparisons with the reference values can be carried out by an experienced veterinary biochemist.

Fitness profiles

Since early man first made the fundamental discovery that one horse can run faster than another horse, an enormous amount of effort and ingenuity has been expended in trying to figure out which one is which. Naturally, in due course attention turned to analysis of the blood, particularly haematology. Early studies appeared to suggest that as a horse becomes fitter, the PCV increases. Unfortunately, later, better controlled experiments which eliminated the effects of the horses' anticipating having needles stuck in their necks, demonstrated that the changes observed were in fact due to increasing excitability/apprehension and consequent splenic contraction, not to athletic fitness as such. The next idea was that perhaps haemoglobin might be a better measurement – but of course PCV and haemoglobin are simply two ways of measuring exactly the same thing. The same applies to erythrocyte sedimentation rate – in the horse, this crude measurement is almost entirely a factor of the PCV.

Plasma enzymes seemed like a good idea. However, one suggestion that AST increases in the early part of training before falling again to stabilize as full fitness is achieved appeared to have more to do with a couple of horses in the small group under investigation being over-exerted in the early stages and suffering some muscle damage. Studies involving horses which suffered no muscle injury reveal no change in plasma enzymes during training.

One difficulty with haematological or biochemical investigations in the horse is that very small events can lead to very marked changes in certain analytes – more marked than may occur with strenuous exertion or even illness. In a healthy thoroughbred, the PCV can increase from 0.32 to 0.40, the plasma protein concentration from 77 to 88 g/l and the plasma AST activity from 170 to 250 iu/l, due to nothing more than starting to eat a feed of hay. The plasma potassium concentration may be 3.3 mmol/l after a period of box rest, but a few minutes later it may be 4.5 mmol/l, due solely to the horse having been pursued five times round the loosebox at a walk before the headcollar could be fitted. Studies which take care to eliminate all these little management effects, and the effects of excitement, apprehension, stress, injury or illness, demonstrate that there is no 'routine' blood analyte which varies at all with athletic fitness, or which is capable of distinguishing between a fast horse and a slow one.

This, of course, does not prevent trainers from insisting on 'having the bloods done', and investing in all sorts of patent nostrums to increase the 'blood count' – in spite of the fact that nutritional deficiency anaemia simply does not happen in well-cared-for horses on a good quality diet. Some training yards even boast their own haematology laboratories. If a client is of this mind there may be little point in arguing, but the best that can be said for the exercise is that (if the analytical procedures are reliable, which is not always the case) it may sometimes allow a mild viral infection to be identified in its early stages, or mild muscle damage to be spotted. It is, however, a good idea not to be swayed by information of this nature when visiting the bookmaker.

Pre-anaesthetic screening

It is instructive to consider the equivalent position in human medicine. Do anaesthetists or surgeons dealing with human patients (in the NHS or in private medicine) routinely request biochemistry or haematology analyses in well individuals scheduled for elective surgery? The answer is no. Neither the NHS nor the private health insurance companies regards this as clinically justifiable, and neither is prepared to fund such screening as an indiscriminate routine. In this situation it is incumbent on the veterinary surgeon to consider his position very carefully. Clients whose pets are due for an anaesthetic can often be vulnerable and anxious, and look to their vet to advise them disinterestedly. The inclusion of an option for 'routine' blood testing on all anaesthetic consent forms can come uncomfortably close to moral blackmail – once faced with the suggestion, the client may feel very guilty if he refuses to take up what appears to be a recommendation from the professional he is trusting with his pet's welfare. Bear in mind that there is absolutely no evidence that indiscriminate 'routine' pre-anaesthetic testing makes any difference whatsoever to the incidence of anaesthetic complications or deaths, and take care not to allow sales pitches for point-of-care analysers to drive what should be a medical decision.

That is not to deny that there are occasions where pre-anaesthetic investigation is genuinely indicated. The most common of these is the elderly dog or cat requiring dental treatment, and where there are features of the history or even the patient's demeanour which raise concerns about possible renal problems. However, the cardinal rule is to proceed according to the findings of the pre-anaesthetic history-taking and clinical examination, which should never be skimped. If something emerges which gives genuine cause for concern, then of course the recommendation that this should be followed up before proceeding with the surgery is reasonable. If not, then there is enough work around that needs doing without inventing it.

The question of 'defensive medicine' is sometimes raised in this context, but it seems inconceivable that a veterinary surgeon could be held to be negligent for failing to go well beyond what would be standard procedure in the equivalent situation in human medicine in the UK. Neglecting the pre-anaesthetic clinical examination and missing something which should have been picked up clinically is where the main danger of litigation lies.

If a pre-anaesthetic profile is considered necessary, which tests should be included? To a large extent this question answers itself – choose the profile which seems most appropriate with regard to the clinical reason for doing the screen. This often translates into the small animal core panel detailed on p. 212; however, it is not always quite that straightforward. For most of the analytes in that panel, an abnormality is either important enough to be acted upon (such as abnormal urea and creatinine), or incidental enough to be ignored (such as signs of infection in a patient already known to have gross stomatitis). However, the unexpected finding of abnormal liver enzymes – raised or even quite high ALT and/or ALP – can pose a real problem. Does this animal have a serious liver condition, perhaps a liver tumour, which is clinically inapparent? Or is this perhaps a relatively benign hepatopathy such as is known to occur in some elderly dogs? Having found the abnormality, what and how much follow-up investigation is now appropriate? How does this affect the original plan to carry out much-needed dental treatment? This is not an especially uncommon scenario, and there is no really easy answer. It is therefore worth considering whether inclusion of liver enzymes in this situation is appropriate. If you don't know what to do with the answer, maybe you shouldn't be asking the question.

Timing of pre-anaesthetic profiling is considered in more detail on p. 310. This is not an emergency investigation, and the use of point-of-care analysers is inappropriate. The aim should be to have the results available at least 24 hours before the scheduled time of surgery to allow due consideration of the implications and an unhurried change of plan if indicated.

Geriatric screening

The position with the elderly animal is similar to the pre-anaesthetic screen. There is absolutely no sign of the NHS calling up all senior citizens for a 'routine blood screen'. Specific screening programmes do of course exist – mammography, cervical smears, coronary thrombosis risk factor analysis, for example – but all these address well-researched and well-defined risks. Some private health care providers do market 'well person' screens of one sort or another (often pitched at the middle-aged well-to-do businessman with a weight problem and a penchant for liquid lunches), but these are not generally recommended to their elderly patients by GPs. A 'check-up' *clinical* examination may be well worth suggesting to owners of genuinely geriatric pets – especially if they are not being seen regularly for booster vaccinations. However, even there, it is important to have a realistic idea of what constitutes 'geriatric'. The target patient is in the age group equivalent to a human in their 70s or 80s, not the 50–60 year old.

If a problem is identified during such an examination, then it should be investigated in the same way as if the animal had been presented for that complaint by the owner, and the choice of what, if any, laboratory investigations are appropriate should be made on that basis. All the stories about pets with unsuspected diabetes mellitus being identified on 'geriatric screening' are actually instances of a polydipsia/polyuria problem being identified at a geriatric clinical consultation, and being appropriately investigated. If a pet checks out as clinically well in every way, there is no justification for recommending biochemistry or haematology tests. The chances of identifying a treatable problem which is completely inapparent clinically are remote in the extreme.

Selling pet accessories is one thing – most people are well able to judge for themselves whether their pet really needs a new collar or a catnip mouse. However, when it comes to clinical matters it is essential to be really sure that you recommend only investigations and treatments which will be of benefit to the patient. In this area clients need and expect professional advice, and any tendency to see the clinical service as just another 'marketing opportunity' can only be deleterious to the profession's standing in the eyes of the public.

Practical pattern recognition

This is a skill which is best learned by doing. The more clinical pathology reports you scrutinise, the better you will be at it. Thus, rather than attempting further explanations, generalizations and rationalizations, the remainder of this chapter is devoted to a series of example cases. The general format is that a patient is presented with certain signs and a certain history, and the most appropriate diagnostic panel is chosen from those detailed earlier in the chapter.

One of the first things to realize is that when lecturers speak about the 'typical' presentation of such-and-such, what they really mean is the absolutely perfect case which shows *all* the features associated with the condition. Unfortunately such cases are not actually typical. Only a minority of patients have read every single page of the book. Nevertheless, it is instructive to look at some of these 'typical' patterns in the first instance, as a baseline for comparison.

The following cases cover a fairly wide range of patterns which may be commonly encountered. They have been selected because the haematology and biochemistry part of the pattern is pretty classic, even though the clinical presentation may not always be so 'typical'. In some cases the pattern on its own is diagnostic, while in others it is merely suggestive, and further investigation will be required. Some indication of where to go next is given for each case.

A useful approach is to cover over the lower part of each page and try to figure out the salient points yourself, before reading further. The cases may also be used as a reference for cases you have encountered yourself – the closer the pattern resembles the 'typical' one, the more likely it is that the condition involved is the same. The importance of examining the *whole* pattern cannot be overemphasized. It will be noted that some of the laboratory patterns are in fact very similar – but in these cases crucial aspects of the clinical histories (and this includes the breed, sex and age of the patient as well as the presenting signs) are quite different. In the same way some of the clinical presentations are very similar, but the laboratory patterns are quite different.

Most of the cases are small animal ones, because small animal patients seem to have a much wider range of diagnostically significant patterns than large animals.

Case 15.1

Patient details: Labrador-type dog, neutered male, 12 years old.

Main presenting signs: Dull and listless, poor appetite, drinking a lot, urinating indoors. Seems to have lost weight.

Polydipsia/polyuria panel

Biochemistry			Haematology			
Total protein	72 gl		PCV	0.33		
Albumin	26 gl		Hb	10.8 g/100 ml	}	low
Globulin	46 g/l		RBC count	5.25 × 10^{12}/l		
Calcium	1.87 mmol/l	low	MCV	62.9 fl		low
Urea	48.2 mmol/l	high	MCHC	32.7 g/100 ml		
Creatinine	503 µmol/l	high	Total WBC count		9.3 × 10^9/l	
Glucose	4.1 mmol/l		Band neutrophils	0%	0 × 10^9/l	
Cholesterol	6.2 mmol/l		Adult neutrophils	74%	6.9 × 10^9/l	
ALT	84 iu/l		Eosinophils	1%	0.1 × 10^9/l	
ALP	367 iu/l	raised	Lymphocytes	19%	1.8 × 10^9/l	
			Monocytes	6%	0.6 × 10^9/l	raised

Film comment. RBCs: normocytic, normochromic, non-regenerative

WBCs: normal

Platelets: adequate

Pattern suggests: Chronic renal failure, quite severe. Likely to be chronic interstitial nephritis, approaching end-stage kidney.

Salient points: Main findings are urea and creatinine quite markedly raised, demonstrating renal failure. Chronicity is confirmed by the history, and by the slight, non-regenerative anaemia. Slight hypocalcaemia is consistent with secondary renal hyperparathyroidism, and the ALP could relate to consequent skeletal changes. There is no neutrophilia evident in this case, but it is not an uncommon feature where uraemic stomatitis and gastritis are present.

What to do next: No further confirmatory tests required, definite confirmation of aetiology could only be gained by renal biopsy, which is not necessarily a good idea. Phosphate estimation could help clarify the extent of the hyperparathyroidism.

Case 15.2

Patient details: Labrador-type dog, neutered male, 12 years old.

Main presenting signs: Dull and listless, poor appetite, drinking a lot, urinating indoors. Seems to have lost weight.

Polydipsia/polyuria panel

Biochemistry			Haematology			
Total protein	78 g/l		PCV		0.37	
Albumin	31 g/l		Hb		12.3 g/100 ml	
Globulin	47 g/l		RBC count		$5.41 \times 10^{12}/l$	
Calcium	2.24 mmol/l		MCV		68.4 fl	
Urea	39.6 mmol/l	high	MCHC		33.2 g/100 ml	
Creatinine	215 µmol/l	raised	Total WBC count		$19.2 \times 10^9/l$	raised
Glucose	5.2 mmol/l		Band neutrophils	0%	$0 \times 10^9/l$	
Cholesterol	5.9 mmol/l		Adult neutrophils	74%	$14.2 \times 10^9/l$	raised
ALT	392 iu/l	raised	Eosinophils	1%	$0.2 \times 10^9/l$	
ALP	2435 iu/l	high	Lymphocytes	9%	$1.7 \times 10^9/l$	
			Monocytes	16%	$3.1 \times 10^9/l$	high

Film comment. RBCs: normal
WBCs: normal
Platelets: adequate

Pattern suggests: Possible abdominal neoplasia.

Salient points: Renal function is impaired, but there is also evidence of liver damage, indicating a disseminated condition. The age, the low-normal PCV and the chronic history are consistent with neoplasia. The somewhat pre-renal pattern in the urea/creatinine and the fact that the ALP activity is about ten times the ALT activity are typical features, probably a consequence of metabolic effects of tissue breakdown. The neutrophilia could simply reflect some non-specific inflammation/infection, but the fairly marked monocytosis, while again a non-specific finding, is quite often seen in association with neoplasia.

What to do next: Further clinical pathology investigation may be relatively unrewarding – even liver function tests such as bile acids may be ambiguous, as there may well be sufficient functioning liver tissue remaining to give unremarkable results – the normal albumin and absence of jaundice could suggest this. Diagnostic imaging – radiography or ultrasound – may reveal more. An exploratory laparotomy and biopsy of any suspicious lesions would be theoretically ideal, but may not be in the best interests of the patient.

Case 15.3

Patient details: Cavalier King Charles spaniel, neutered female, 9 years old.

Main presenting signs: Poor exercise tolerance, coughing, possibly some ascitic fluid present but nothing on paracentesis. Rather pale.

Core panel

Biochemistry			Haematology			
Total protein	65 g/l		PCV	0.48		
Albumin	26 g/l		Hb	16.7 g/100 ml		
Globulin	39 g/l		RBC count	$6.84 \times 10^{12}/l$		
Urea	28.4 mmol/l	high	MCV	70.2 fl		
Creatinine	166 µmol/l	raised	MCHC	34.8 g/100 ml		
ALT	116 iu/l	raised	Total WBC count		$15.6 \times 10^9/l$	
ALP	523 iu/l	high	Band neutrophils	2%	$0.3 \times 10^9/l$	
			Adult neutrophils	73%	$11.4 \times 10^9/l$	raised
			Eosinophils	1%	$0.2 \times 10^9/l$	
			Lymphocytes	20%	$3.1 \times 10^9/l$	
			Monocytes	4%	$0.6 \times 10^9/l$	raised

Film comment. RBCs: normal
WBCs: normal
Platelets: adequate

Pattern suggests: Decompensating congestive heart failure.

Salient points: The diagnosis would be strongly suspected from the history, especially as a very high percentage of this breed suffer from this problem in middle/old age. The urea/creatinine pattern is clearly pre-renal/circulatory, and the liver enzymes are suggestive of liver congestion. The haematology is unremarkable; the slight neutrophilia/monocytosis would be consistent with mild inflammation. There is no anaemia, which suggests that any pallor must be circulatory. Note that the biochemistry pattern is not very dissimilar to Case 15.2 – there is quite some overlap between these two patterns, and sometimes the distinction is more on the clinical presentation than the actual results.

What to do next: Cardiology work-up is more appropriate than further laboratory investigations.

Case 15.4

Patient details: German shepherd dog, entire male, 6 years old.

Main presenting signs: Sudden onset collapse, panting, high temperature, possibly jaundiced but mucous membranes very red. Has fitted once.

Fits/faints/collapse panel

Biochemistry			Haematology			
Total protein	82 g/l	raised	PCV		0.57	
Albumin	34 g/l		Hb		19.2 g/100 ml	
Globulin	48 g/l		RBC count		7.78×10^{12}/l	
Sodium	144 mmol/l		MCV		73.3 fl	
Potassium	5.2 mmol/l		MCHC		33.7 g/100 ml	
Calcium	2.68 mmol/l		Total WBC count		12.8×10^9/l	
Urea	46.3 mmol/l	high	Band neutrophils	4%	0.5×10^9/l	
Creatinine	395 µmol/l	high	Adult neutrophils	81%	10.4×10^9/l	raised
Glucose	6.8 mmol/l	raised	Eosinophils	3%	0.4×10^9/l	
Bilirubin	62 µmol/l	high	Lymphocytes	6%	0.8×10^9/l	low
ALT	422 iu/l	high	Monocytes	6%	0.8×10^9/l	raised
ALP	2879 iu/l	high				

Film comment: RBCs: normal
WBCs: normal
Platelets: adequate

Pattern suggests: Possible acute poisoning.

Salient points: Both renal dysfunction and hepatocellular damage/dysfunction are evident, suggesting a generalized pathology involving more than one organ system. The acute onset, the absence of anaemia and the relatively young age of the patient all argue against neoplasia as an explanation for these findings. The dog seems somewhat dehydrated, but electrolyte concentrations are normal. The glucose and the white cell pattern are probably stress-related.

What to do next: This pattern is often seen where the history is consistent with exposure to 'garden centre' type poisons – weedkillers, pesticides, etc. Urine γGT measurement may confirm acute nephrotoxicity. If there is known access to a particular compound, then specific treatment may be possible, but even if stomach contents can be obtained for toxicology the results may not be available for some time. Random searches for 'poison' without any clue what you are looking for are invariably unrewarding. These cases are best treated symptomatically – induce vomiting if possible to eliminate any poison still in the stomach, and institute full supportive therapy (intravenous fluids, antibiotic cover, anti-inflammatory medication, sedation if necessary). The prognosis is guarded to fair in an otherwise healthy individual.

Case 15.5

Patient details: Standard poodle, entire female, 4 years old.

Main presenting signs: Dull and depressed off and on for a couple of weeks, poor appetite, not polydipsic. Collapsed this morning. Seems pale, poor capillary refill time, not pyrexic.

Fits/faints/collapse panel

Biochemistry			Haematology			
Total protein	93 g/l	high	PCV		0.37	
Albumin	42 g/l	raised	Hb		12.8 g/100 ml	
Globulin	51 g/l	raised	RBC count		5.34×10^{12}/l	
Sodium	128 mmol/l	low	MCV		69.3 fl	
Potassium	9.4 mmol/l	high	MCHC		34.6 g/100 ml	
Calcium	3.19 mmol/l	raised	Total WBC count		10.8×10^9/l	
Urea	26.3 mmol/l	high	Band neutrophils	0%	0×10^9/l	
Creatinine	192 µmol/l	high	Adult neutrophils	42%	4.5×10^9/l	
Glucose	3.6 mmol/l	low	Eosinophils	14%	1.5×10^9/l	raised
ALT	74 iu/l		Lymphocytes	44%	4.8×10^9/l	
ALP	211 iu/l		Monocytes	0%	0×10^9/l	

Film comment. RBCs: normal
WBCs: normal
Platelets: adequate

Pattern suggests: Addison's disease.

Salient points: The low sodium/high potassium are essentially pathognomonic under the circumstances. The only other condition which might produce these results is acute renal failure, and both the relatively chronic history and the relatively unremarkable urea and creatinine argue against this. The proteins suggest quite severe dehydration, and the urea/creatinine pattern is consistent with a pre-renal/circulatory effect. The rather low PCV suggests that the dehydration may be masking a significant anaemia, while the eosinophilia, the hypercalcaemia, the slight hypoglycaemia and the relatively low neutrophil and high lymphocyte counts are all 'typical' of Addison's disease.

What to do next: This is an *EMERGENCY*, because that potassium concentration is close to being incompatible with life. Immediately start an isotonic saline i/v drip with a fast infusion rate. In this case confirmatory tests are scarcely needed, though you could telephone the lab and ask if they can do an emergency cortisol on the sample they already have. A rock-bottom result in an animal so metabolically stressed is pathognomonic. In a less clear-cut case it is essential to do an ACTH stimulation test before beginning steroid treatment, but as soon as the second sample has been collected, add soluble dexamethasone to the drip at a dose rate of 2 mg/kg. This takes care of emergency treatment, and when the dog is stable she can be gradually switched to permanent maintenance therapy.

Case 15.6

Patient details: Dachshund, entire female, 9 years old.

Main presenting signs: Drinking a lot and panting, good appetite. Overdue for season. 'Pot-bellied' appearance, bald patches on flanks.

Polydipsia/polyuria panel

Biochemistry			Haematology			
Total protein	72 gl		PCV	0.57		
Albumin	28 gl		Hb	19.7 g/100 ml		
Globulin	44 g/l		RBC count	$7.66 \times 10^{12}/l$		
Calcium	2.14 mmol/l		MCV	74.4 fl		
Urea	3.2 mmol/l		MCHC	34.6 g/100 ml		
Creatinine	74 µmol/l		Total WBC count		$11.3 \times 10^9/l$	
Glucose	6.2 mmol/l	raised	Band neutrophils	0%	$0 \times 10^9/l$	
Cholesterol	12.7 mmol/l	high	Adult neutrophils	84%	$9.5 \times 10^9/l$	
ALT	153 iu/l	raised	Eosinophils	0%	$0 \times 10^9/l$	
ALP	1468 iu/l	high	Lymphocytes	6%	$0.7 \times 10^9/l$	low
			Monocytes	10%	$1.1 \times 10^9/l$	raised

Film comment. RBCs: normal
WBCs: normal
Platelets: adequate

Pattern suggests: Cushing's disease.

Salient points: This condition is very common in this breed, particularly in bitches, and the clinical presentation is very suggestive. The Cushing's pattern in the results is 'classic' – low-normal urea, raised glucose, moderately high cholesterol, raised ALT with ALP relatively high, PCV over 0.50, eosinopenia, lymphopenia and monocytosis.

What to do next: Although the diagnosis seems obvious, the treatment for this condition is potentially extremely toxic and should never be initiated without confirmation. An ACTH stimulation test is the next step, and if that is indisputably diagnostic it may not be necessary to do any more. If the ACTH stimulation results are inconclusive, a low dose dexamethasone test should be carried out.

Case 15.7

Patient details: Dobermann pinscher, neutered male, 3 years old.

Main presenting signs: Overweight and reluctant to exercise. Doesn't eat a great deal. Coat poor, some hair loss, patches of seborrhoea.

Skin presentation panel

Biochemistry			Haematology			
Total protein	78 g/l		PCV		0.32	
Albumin	31 g/l		Hb		10.6 g/100 ml	low
Globulin	47 g/l		RBC count		4.68×10^{12}/l	
Calcium	2.57 mmol/l		MCV		68.4 fl	
Urea	6.1 mmol/l		MCHC		33.1 g/100 ml	
Creatinine	83 μmol/l		Total WBC count		8.4×10^9/l	
Cholesterol	23.7 mmol/l	high	Band neutrophils	0%	0×10^9/l	
CK	428 iu/l	high	Adult neutrophils	72%	6.0×10^9/l	
AST	112 iu/l	raised	Eosinophils	3%	0.3×10^9/l	
ALT	68 iu/l		Lymphocytes	23%	1.9×10^9/l	
ALP	127 iu/l		Monocytes	2%	0.2×10^9/l	

Film comment. RBCs: normocytic, normochromic, non-regenerative

WBCs: normal

Platelets: adequate

Pattern suggests: Hypothyroidism.

Salient points: The age, breed and clinical presentation are all suggestive of hypothyroidism, and the very high cholesterol and mild, non-regenerative anaemia are extremely 'typical'. The elevated CK is another feature which is sometimes seen.

What to do next: This has all the hallmarks of an 'obvious' hypothyroid case, and there is an excellent chance that a single free-T$_4$ or even total-T$_4$ will be diagnostic. Failing that, a TRH stimulation test would be the most definitive test, but as the dog is only 3 years old and the probability of hypothyroidism is high, thyroglobulin autoantibody estimation might be worth considering.

Case 15.8

Patient details: Medium-sized non-pedigree dog, entire female, 8 years old.

Main presenting signs: In season 3 weeks ago, now depressed, not interested in food and very polydipsic.

Polydipsia/polyuria panel

Biochemistry			Haematology			
Total protein	67 g/l		PCV	0.52		
Albumin	26 g/l		Hb	17.6 g/100 ml		
Globulin	41 g/l		RBC count	7.04×10^{12}/l		
Calcium	2.24 mmol/l		MCV	73.9 fl		
Urea	6.4 mmol/l		MCHC	33.8 g/100 ml		
Creatinine	59 µmol/l		Total WBC count		16.2×10^9/l	
Glucose	27.8 mmol/l	high	Band neutrophils	0%	0×10^9/l	
Cholesterol	13.2 mmol/l	high	Adult neutrophils	83%	13.4×10^9/l	raised
ALT	225 iu/l	raised	Eosinophils	0%	0×10^9/l	
ALP	2047 iu/l	high	Lymphocytes	11%	1.8×10^9/l	
			Monocytes	6%	1.0×10^9/l	raised

Film comment. RBCs: normal
WBCs: normal
Platelets: adequate

Pattern suggests: Diabetes mellitus, almost certainly an insulin-resistant type II associated with high progesterone.

Salient points: The marked hyperglycaemia is pathognomonic under the circumstances. The high cholesterol and the (probable) fatty change in the liver are also typical of diabetes mellitus. The haematology is essentially unremarkable, but there is some suggestion of infection/inflammation. Note that without the glucose result this pattern looks quite similar to Case 15.7, and if that test is not done one might be tempted to consider Cushing's disease.

What to do next: Much depends on the clinical condition. Ideally a spay should be scheduled as soon as possible to remove the source of the insulin antagonism, and with luck the diabetes may gradually resolve. However, if the bitch is too unwell for immediate surgery then insulin treatment should be instituted – even if this is unsuccessful in achieving glycaemic control, it will almost certainly lead to sufficient clinical improvement to allow surgery to go ahead. A proportion of cases become non-insulin-dependent in the weeks following surgery, but some require maintenance on insulin.

Case 15.9

Patient details: Medium-sized non-pedigree dog, entire female, 8 years old.

Main presenting signs: In season 3 weeks ago, now depressed, not interested in food and very polydipsic.

Polydipsia/polyuria panel

Biochemistry			Haematology				
Total protein	97 g/l	high	PCV		0.44		
Albumin	23 g/l	low	Hb		14.8 g/100 ml		
Globulin	74 g/l	high	RBC count		6.54×10^{12}/l		
Calcium	2.09 mmol/l		MCV		67.3 fl		
Urea	2.7 mmol/l	low	MCHC		33.6 g/100 ml		
Creatinine	74 µmol/l		Total WBC count		31.6×10^9/l		
Glucose	5.7 mmol/l		Band neutrophils	0%	0	$\times 10^9$/l	
Cholesterol	6.8 mmol/l		Adult neutrophils	81%	25.6	$\times 10^9$/l	high
ALT	64 iu/l		Eosinophils	0%	0	$\times 10^9$/l	
ALP	747 iu/l	high	Lymphocytes	8%	2.5	$\times 10^9$/l	
			Monocytes	11%	3.5	$\times 10^9$/l	high

Film comment. RBCs: normal
WBCs: normal
Platelets: adequate

Pattern suggests: Pyometra.

Salient points: The marked neutrophilia (and monocytosis) are extremely suggestive of pyometra in the context of a polydipsic bitch with a history of recent oestrus. The marked hyperglobulinaemia is also consistent with gross sepsis, and the depressed urea concentration and moderately raised ALP are also frequent features of this condition. Note that while diabetes mellitus can also present in the post-oestrus period, this bitch is not diabetic.

What to do next: Surgery. The presentation is very straightforward, there are no obvious complications, and the sooner a bitch like this is operated on the better.

Case 15.10

Patient details: Bulldog, entire male, 9 years old.

Main presenting signs: Weight loss for a couple of months, fussy appetite, possibly slightly polydipsic but nothing much. Looks pale, a few petechial haemorrhages seen.

Core panel

Biochemistry			Haematology			
Total protein	102 g/l	high	PCV	0.28		
Albumin	11 g/l	low	Hb	9.4 g/100 ml	} low	
Globulin	91 g/l	high	RBC count	3.79 × 10^{12}/l		
Urea	22.4 mmol/l	high	MCV	73.9 fl		
Creatinine	248 µmol/l	high	MCHC	33.6 g/100 ml		
ALT	77 iu/l		Total WBC count		5.3 × 10^9/l	
ALP	532 iu/l	high	Band neutrophils	0%	0 × 10^9/l	
			Adult neutrophils	77%	4.1 × 10^9/l	
			Eosinophils	0%	0 × 10^9/l	
			Lymphocytes	17%	0.9 × 10^9/l	low
			Monocytes	6%	0.3 × 10^9/l	

Film comment. RBCs: slightly regenerative and slightly hypochromic
WBCs: normal
Platelets: low in number

Pattern suggests: Very probable paraproteinaemia, most probably a plasma cell myeloma.

Salient points: The proteins are spectacularly abnormal. Not only is the abnormality too great to be likely to be caused simply by gross sepsis, there is no sign of sepsis in the white cell picture. The moderate renal dysfunction is also a common finding in myeloma cases. In addition the haematology shows general evidence of bone marrow depression, consistent with the haemopoietic tissue being crowded out by neoplastic cells.

What to do next: Serum protein electrophoresis, to demonstrate a paraprotein. If a paraprotein is found then the presumptive diagnosis is very strong, unless the dog has been out of the British Isles at any time in its life – certain parasitic conditions enzootic in Europe can produce a similar pattern, most notably ehrlichiosis. Bone marrow biopsy would also be informative, but may be unwise in the light of the apparent thrombocytopenia.

Case 15.11

Patient details: Domestic short hair cat, neutered female, 14 years old.

Main presenting signs: Losing weight for several months, drinking a lot, off food now. Occasional diarrhoea. Coat poor, bad mouth.

Polydipsia/polyuria panel

Biochemistry			Haematology		
Total protein	86 g/l	raised	PCV	0.47	
Albumin	21 g/l	low	Hb	16.1 g/100 ml	
Globulin	65 gl	raised	RBC count	10.45×10^{12}/l	
Calcium	2.11 mmol/l		MCV	45.0 fl	
Urea	18.8 mmol/l	raised	MCHC	34.3 g/100 ml	
Creatinine	167 µmol/l		Total WBC count	19.1×10^9/l	
Glucose	7.1 mmol/l	raised	Band neutrophils	0%	0×10^9/l
Cholesterol	4.5 mmol/l		Adult neutrophils	71%	13.6×10^9/l
ALT	189 iu/l	raised	Eosinophils	9%	1.7×10^9/l raised
ALP	267 iu/l		Basophils	0%	0×10^9/l
			Lymphocytes	14%	2.7×10^9/l
			Monocytes	6%	1.1×10^9/l raised

Film comment. RBCs: normal
WBCs: normal
Platelets: adequate

Pattern suggests: Hyperthyroidism.

Salient points: Although the clinical history might have suggested chronic renal dysfunction, the urea is only slightly raised and the normal creatinine indicates this is a pre-renal effect – probably a circulatory/cardiac effect due to thyrotoxic cardiomyopathy. Most hyperthyroid cats are polyphagic, but not all, and a poor appetite should not be seen as excluding the diagnosis (neither should inability to palpate an enlarged thyroid gland). The raised ALT is very typical of the hyperthyroid cat, as is the high/normal PCV and the eosinophilia. The protein pattern and the monocytosis are consistent with the inflammation associated with chronic gingivitis, and the raised glucose is just a stress effect.

What to do next: Measure total-T_4. This will almost certainly be high. If this is not conclusive one could consider a T_3 suppression test. With an atypical clinical presentation, trial therapy with carbimazole is probably unwise at this stage.

Case 15.12

Patient details: Birman cat, entire female, 10 months old.

Main presenting signs: Undersized compared to littermate in same household, seems thin and somewhat pot-bellied. Poor appetite, occasional diarrhoea.

Core panel							
Biochemistry			**Haematology**				
Total protein	93 g/l	high	PCV	0.28			low
Albumin	16 g/l	low	Hb	9.7 g/100 ml			
Globulin	77 g/l	high	RBC count	5.86×10^{12}/l			
Urea	12.2 mmol/l		MCV	47.8 fl			
Creatinine	154 µmol/l		MCHC	34.6 g/100 ml			
Bilirubin	26 µmol/l	raised	Total WBC count			18.6×10^9/l	raised
ALT	282 iu/l	raised	Band neutrophils	0%	0	$\times 10^9$/l	
ALP	264 iu/l		Adult neutrophils	79%	14.7	$\times 10^9$/l	raised
			Eosinophils	4%	0.7	$\times 10^9$/l	
			Basophils	0%	0	$\times 10^9$/l	
			Lymphocytes	15%	2.8	$\times 10^9$/l	
			Monocytes	2%	0.4	$\times 10^9$/l	

Film comment. RBCs: slightly regenerative and slightly hypochromic
WBCs: normal
Platelets: low in number

Pattern suggests: Feline infectious peritonitis.

Salient points: Clinical FIP is commonest in young pedigree cats, and while the protein pattern seen here might merely suggest chronic gingivitis in an older animal, this is unlikely in a youngster (as is a para-proteinaemia). The slight jaundice and elevated ALT are also quite suggestive of FIP, and the slight anaemia and neutrophilia also fit the picture.

What to do next: If there is any ascitic fluid to be had, analysis of that (especially protein composition) might be sufficient to confirm the diagnosis. If not, a high FIP (coronavirus) antibody titre could be considered confirmatory under the circumstances. However, dissuade the owner from testing the healthy littermate – he almost certainly has a positive titre too, as the entire litter will have been in contact with the virus, but antibody in a clinically healthy individual is indicative of no more than exposure, it is unusual for two kittens in a litter to go down with clinical disease, and a positive result can serve no purpose but to spread unnecessary alarm and despondency.

Case 15.13

Patient details: Springer spaniel, neutered female, 4 years old.

Main presenting signs: Slightly off colour for a few days, now pale and weak with very poor exercise tolerance. High temperature, panting. Haematuria, enlarged spleen.

Core panel

Biochemistry			Haematology			
Total protein	68 g/l		PCV		0.12	
Albumin	33 g/l		Hb		3.7 g/100 ml	low
Globulin	35 g/l		RBC count		1.24 × 10¹²/l	
Urea	5.6 mmol/l		MCV		96.8 fl	high
Creatinine	43 μmol/l		MCHC		30.8 g/100 ml	
Bilirubin	16 μmol/l	raised	Total WBC count		15.7 × 10⁹/l	
ALT	25 iu/l		Band neutrophils	3%	0.5 × 10⁹/l	
ALP	96 iu/l		Adult neutrophils	78%	12.2 × 10⁹/l	raised
			Eosinophils	2%	0.3 × 10⁹/l	
			Lymphocytes	13%	2.0 × 10⁹/l	
			Monocytes	4%	0.6 × 10⁹/l	raised

Film comment. RBCs: moderately regenerative, one or two nRBCs seen. Slightly hypochromic, target cells and spherocytes present.
WBCs: normal
Platelets: low in number

Pattern suggests: Autoimmune haemolytic anaemia.

Salient points: The anaemia is very severe, and regenerative. Haemolysis is suggested by the absence of hypoalbuminaemia (making blood loss less probable), the slight jaundice, and the fact that the RBC picture is perhaps somewhat less regenerative than one might expect considering the severity of the anaemia. The reported 'haematuria' in fact proved to be haemoglobinuria. This breed of dog is very prone to AIHA at about this age. Splenomegaly is commonly seen in AIHA as the spleen is involved in the haemolytic process, and thrombocytopenia is also encountered as most cases are reacting against both red cells and platelets, though to different degrees in the different conditions. PFK deficiency, another possibility in this breed, is not usually such a severe presentation.

What to do next: A Coombs' test might confirm the diagnosis, but false negatives do occur and it is questionable whether it is worth further investigation in such a classic presentation. In any case, the anaemia is so severe that initiation of treatment must be the first priority. If the PCV shows signs of falling below 0.10, a transfusion should be considered.

Case 15.14

Patient details: German Shepherd dog, entire male, 11 years old.

Main presenting signs: Collapsed last night, pale and panting, but relatively normal this morning. This is the third and worst episode within a month.

Fits/faints/collapse panel

Biochemistry			Haematology			
Total protein	68 g/l		PCV	0.22		
Albumin	33 g/l		Hb	6.9 g/100 ml	}	low
Globulin	35 g/l		RBC count	$2.33 \times 10^{12}/l$		
Sodium	152 mmol/l		MCV	94.4 fl		high
Potassium	4.8 mmol/l		MCHC	31.4 g/100 ml		
Calcium	2.44 mmol/l		Total WBC count		15.7 × 10⁹/l	
Urea	5.6 mmol/l		Band neutrophils	3%	$0.5 \times 10^9/l$	
Creatinine	43 μmol/l		Adult neutrophils	78%	$12.2 \times 10^9/l$	raised
Glucose	6.4 mmol/l	raised	Eosinophils	2%	$0.3 \times 10^9/l$	
Bilirubin	16 μmol/l	raised	Lymphocytes	13%	$2.0 \times 10^9/l$	
ALT	25 iu/l		Monocytes	4%	$0.6 \times 10^9/l$	raised
ALP	96 iu/l					

Film comment. RBCs: moderately regenerative, one or two nRBCs seen. Slightly hypochromic. Many poikilocytes, esp. burr cells, but normal cells also present

WBCs: normal

Platelets: low in number

Pattern suggests: Ruptured abdominal neoplasm, probably splenic.

Salient points: Note that with the exception of some subtle differences in red cell appearance, the results are very similar to those of Case 15.13. The distinction is almost entirely in the history and presenting signs. AIHA is less common at this age, and is much less likely to present as recurrent collapse with spontaneous recovery. GSDs are especially prone to haemangiosarcomas and haemangiomas of the abdominal organs, especially the spleen and liver, and there is no sign here of liver damage. The normal albumin and relatively modest degree of regeneration are due to the fact that the blood is not being lost from the body but is reabsorbed through the peritoneum (hence the spontaneous recovery), the thrombocytopenia to the fact that a substantial proportion of the body's platelet stores are in the spleen, and the jaundice to the fact that blood subjected to this traumatic extravascular recycling is prone to haemolyse.

What to do next: Paracentesis to check for blood, followed by an exploratory laparotomy. It is vital for an accurate prognosis to obtain histological confirmation of the nature of any mass removed.

Case 15.15

Patient details: Irish setter, entire female, 7 years old.

Main presenting signs: In season 3 weeks ago. Now lacking in energy, poor exercise tolerance, bruising visible inside thighs and on gums. Rather pale. High temperature.

Core panel

Biochemistry		Haematology			
Total protein	66 g/l	PCV	0.19		
Albumin	31 g/l	Hb	6.2 g/100 ml	}	low
Globulin	35 g/l	RBC count	$2.79 \times 10^{12}/l$		
Urea	6.1 mmol/l	MCV	68.1 fl		
Creatinine	78 μmol/l	MCHC	32.6 g/100 ml		
ALT	36 iu/l	Total WBC count	1.6	$\times 10^9/l$	low
ALP	118 iu/l	Band neutrophils	0%	0	$\times 10^9/l$
		Adult neutrophils	16%	0.3	$\times 10^9/l$ low
		Eosinophils	0%	0	$\times 10^9/l$
		Lymphocytes	83%	1.3	$\times 10^9/l$
		Monocytes	1%	0.02	$\times 10^9/l$

Film comment. RBCs: non-regenerative, normochromic
WBCs: normal morphology
Platelets: none seen

Pattern suggests: Bone marrow aplasia.

Salient points: Erythrocytes, granulocytes and platelets are all markedly depressed, and there is no sign of red cell regeneration. The time-scale of the process is consistent with a single insult to the bone marrow, with the shorter-lived elements (platelets and granulocytes) disappearing first, causing petechiation and pyrexia, before the anaemia becomes critical. Situations where the bone marrow is being infiltrated by tumour cells (e.g. lymphosarcoma) may appear similar, but there is often some evidence of red cell regeneration in these cases. It transpired that this bitch had been involved in a mismating three weeks earlier, and had been injected with oestradiol to prevent pregnancy.

What to do next: Bone marrow biopsy to distinguish definitively between aplasia and neoplasia. However, this is not without difficulties, particularly in a markedly thrombocytopenic patient, and it is preferable to refer a case like this to a specialist centre.

Case 15.16

Patient details: Angloarab hunter, entire female, 6 years old.

Main presenting signs: No energy, reluctant to go forward, pulls up early in the day. Slight colic a couple of weeks ago. No diarrhoea.

Core panel

Biochemistry			Haematology			
Total protein	56 gl	low	PCV	0.33		low
Albumin	38 g/l		Hb	12.1 g/100 ml		
Globulin	18 g/l	low	RBC count	$6.75 \times 10^{12}/l$		
Urea	6.3 mmol/l		MCV	48.9 fl		
CK	569 iu/l	raised	MCHC	36.7 g/100 ml		
AST	346 iu/l		Total WBC count		$5.2 \times 10^9/l$	
γGT	32 iu/l		Band neutrophils	0%	$0 \times 10^9/l$	
			Adult neutrophils	47%	$2.4 \times 10^9/l$	low
			Eosinophils	2%	$0.1 \times 10^9/l$	
			Lymphocytes	50%	$2.6 \times 10^9/l$	
			Monocytes	1%	$0.05 \times 10^9/l$	

Film comment. RBCs: normocytic, normochromic
WBCs: normal morphology
Platelets: adequate

Pattern suggests: Virus infection/post-viral syndrome

Salient points: Markedly low globulins and neutropenia are common features of viral infections in the horse, particularly associated with the poor performance syndrome which can follow a viral infection. There has been some suggestion of possible enterovirus (coxackievirus) involvement, but the virus(es) concerned are usually not identified. The CK increase is only slight, and there is unlikely to be sufficient muscle damage to affect performance. The slightly depressed PCV is consistent with a somewhat debilitated horse; it should not be regarded as anaemia as such.

What to do next: Rest and *light* exercise are the best approach; most cases return to normal gradually but may deteriorate if forced to exercise strenuously. The use of levamisole (off data sheet) may be considered.

Case 15.17

Patient details: Highland pony, 24 years old, neutered male.

Main presenting signs: Presented in February, having lost more weight than usual while at grass over the winter, and having just developed oedema of the prepuce and ventral abdomen. On examination the pony was dull, and the tail and perineum were stained by loose faeces

'Sick horse' panel

Biochemistry			Haematology		
Total protein	42 g/l	low	PCV	0.28	
Albumin	13 g/l	low	Hb	10.8 g/100 ml	low
Globulin	29 g/l		RBC count	5.20 × 10^{12}/l	
Urea	4.8 mmol/l		MCV	53.8 fl	
Creatinine	102 µmol/l		MCHC	38.6 g/100 ml	
Glucose	4.7 mmol/l		Total WBC count	9.9 × 10^9/l	
T. glycereol	12.0 mmol/l	high	Band neutrophils	0% 0 × 10^9/l	
CK	203 iu/l		Adult neutrophils	68% 6.7 × 10^9/l	
AST	251 iu/l		Eosinophils	2% 0.2 × 10^9/l	
ALP	668 iu/l	raised	Basophils	3% 0.3 × 10^9/l	
GDH	29 iu/l	raised	Lymphocytes	27% 2.7 × 10^9/l	
γGT	42 iu/l		Monocytes	0% 0 × 10^9/l	

Film comment. RBCs: normocytic, normochromic
WBCs: normal
Platelets: adequate

Pattern suggests: Protein-losing enteropathy.

Salient points: The hypoalbuminaemia is severe and becoming dangerous. Intestinal protein loss is overwhelmingly probable from the clinical evidence of diarrhoea, the absence of a raised globulin concentration, the absence of any real evidence of renal or hepatic problems, and simply on statistical grounds (PLE is by far the commonest cause of hypoalbuminaemia in the horse). The raised ALP is probably due to intestinal damage, and the GDH is only marginal. There is also a fairly marked hyperlipidaemia, which suggests the pony has not eaten for several days, and the situation is becoming critical.

What to do next: Definite aetiological diagnosis is often impossible in this type of case (though parasite involvement is often suspected), and treatment becomes the main priority. Stopping the diarrhoea is the most important thing, closely followed by reversing the hyperlipidaemia. Bowel sedatives and adsorptive agents are the main things; this is not an infectious condition and antibiotics are contraindicated. High-carbohydrate feed may be sufficient to deal with the hyperlipidaemia, but if not, i/v heparin is indicated. (This pony made a full recovery on kaolin and pectin (Kaogel: Pharmacia & Upjohn) and tincture of chloroform and morphine (Chlorodyne), heparin was not needed as he voluntarily ate soaked sugar beet pulp. Ivermectin was also administered. He was eventually switched to permanent codeine therapy at 300 mg twice daily in conjunction with regular anthelmintic treatment. He remained well with normal faeces until dying of an unrelated illness at the age of 33 years. No post-mortem examination was carried out.)

IV

Practical Laboratory Medicine

16 Sample Collection and Use of External Laboratories

Any laboratory result is only as good as, firstly, the sample which is being analysed and secondly, the laboratory which is analysing it. Meticulous care is therefore required at all stages to ensure that results obtained are of maximum reliability for diagnostic purposes.

Sample collection

Many people fail to appreciate the necessity of collecting a *good quality* sample. It is not enough simply to succeed in transferring a small quantity of red fluid from the patient's veins into a sample bottle: most of the problems caused by poor sample quality are only evident in the laboratory and these are often not appreciated by the person collecting the sample.

Sample processing

Blood samples are extremely perishable, and do not take at all kindly to being left in a coat pocket or a car boot for hours (let alone days!). It is vital that samples are either analysed promptly, or else are promptly and correctly processed for any travelling or storage which might be necessary.

Laboratory reliability

This aspect requires careful consideration irrespective of whether tests are being done in the practice side-room or referred to a professional laboratory. In the case of analyses carried out in the practice, the ultimate responsibility for ensuring accuracy and reliability rests firmly at the door of the supervising veterinary surgeon, and this aspect is considered in detail in Chapters 17 and 18. However, it is also the responsibility of the veterinary surgeon to make an intelligent, critical assessment of the service provided by the referral laboratory and to choose wisely when deciding whom to trust with his patients' samples.

Sample collection

Blood

Site

In nearly all species the jugular vein is the site of choice. The only exceptions are pigs, where the anterior vena cava is usually used (or an ear vein in large individuals), rabbits, where the ear vein may again be used, *large* dogs with short, thick necks and lots of hair and loose skin (such as Old English sheepdogs or Newfoundlands) where the cephalic vein may occasionally be easier, and cattle, where the tail vein provides a useful alternative to the jugular in animals standing in stalls. Jugular blood sampling in small animals is not nearly so commonly performed as it ought to be, which is unfortunate as it is probably the single most effective way to improve sample quality (see p. 258).

Equipment

Always use a new disposable needle for each venepuncture. 20G 1″ needles are generally best, although a 19G may be preferred if a sample volume of 20 ml or more is required, and a 21G may be better in kittens, small cats or very small puppies. Smaller needles tend to lead to haemolysis of the sample, and larger needles predispose to haematoma formation as well as increasing the likelihood of the patient resenting the procedure and becoming needle-shy. Four types of blood collection vessel are available.

Screw-topped tubes

These are made by a variety of manufacturers, and conform to a standard colour-code to indicate which anticoagulant or preservative they contain:

Pink: EDTA, for routine haematology
Mauve: Citrate, for coagulation tests (prothrombin time, etc.)
Orange: Heparin, for plasma for general biochemistry
Yellow: Fluoride, for glucose measurement
White: No additive, for clotted blood (serum harvesting). Note that while tubes with anticoagulant may be (and usually are) plastic, tubes for clotted blood must be glass.

Brands with actual screw-threaded caps are more secure than those with push-on caps.

A particular subset of this type of tube is the *gel tube*, a range of small collection tubes suitable for use with dual-purpose high-speed (microhaematocrit) centrifuges. These have a nominal volume of 1.5 ml blood, and contain a separation gel specifically designed for use with these centrifuges. The (brown-coded) tubes for serum separation (clotted blood) are plastic, but have a special coating which makes them equivalent to glass tubes for this purpose. Points to watch out for are the small volume – it may be necessary to use two tubes for patients with particularly high PCVs – and the fact that they are intended only for use in high-speed centrifuges. The gel does not function well in an ordinary bucket centrifuge such as will be used by a referral laboratory; therefore only use a gel tube if you definitely intend to spin it yourself. Once spun, the gel holds the separation very well, and it is possible to post the tubes as they are, without transferring the serum or plasma to a separate tube.

Method.   Before you begin, lay out the collection tube(s) conveniently to hand with their tops off. Use a new disposable syringe to aspirate the blood, choosing the size according to the total volume required for all tests. Venepuncture is made easier by using the syringe as a handle to control the needle, and as the needle penetrates the skin the application of a slight back pressure to the plunger helps to 'feel' when the needle enters the vein. This is confirmed by the free flow of blood into the syringe. Continue to aspirate until the desired volume is in the syringe, then withdraw the needle from the vein, replace the needle guard and *remove the needle from the syringe. Quickly* transfer the blood into the open tubes, taking care not to overfill, and immediately cap the tubes and mix by repeated inversion (not shaking), unless you want clotted blood. See p. 41 regarding the importance of prompt mixing of blood with anticoagulant.

The tube you are most anxious to prevent clotting is the EDTA one. If you have an assistant capping and mixing tubes as you fill them, fill this one *first*. However, if you are working single-handed, work as quickly as you can and fill the EDTA tube *last*, then immediately cap it and mix it before attending to any of the others. Blood being agitated in the syringe is less likely to start clotting than blood stationary in an unmixed tube.

When capping tubes, make sure the right cap goes on the right tube. Not only is the retention of the colour-coding on the cap important, but mixing the caps could introduce traces of the wrong additive into a sample, with deleterious consequences for the analysis.

Advantages.   These tubes are cheap, they are available in a wide variety of sizes including very small paediatric sizes, and where three or more different tubes are required it is easy to fill all of them from a single syringe. This is probably the method of choice for small animal use.

Disadvantages.   These are less suitable for use in large animals, as they depend on having somewhere reasonably safe where they can be laid out with their tops off before the sample is actually collected – rain, wind and the absence of a flat surface are serious drawbacks. Any delay during sample collection is also quite serious, as the blood is initially collected into a plain syringe and will therefore clot unless quickly transferred, and it is easy to knock these tubes over while filling them, and spill the sample. The addition of the syringe to the price means they are not quite as cheap as they first appear.

Warning. The procedure whereby blood is dripped into the tubes from the end of a needle with no syringe being used should be avoided for a number of reasons.

(1)   The quality of the sample will be much poorer due to the prolonged haemostasis needed. This is partly due to increased haemolysis (and fragmentation of the white cells), but another important factor is that during the extended period of venous stasis, water and small molecules migrate out through the vein wall thus changing the concentrations of most things which might be measured on the sample.

(2)   Safety – it is virtually impossible to avoid getting blood (potentially infective?) over your hands and the outside of the sample tube (which makes it difficult to write on or to read).

(3)   Samples collected this way frequently clot shortly afterwards – although the blood goes directly into the tube with the anticoagulant, it is the time before it is capped and mixed which is important, and this is usually too long.

(4)   It is often difficult to collect the full volume of blood required as the needle often becomes blocked by clots.

(5)   The sample is easily contaminated by dirt, hair and/or rain.

(6)   Animal handling can be difficult because of the time taken.

(7)   If the animal escapes with the needle in the vein, a blood-bath may ensue (a needle/syringe combination will either stay put with no blood leakage until the animal is caught, or it will fall out in its entirety, in which case it is easier to find than a needle alone and again little blood will escape).

(8)   A larger needle is often necessary and so haematomas are more likely.

(9)   Many owners become upset at the sight of free-flowing blood.

Evacuated glass tubes ('Vacutainer')

Method. These tubes require a special double-pointed needle which is screwed into a holder before use. *It is essential to use a new, clean needle for each animal.* 'Safety' needles with rubber sleeves are available which prevent blood dripping into the holder or elsewhere when the collecting tube is not attached. These are not generally used in veterinary practice as the risk to the operator when handling non-human blood is low compared with risks from human blood. However, it is still bad practice to make a habit of splashing blood around, and to prevent this it is usual to push the rubber bung of the tube part-way on to the needle (*without* penetrating the seal) before performing the venepuncture (see Fig. 16.1). This prevents blood splashes building up on the reusable holder, but means (as with the safety needles) that you have no evidence that you are in the vein until you push the tube right home and break the

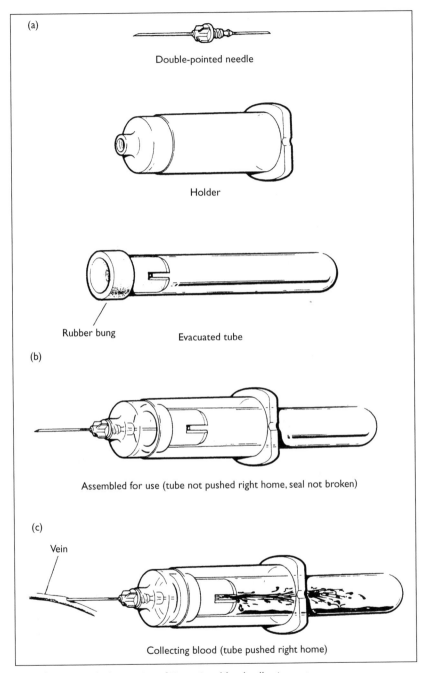

(a)

Double-pointed needle

Holder

Rubber bung   Evacuated tube

(b)

Assembled for use (tube not pushed right home, seal not broken)

(c)

Vein

Collecting blood (tube pushed right home)

Fig. 16.1   Method of operation of Vacutainer blood collection system.

seal. It is therefore particularly important to be sure of hitting the vein cleanly every time. Once the needle is in the vein the tube is simply pushed forward in the holder so that the needle penetrates the seal and the tube fills with blood automatically. If you need more than one tube from the same animal, e.g. heparin and EDTA, wait until the blood has stopped flowing, pull the tube away from the end of the needle (it will reseal automatically) and replace with the second tube without removing the needle from the vein. It is virtually impossible to avoid dripping blood on to the needle holder at this point unless a safety needle is used. When the last tube has been filled, withdraw needle, holder and all from the vein before removing the tube from the needle. This procedure eliminates any residual vacuum from the tube which might cause haemolysis, and it is usually wise to puncture the tops of any earlier tubes once more for the same purpose, especially any which are obviously underfilled. Then replace the needle guard, unscrew the needle, and replace it with a new one if another animal is to be sampled. It is particularly important to ensure safe disposal of these double-pointed needles as there is always one unguarded point left exposed.

Advantages.   As the blood goes straight into the anticoagulant, samples are much less liable to clot, no syringe is needed, and it is not necessary to lay out a neat row of tubes (they can be used straight from a pocket and, as they self-seal instantly, can be dropped straight back in – but be careful to identify tubes after each animal). The main advantage, however, is that the tubes fill themselves without having to pull back on a plunger, which can be a real boon when a large number of animals has to be sampled. This system's particular use (though it is not unsurpassed) is for herd or flock sampling exercises in large animals, especially where only one tube is required from each animal.

Disadvantages.   This is the most expensive of all the systems. It is also very prone to haemolysis as the fierce vacuum needed to ensure that the tube fills causes a lot of turbulence and some very fast-flowing blood. If the needle misses the vein, or the vein is lost during collection, it is easy to lose the vacuum while searching for the vein, rendering the tube useless. The double-pointed needle can be dangerous, and changing needles between animals is time-consuming unless a helper can be found. The glass tubes (essential to hold the vacuum under storage) break more easily and more dangerously than plastic ones. For some reason, the colour codings which signify the anticoagulant contained in the tube are *not* the same as the standard colour codes used in all the other systems. This can cause serious confusion to the unwary, in particular because the red/orange colour which means 'heparin' in the standard codes means 'plain' (i.e. for clotted blood) in Vacutainer language. Beware particularly when laboratories specify their sample requirements by colour.

The Vacutainer system is really *quite unsuitable* for small animal use. The vacuum tends to collapse the smaller, thin-walled veins, the tubes are hard to fill, and dog and cat blood is in any case much more prone to haemolysis than horse or ruminant blood. Small animal veins are harder to find than large animal veins, and the patients are more prone to wriggling, which means that the incidence of lost vacuums is much higher. Small-volume 'paediatric' Vacutainers are sometimes used, but these suffer from some of the same problems, and frequently collect insufficient blood for the tests required. This system is also to be avoided for haematology samples in any species.

Vacutainers should not be uncapped and used as ordinary sample tubes with a syringe, as the rubber bung will not remain in place when it is replaced due to air compression inside the tube, using them this way is also needlessly expensive.

Note: Vacutainers are often supplied with no labels, with the intention that a uniquely identified coded label (supplied in the same box) be applied after filling. It is necessary to record separately the identity of the animal which corresponds to the label code. This system must be followed even when using these tubes for diagnostic work (rather than for *Brucella* testing), or else a blank label with the animal's identity written on must be used. It is quite unsatisfactory to try to write on the rubber bung (which may be discarded soon after the tube reaches the lab), and attempts to write directly on to the glass are almost always illegible.

Plastic blood collecting syringes ('Monovette')

Method.   These are essentially syringes which are designed to be comfortable for aspirating (rather than injecting) and which contain anticoagulant. They convert directly to sample containers by replacing the needle with a small cap, and unscrewing and discarding the plunger. The method is basically the same as for an ordinary syringe, except that there is, of course, no need to lay out the collection tubes, and where more than one tube is required it is necessary to detach the first at the Luer fitting and re-attach the second without removing the needle from the vein (or perform more than one venepuncture, which won't please the patient!). As the Luer holes are so small the tubes can be laid aside or even put briefly into a pocket as they are filled. Very little leakage will occur, and they can all be capped and the plungers removed after the last one has been filled and the needle is out of the vein. Although the tubes for clotted blood are plastic, they are specially coated, and function like glass tubes for serum separation.

Advantages.   The tubes are fairly cheap, and it is not necessary to buy special needles – the usual ones will fit. Samples are unlikely to clot as the blood goes straight into the anticoagulant, there is no vacuum to lose or to haemolyse the blood, and the 'feel' of a syringe which helps find the vein is still there. The syringes are more comfortable to use than those designed for injecting. This is probably the system of choice for horse and for farm work where very large numbers of samples are not being collected and where avoidance of haemolysis is important (e.g. haematology and diagnostic biochemistry, as opposed to serology).

Disadvantages.   The range is rather lacking in true paediatric tubes and the smaller ones are less convenient than they might be for small animal use. Unless a special valve is used on the end of the needle, the process of changing tubes with the needle still in the vein is awkward and inevitably leaves some blood on the fingers. Although they are not as vulnerable as screw-top tubes, accidents can happen until they are capped and the plunger removed (unlike evacuated tubes, which are safe as soon as they are filled).

Convertible syringe/evacuated tubes ('S-Monovette')

This system combines the best features of evacuated glass tubes and blood collecting syringes, and can be used as either. It is the system of choice in human medicine. Its design is shown in Fig. 16.2. It requires special double-pointed needles similar to Vacutainer needles, but the second point is permanently enclosed in the holder which is part of the needle assembly, and therefore much safer. Instead of a Luer fitting on the syringe there is a rubber cap so that the syringe is sealed (like a Vacutainer) except when the needle is piercing it, and the second needle point has a rubber sleeve which prevents any blood passing through the needle unless the sleeve is pushed back by the rubber syringe cap. When the needle is fitted to the syringe the needle holder locks positively on to the syringe head forming a rigid unit. The 'S' in the name stands for 'safety', as it is virtually impossible to get blood on your hands when using this system.

Method.   As syringe: Fit the needle to the syringe as if it were an ordinary Monovette (or syringe) and proceed in the same way. If more than one tube is required the size of the needle holder and the locking system make it very easy to remove the first tube and attach another without disturbing the needle, and each tube seals automatically as soon as it is detached. Once all the tubes have been filled and the needle (with holder still attached) discarded as if it were an ordinary needle, the plungers can be unscrewed and discarded – but even if a plunger is depressed by accident the tube is sealed and will not leak.

As evacuated tube: Before using, the plungers of all tubes which will be required should be pulled back until they click into the bottom of the 'syringe', and then broken off. This creates a vacuum inside the tube. As these tubes are plastic, not glass, the vacuum is not stable for very long, but tubes may be prepared a few hours in advance, by lay staff if necessary. Perform the venepuncture using the needle (with holder) alone, then clip the pre-evacuated tube on to the holder (which allows the second point of the needle to pierce the rubber cap) and allow it to fill. (As with the Vacutainer, there is no way of knowing whether or not you are in the vein until the seal is pierced, and it is easy to lose the vacuum while looking for the vein if you are not.) Further tubes

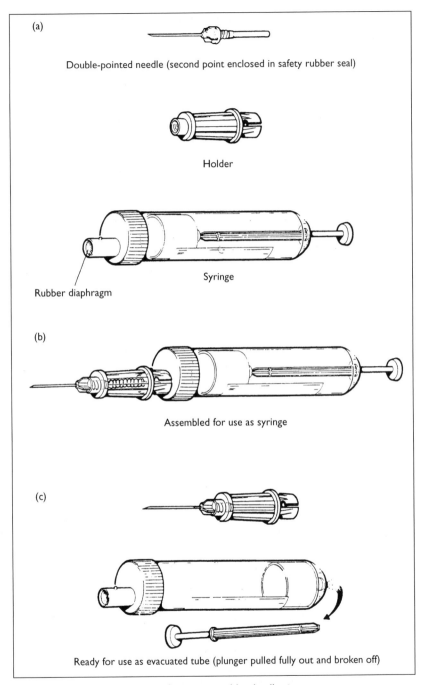

(a)

Double-pointed needle (second point enclosed in safety rubber seal)

Holder

Rubber diaphragm

Syringe

(b)

Assembled for use as syringe

(c)

Ready for use as evacuated tube (plunger pulled fully out and broken off)

Fig. 16.2 Methods of operation of S-Monovette blood collection system.

are filled simply by removing one and attaching the next. When all the tubes have been filled it is only necessary to replace the guard on the needle and discard it. However, as with Vacutainers, any tube which has not filled completely should have its cap pierced once more to release any residual vacuum.

Advantages.   Numerous. The user has the choice as to whether the convenience of the evacuated tube or the much less traumatic syringe aspiration is preferable for each individual circumstance. Samples are very unlikely to clot, and all tubes are sealed the moment the needle is detached, even if the syringe method has been used. The needle, although double-pointed, is as safe as a single-pointed needle, there is no need to fiddle with reusable needle-holders, and the needle/holder/tube assembly is as rigid as an ordinary needle and syringe. Blood splashing or spilling simply does not happen.

Disadvantages.   The system is more expensive than either the screw-topped tube or the Monovette, although it is comparable in price to the Vacutainer (cheaper where one needle is used for two or three tubes as it is the needles which are expensive rather than the tubes, but do *not* be drawn into reusing the needles for more than one patient). Like the ordinary Monovettes, the availability of small-volume tubes is rather limited, making the system less suitable for small animal work. Also, *Brucella*-testing laboratories are used to receiving Vacutainers, and may prefer not to be sent 'non-standard' tubes. However, taken simply on its merits, this system is the most versatile and easy to use of all four options, as well as being by far the least messy.

General points regarding technique

(1)   Appropriate restraint is very important. An experienced handler is invaluable, but if you must use the owner to restrain an animal it is essential to give him or her clear and specific instructions. The aim should be to hold the *relaxed* animal gently but firmly in the optimum position. It is very difficult to bleed a kicking and struggling patient even with forcible restraint, and the resulting sample quality is usually poor.

(2)   It is always easier to hit the vein if the hair is clipped (electric clippers are much more satisfactory than curved scissors). However, hair takes some time to grow and owners often don't appreciate the bald patch – especially on a show animal. Once you are well practised in the technique you will find that clipping is only necessary with particularly difficult animals – short hair can be damped down with spirit, and long hair too after a parting has been made directly over the vein, or the whole procedure can be carried out entirely by touch.

(3)   There is some controversy over the efficacy of surgical spirit in sterilizing the skin before venepuncture. If a new sterile needle is used every time the incidence of abscess formation is virtually negligible even if no disinfectant is used, and it is noticeable that when a needle is inserted through

skin which is *wet* with spirit the animal often flinches as the spirit stings. However, owners often expect visible sterile precautions, and the spirit is very useful to 'lay' the hair and improve visualization of the vein. The sting reaction can be avoided by allowing the spirit to dry before inserting the needle.

(4)   The importance of using minimal venous stasis cannot be overstressed, as the composition of blood which has been held static in a vein for even a short period will alter significantly. Correct practice is to release the vein and allow the blood to flow freely for a few seconds after the vein has been penetrated and before either continuing to aspirate with a syringe or puncturing the seal of an evacuated tube. In small animals this may not be practical as the vein may collapse, blocking the needle, and in this case all that can be done is to collect the sample as quickly as possible after the vein has been occluded – preferably again allowing a few seconds of free blood flow after the needle has been inserted and before re-occluding the vein.

(5)   It is good practice to apply pressure over the site of venepuncture with a clean piece of cotton wool as the needle is withdrawn, and to keep it there for half a minute or so. However, pressure *proximal* to the puncture site is worse than none at all, and if the animal moves it may be better to move the pressure distally or abandon it entirely rather than risk *causing* a haematoma in this way. If you are using screw-top tubes the necessity for immediately filling, capping and mixing the tubes at this point conflicts with careful attention to haemostasis, and so the person holding the animal must be instructed to carry out this procedure correctly.

(6)   Cold water is best for removing fresh bloodstains from the patient, operator or sample tubes – spirit is useless for this. If there is any blood on the tube labels, the tubes should be run under the cold tap (or dipped in the water bucket) and towel-dried before attempting to write on them. Make sure they are securely sealed first!

Sample volume

Haematology

It is essential that *EDTA* tubes are filled with exactly the right amount of blood specified on the label. If too little blood is collected the resulting high EDTA concentration will damage the cells; if the tube is overfilled, the blood will probably clot. Take care to examine the labels of screw-topped tubes before using, as 5 ml and 2.5 ml (and 1 ml and 0.5 ml) tubes are superficially similar; 2.5 ml is sufficient for general haematology and should generally be considered the minimum. The larger (5 ml) tubes are seldom, if ever, required. It is possible to carry out general haematology on the small paediatric (1 ml and 0.5 ml) tubes, but these should be reserved for very small patients only, as results from these tubes are known to be much less precise than from standard size tubes.

This is because of the greatly magnified effect of small cumulative mixing errors during the laboratory procedures. In addition, the poorer mixing mechanics of the small tubes make the blood more likely to clot. With EDTA tubes, as with all other anticoagulants, it is important to check that tubes are not past their expiry dates. These prepared tubes do not last indefinitely, and outdated anticoagulant can lead to some very strange results. Avoid buying in excessively large stocks even if it seems like a bargain.

Biochemistry

Volume requirements are less critical, although it is unwise to put much less than half the nominal amount of blood into a *heparin* tube. Modern biochemistry analysers can do a surprisingly large number of tests on a relatively small volume, and sometimes actual ability to handle the sample becomes more of an issue than how much is needed for the analysis. Very small volumes can also be a problem due to the disproportionate effects of evaporation. 2 ml of blood is usually enough for a wide range of tests, and even the 1.5 ml gel tubes for use with microhaematocrit centrifuges seldom prove insufficient.

Remember, however, that clotted blood yields less serum than the equivalent volume of heparinized blood will yield plasma, and that the high PCVs of very excited horses and some breeds of dog will also reduce serum or plasma yield. For glucose estimation, only a small volume of *fluoride/oxalate* blood is required and 1 ml tubes are quite sufficient. Exact adherence to the nominal blood volume is not critical, but extreme over- or underfilling should be avoided. Remember that the small fluoride/oxalate (and EDTA) tubes are very prone to clot, so take care to fill and *mix* them very quickly after the sample has been collected.

Haemolysis

Causes include:

(1)   Drawing back too hard on a syringe while using too small a needle.
(2)   Vacutainers.
(3)   Fluoride tubes, because the fluoride 'poisons' red cell metabolism and cell deterioration begins immediately. These tubes should always be separated as soon as possible – avoid posting whole fluoride blood.
(4)   Wet syringes and/or needles, or rain entering the collection tube.
(5)   Losing the vein half-way through and applying negative pressure to blood already in syringe while searching for the lost vein.
(6)   Squeezing blood through the needle into the sample tube – always remove the needle first.
(7)   Violent shaking – repeated inversion is sufficient for mixing.
(8)   Use of uncoated plastic tubes for clotted blood.

(9)   Lipaemic samples (see below).
(10)   Time, especially if the sample is not refrigerated.
(11)   Freezing of the sample.

Patients with acute haemolytic anaemia will also have haemolysed plasma and as this is intravascular haemolysis it cannot be prevented. It should be obvious from the haematology results when this has occurred.

Effects:

(1)   Very poor haematology results, especially poor cell morphology.
(2)   Erroneous biochemistry results due to red colour in plasma.
(3)   Falsely high results for biochemical constituents which are much higher in concentration intracellularly than in the plasma: K^+, Mg^{2+}, AST, etc.

Lipaemia

This is not a sampling or sample handling problem, it is a feature of the patient. In horses it is a serious clinical finding (see p. 133) which should never be ignored. In small animals, especially dogs, it is less of a concern; indeed it is quite often encountered in animals with apparently very little wrong with them. It becomes a sample processing problem because the white opacity interferes with photometric analysis, and in marked cases biochemistry results may be unobtainable.

The one readily identifiable cause of lipaemia in small animals is uncontrolled diabetes mellitus. Fortunately, this is usually fairly easy to confirm or deny, either using a glucose meter (glucose meters are more able to cope with lipaemic samples than transmission/absorbance photometers and, as they are designed for whole blood use, haemolysis is not a particular problem either) or by collecting a urine sample. In non-diabetic individuals lipaemia often seems fairly random, though it is disproportionately common in the schnauzer breed of dog. There is often a correlation with obesity, and some authors also report a correlation with Cushing's disease or hypothyroidism. However, the majority of Cushing's and hypothyroid cases are not lipaemic, and many extreme lipaemias seem to have no readily identifiable cause.

The white milky opacity is caused by the presence of triglycerides in the plasma. Free triglycerides remain in suspension on standing, but triglycerides in the form of chylomicrons will rise to the top (like the cream on a bottle of milk) leaving relatively normal plasma underneath. In carnivores a degree of lipaemia is fairly normal a couple of hours after a meal due to absorption of fats from the small intestine, which is a good reason for avoiding the post-prandial period for routine blood sampling. However, this type of lipaemia is usually fairly trivial, and the really marked white opacities are far more likely to have come from mobilization of fat deposits. Thus prolonged 'starving' to eliminate problem lipaemia is not necessarily the best approach.

There are a number of tricks to deal with a lipaemia problem.

(1)   Always separate lipaemic samples as soon as possible. Lipaemia seems to promote red cell fragility, and lipaemic samples haemolyse readily. If this happens there is probably nothing that can be done to rescue the situation, as even if the lipaemia can be dealt with, the haemolysis itself will prevent analysis.

(2)   Take a larger than usual volume of sample – a 5 ml tube is a good idea. The reason is that if a good volume of plasma can be obtained, and the lipaemia is caused by chylomicrons which rise to the surface on standing, there might be enough clear plasma in the bottom of the tube to enable the analysis to be done. However, there is little chance of this from a small-volume sample.

(3)   Once the plasma is separated, let the tube stand in the fridge overnight – or even for 48 hours (you can do this yourself or ask your laboratory to do it – most laboratories will try this routinely with lipaemic samples that look as if they may be going to settle). If the bottom of the tube does clear, *carefully* pass a pipette through the creamy layer and aspirate the clear plasma for analysis.

(4)   Proprietary 'lipo-clear' preparations are available to dissolve lipaemia in plasma samples. However, they do seem to cause some alteration to the results obtained, and they are best reserved for cases where there is a pressing need for at least an approximate result. For routine case work-up it is better to try other ways round the problem.

(5)   Sometimes a second sample taken a few days (or even better, a couple of weeks) later will prove to be perfectly all right, so if there is no great urgency it is often worth simply waiting.

(6)   Intravenous heparin will usually clear lipaemia *in vivo* by potentiation of lipoprotein lipase, and this is the treatment of choice for hyperlipidaemic horses. In small animals it can be used as a means of obtaining a usable sample. Heparin is injected i/v at a dose rate of 100 iu/kg bodyweight, and the sample collected 15 minutes later. It is fairly rapidly metabolized, and haemostatic problems have not been reported with this procedure (though one allergic reaction is recorded). It is even possible to repeat the injection within a couple of hours if a dynamic test is being performed.

Lipaemia interferes with analysis by changing the optical density of the solution. Effects are most obvious in the protein analyses – total protein often appears improbably high, and the same may be true of albumin. Haemoglobin estimation is also seriously affected, with the result that an impossibly high MCHC is reported.

Waste disposal

Used needles must be put in a rigid, securely closed disposable container (e.g. Cin-bin, Dispo-safe, etc.), preferably after replacing the needle guard. Everything else is treated as contaminated clinical waste.

Jugular blood sampling in small animals

In cats and in all but the largest breeds of dog the cephalic (and saphenous) veins are really too small and thin-walled for blood sampling. If you aspirate too strongly with a syringe (or, even worse, use an evacuated tube) these veins collapse flat and blood flow stops, and it is often very difficult to collect the sample volume required before everything in your syringe simply clots. Monovettes can help, but the sizes available are usually unsuitable for very small dogs and cats, and it can be tricky changing syringes if more than one tube is wanted. Drip-bleeding is sometimes used in an attempt to overcome the problem, but this is a very unsatisfactory technique and should be avoided whenever possible (see p. 246). Animal restraint is also a problem with cephalic samples. Many dogs resent sitting with one forepaw in the air and begin to fidget, and as the venepuncture is performed there is often (especially with cats) a sudden withdrawal reflex which causes the needle to slip out and the vein to 'blow'.

In contrast, the jugular vein is large enough, even in cats, for up to 5 ml of blood to be aspirated in just a few seconds. This minimizes venous stasis and haemolysis, and allows the sample to be transferred to the anticoagulant before it begins to clot. The period of restraint is much shorter and many animals seem to resent the actual position rather less. Withdrawal reflex from the needle occurs much less frequently, and even when it does happen the needle usually stays in the vein. Lastly, a patient which has been sampled from the jugular vein still has two untouched cephalic veins if i/v injection is subsequently required. (The cephalic vein is still the best site for injection because peri-vascualr injection is much more easily seen, and a foreleg is a good place to secure a needle or cannula. Even the thinnest-walled vein will not collapse when you are putting something *in*.)

The usual method of restraint is to have the patient held in a sitting position on the examination table (or even on the floor for a large dog which is nervous on the table) with the head about 45° above the horizontal and turned slightly away from the side of the venepuncture (Fig. 16.3). The vein is raised by placing the left thumb in the lower angle of the jugular groove and can then be located either visually or by palpation with the left forefinger. See also the general points listed on p. 252. It helps to stabilize the vein by laying the left forefinger parallel and to the left of it so that it cannot be pushed aside by the needle point. The needle is inserted point upwards and angled very slightly from right to left so that the vein is fixed between the needle and the left forefinger. As the needle penetrates the skin the syringe plunger is pulled back slightly using the fourth and fifth fingers of the right hand to create a slight vacuum, which makes it very easy to feel when the needle enters the vein. It is preferable to release the venous stasis (left thumb) for a couple of seconds before collecting the sample. As the vein will not collapse even with quite strong back-pressure on the syringe plunger, the required volume of blood can be collected very quickly.

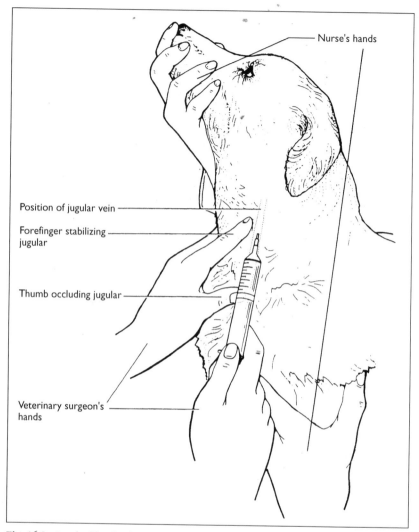

Nurse's hands

Position of jugular vein

Forefinger stabilizing jugular

Thumb occluding jugular

Veterinary surgeon's hands

Fig. 16.3   Jugular blood collection in the dog.

This method of restraint can also be used with very tractable cats, but an alternative technique, which is also useful for small dogs with a tendency to wriggle, is to lay the animal on its side on the examination table with the head extended dorsally. Two helpers are preferable for this procedure, and a small sandbag placed under the neck will help locate the vein. A third possibility (for cats) is to have the seated helper restrain the cat upside-down on his or her lap with the head extending just beyond the helper's knees. It is possible to do this with the cat wrapped in a towel, but specially-made zipped canvas bags are a real advantage. The helper has to confine all four legs and raise the vein, while the person taking the sample kneels in front and positions the head with the left hand. In this method the point of the needle is towards the heart rather than the head, but this is unimportant.

Urine

In direct contrast to human medicine, urine samples are much less easy to obtain than blood samples. Urine collection therefore takes its more appropriate place as a secondary technique in veterinary medicine, used to provide extra information which cannot be obtained from a blood sample, generally after the need for this information has been demonstrated by abnormal blood results. It is not the first line of attack it sometimes becomes (due to ease of sample collection) in human patients. The urine collection method of choice varies with species, as does ease of collection.

Dogs

Male.   Collection is quite easy. The dog may be walked on a lead and a collection vessel (e.g. kidney dish) interposed when he begins to urinate, or else the bladder may be catheterized (which is not difficult even in unsedated dogs).

Female.   Bitches urinate less readily and often squat very low. A flat, shallow collection vessel is an advantage. Bladder catheterization of conscious bitches is difficult.

Cats

Both sexes can be very difficult. Very tolerant individuals may allow a small pot to be placed under them when they are using a litter tray, which will give a fairly clean sample, but this requires guile and vigilance. Often the only practical method is to keep the cat confined with a clean *empty* litter tray or in a clean empty cage with suitable drainage. Samples collected in this way are frequently contaminated. Catheterization of cats is virtually impossible without a general anaesthetic.

Horses

Male.   Collection during natural urination is not usually difficult, but requires patience. Many horses will urinate when first introduced to a freshly bedded loosebox. Alternatively, urine collection harnesses are quite easy to make, but many horses require training to accept these. Tranquillization is necessary before attempting catheterization in stallions and geldings (to relax the penis) and is not recommended unless absolutely unavoidable.

Female.   Again collection during natural urination is fairly easy. Urine collection harnesses for mares are more complicated than for geldings, but catheterization of unsedated mares is quite feasible once the technique has been mastered and provided adequate restraint is available.

Farm animals

The only practical method is simply patience, and having a bucket ready at the crucial moment.

Cystocentesis

This is the technique of passing a needle directly into the bladder through the abdominal wall. It is usually reserved for relieving bladder pressure in severe cases of urethral obstruction. The use of an invasive procedure of this type is very seldom justified simply to secure a urine sample.

Owner-collected samples

It is quite feasible to ask an owner to collect a urine sample, particularly if the sample is not required with any great urgency. However, it is necessary to assure yourself that the owner is competent and not over-fastidious (particularly where small animals are concerned), and to give clear instructions on how to proceed. It is preferable to supply the owner with suitable containers so that you can rely on their cleanliness – several diagnoses of 'diabetes mellitus' have been traced back to unwashed ice cream cartons! Consider also whether an owner-collected sample (perhaps collected in the evening) will be adequately fresh for your purposes by the time it is delivered.

Collection vessels

It is essential that all containers used for urine collection are *clean* and *dry* – this applies to kidney dishes and buckets as well as to the final container. For routine purposes 5 ml or so of urine is adequate, but samples of 15–20 ml in a standard 30 ml universal bottle are easier to handle so far as immersing multiple test strips is concerned. It is important to keep urine samples tightly capped to aid preservation.

Faeces

Where only small quantities are required (e.g. occult blood) a rectal swab is the best method. Where larger quantities are needed these can be obtained *per rectum* from large animals; in small animals, collect (or instruct the owner to collect) freshly passed, uncontaminated faeces which you are *certain* came from the animal in question. Faeces contaminated with earth, grass, bedding or cat litter are not suitable. Always use a clean, dry, wide-mouthed pot for faeces collection – faecal samples are very difficult to remove from narrow-necked bottles, and rectal gloves are not sample containers. Again, it is best to give the owner a suitable container if they are asked to collect the sample.

Other body fluids

Peritoneal fluid

This is not difficult to collect when present in abnormal quantities. It is usually collected from a standing animal. The site of choice is as low down on the abdomen as possible, somewhat to the right of the mid-line (to avoid both the spleen and the falciform fat). Clip up a small area of skin, clean and disinfect as for a surgical operation. Local anaesthetic may be used but is not absolutely necessary. Choose a needle which is long enough to reach the abdominal cavity of the species in question (in horses with ventral oedema a very long needle may be needed); 20G or 21G is quite large enough. It is most satisfactory simply to insert the needle alone and allow the fluid to drip into a collecting tube under its own pressure. Aspiration with a syringe often causes omental fat or intestine to be drawn against the end of the needle, blocking it. If problems are encountered obtaining fluid by this method, there are other tricks to try. One is to restrain the patient on its side and insert needles at four different sites on the abdominal wall – left anterior, left posterior, right anterior and right posterior. Another is to restrain the patient on its back, and pat the abdominal wall gently. This allows the abdominal viscera, which may be blocking the needle, to fall away from the abdominal wall, leaving fluid uppermost. Fluid has to be aspirated with a syringe in this position, but otherwise sampling proceeds as above.

Fluid should be collected into a plain sterile container (glass or plastic). It will not clot, so there is no requirement for an anticoagulant, and as EDTA both interferes with some of the analyses and renders the sample useless for bacteriological culture, it should not be used. Bear in mind that EDTA does not preserve cells, it is merely the anticoagulant which *least damages* cell morphology, and there is no justification for its routine use for non-blood cytology. Some authors have suggested the addition of a small amount of formalin to preserve cytology in fluid samples, but once again this can prevent other analyses such as protein from being carried out, and in fact formalinized samples often seem to have particularly poor cell morphology. 5 ml of fluid ought to be sufficient for all tests which are likely to be required.

Pleural fluid, pericardial fluid and cerebro-spinal fluid

These require specialized sampling techniques which must be mastered before collection is attempted. CSF sampling is carried out under general anaesthesia and should be practised on fresh cadavers before attempting it on a patient.

Sample processing and storage

Samples which are collected because of a need for the results (rather than simply as a means of impressing the owner with your skill and diligence) should not be left to linger and fester in coat pockets, car boots or even fridges. Just as a radiographic procedure is not considered complete until the film has been developed, laboratory sampling procedures are not complete until the sample has been properly dealt with.

Labelling is the first essential, and this should be carried out immediately after collecting the sample. It is not necessary to fill in all the fiddly little boxes printed on many blood collecting tubes. The main essential is to ensure that something is written on the tube which will enable it to be unequivocally matched up with the request form which will accompany it to the laboratory. Ballpoint pens and pencils often write poorly on shiny-surfaced labels, and a fine-pointed, water-resistant marker pen is extremely useful for this job. The *owner's name* is the most usual identification, but where the owner has more than one animal, or where you intend to collect more than one sample from an animal, more detail (*animal identity* or *date/time of day*) will be needed. If there is any possibility of confusion, add also the *nature of the sample*, as things like urine, peritoneal fluid, heparin plasma and fluoride/oxalate plasma may appear grossly similar. Even if the sample is to be individually wrapped with its request form for posting, the labelling should not be omitted. It is unfair (and risky!) to assume that the person opening the package will notice a blank label and rectify it. Be particularly careful with farm animals, or indeed any other situation (such as dog or cat breeders) where one client owns a large number of similar animals. It is absolutely vital both for laboratory records and for your own subsequent reference that you record the animal's own unique identity, either ear tag number or name (it may be necessary to identify a sheep with a spray-on marker). Recording the animal's colour is not sufficient (most Friesians are black and white!), neither is it acceptable to identify the animal by its illness (one hopes it will get better: alternatively, five more like it may be found ill tomorrow!). Even from your own point of view, it is surely desirable to have a definite record of the identity of each patient. It may seem pedantic to belabour these minutiae, but it is a sad fact that every laboratory has its own catalogue of samples rendered useless or even actively misleading by inappropriate or absent identification.

The next step is to fill in a lab request form for the sample. Even if the sample is to be dealt with by your own practice lab, you should have an internal request form to accompany the sample to the lab, as there really is no other way of ensuring that the right tests get done on the right sample (see p. 334). If the correct form is not available it is acceptable to write a letter to accompany the sample (this must include all the information which would normally be entered on a request form), but it is usual to keep a stock of forms to hand for each laboratory you normally deal with. You should not send one of laboratory A's forms to laboratory B, and you should not ask for a test which is not in a laboratory's catalogue unless you have specifically checked that the lab will actually do it. It is discourteous to leave parts of the request form blank: it implies that you have no regard for the ability of the clinical pathologist to help interpret the findings, and it denies laboratory staff the educational opportunities of assessing the full significance of their findings in context. Some of the information is actually necessary for the analysis to be carried out properly. In particular, always ensure that the correct age is filled in – it is absolutely impossible to assess the significance of laboratory findings without having at least some idea of the age of the patient (if the exact age is unknown, at least give some approximate indication). Note also that when the laboratory asks for the species of the patient, they mean the *species* – that is cat, dog, horse, rabbit, tortoise, grey seal, mute swan, rhesus monkey, or whatever. They are not asking for the genus or the family, and while 'canine' or 'feline' are usually unambiguous in companion animal practices (but what does 'Ca' mean?), even 'equine' can cause problems (horse or donkey?), and sesquipedalian obfuscations such as 'chelonion' or 'lagomorph' are simply silly.

Although it may be quite acceptable to ask a nurse to complete the rest of the form, the clinical history should always be entered by the veterinary surgeon, and there is something of an art to doing this effectively. It is not acceptable simply to print out five pages of case records from the computer and staple these to the form – the clinical pathologist just doesn't have time to wade through all that to extract the important information, and may not understand your practice's in-house abbreviations. The best approach is to put yourself in the position of the clinical pathologist. What would *you* like to be told about this animal, in no more than three or four lines? The most important clinical abnormalities, obviously, and also any abnormalities which are *absent* where that is also significant (for example, it can often be illuminating to know that an animal is *not* vomiting, or polydipsic, or coughing, or whatever). The time-course of the condition is also very important. Then, bear in mind the purpose of the request, the question you are asking the laboratory (see p. ix). It is often worth asking this explicitly, as an explicit question is likely to elicit a specific answer, and this can save follow-up phone calls to the laboratory for clarification. Be particularly careful with follow-up requests. 'See previous' may be appropriate if 'previous' was yesterday, and the request is a direct follow-on from that report. However, not only may it not be easy for a laboratory to find a request form from 6 weeks ago, it is pretty much inevitable that the situation will have moved on from then. Always make sure that a clinical history includes the most up-to-date relevant information about the case.

Many laboratory request forms also provide a line to enter differential diagnoses. Note that this means *the conditions you are actually considering in relation to this patient*, including the most obvious one. It doesn't mean 'all the other things it might be, if it isn't what I think it is', and it doesn't mean 'every single possible cause of every single one of this animal's presenting signs'. However, if you already have a confirmed diagnosis and the sample is being sent for some other reason (follow-up, for example), that line should be left blank – the place to write a confirmed diagnosis is in the clinical history section.

It is also important to tell the clinical pathologist about any recent or current treatment which might influence the interpretation of the results.

This doesn't actually take very long to do, and if it is done well then it can save an enormous amount of time later.

If the sample is to be dealt with in the practice, or if your laboratory provides a courier who will be calling later the same day, or if you are arranging another way of hand-delivering the sample to the laboratory (owners may well be willing to do this if a pet is seriously ill), then this may be all you need to do (apart, possibly, from putting the sample and its form in a suitable envelope).

However, if you are sending an owner or someone else to deliver a sample, ensure that the lab is actually open before you send the messenger (it is easy to forget, in the middle of a busy surgery, that it is Saturday, or a Bank Holiday, or 7 o'clock in the evening!), and make sure that he or she knows exactly where to go and who to give the sample to.

If you are posting the sample, or it cannot be delivered or analysed immediately for some reason (because it is Saturday, or a Bank Holiday, or 7 o'clock in the evening) it is certainly possible to do no more than this and either to send it as it is or just leave it lying around until it can be dealt with. However, this course of (in)action is responsible for rendering a horrifyingly large proportion of originally perfectly good samples diagnostically useless. Having taken the trouble to collect your sample, it is always worthwhile to take a little extra trouble to ensure that it arrives at the lab in a fit state to be analysed.

Blood

(1) *Haematology.* The haematological information which is most labile is the morphology of the cells, particularly the white cells. Although dog and cat blood will usually survive overnight in this respect, longer delays (especially involving weekend post) often result in so many degenerate or unrecognizable white cells that a differential count is impossible (see Plate 6b). Horse leucocytes are particularly labile, and a delay of longer than a few hours is likely to destroy their morphology. This can be avoided by making a *good-quality* blood film from the fresh sample and sending that with it. You should also make a smear from any sample which cannot be examined in a practice lab until the next day. The method is detailed on p. 291. Although there is no way of ensuring a reliable numerical platelet count on a sample more than a few hours old, it is much easier to give an intelligent estimate of platelets on a freshly made smear than on a smear of old blood in which the platelets are clumped into 'rafts'. The other obvious alterations with time in a haematology sample are that the erythrocytes swell and the PCV increases slightly, leading to an artificially high MCV and an artificially low MCHC. This effect can theoretically be minimized by leaving the sample exposed to air (leaving the cap off the

tube), but this is impractical. In practice there is little that can be done to preserve the liquid blood for haematology except keep it cool. Whole blood is more stable at +4°C than any other temperature, and so while the sample is on your own premises it should be kept in the fridge. Even refrigerated, however, haematology samples will be deteriorating within 36 hours and are generally useless when over 3 days old.

(2) *Biochemistry.* The main source of sample deterioration, so far as biochemistry tests are concerned, is the red cells, which are simply an unwanted nuisance to be got rid of as soon as possible (see 'Haemolysis', p. 254). The best possible treat you can give your biochemistry sample is to separate it from the red cells immediately after collection and to send only the important bit, the plasma (or serum). If a sample is delayed in the post this will make all the difference between a perfectly usable sample arriving eventually, and a haemolysed mess which is only fit for the bin. Centrifugation is by far the best way of separating plasma, and the possession of a centrifuge for this purpose should be a major priority for all modern practices. The method is detailed on p. 302. It is possible to separate serum from a clotted sample without centrifugation, but for this the blood must be collected into a *glass* tube and allowed to stand at room temperature or better still 37°C for at least 2 hours to allow the clot to form and retract sufficiently. It is best to use a Pasteur pipette to draw off the serum, but it is possible, with care, to pour it into another tube. Obviously with this method it often comes down to sending the blood as it is or missing the post. Horse blood has an unusually high erythrocyte sedimentation rate and a heparinized sample (or one in any other anticoagulant for that matter) which is left upright and undisturbed for about half an hour will settle out so that most of the plasma can be *carefully* pipetted off (not poured). Some cat samples can also be separated in this way.

Whichever method you use, be sure to transfer all necessary sample identification to the plasma/serum tube and also to indicate the nature of the sample (heparin plasma, fluoride/oxalate plasma or serum). Most biochemical constituents are reasonably stable for several days at +4°C, and freezing is usually unnecessary unless samples have to be kept for more than a week. Plasma or serum which has not been centrifuged usually still has a few cells in it and should not be frozen (the lab will centrifuge it on receipt if necessary). *Never attempt to freeze whole blood.*

Note: One enzyme, glutathione peroxidase, is measured not on plasma but on whole blood, and so about 1 ml of the heparinized sample should be taken off into a separate tube before the sample is centrifuged if this test is required.

Urine

There is no reason for not doing dipstix-type tests immediately, and even specific gravity is so easy to measure with a refractometer that there seems very little point in delaying or sending samples elsewhere for these tests. Refrigeration is a two-edged sword as regards urine samples. Sometimes crystals and other sediment components can actually be deleteriously affected by lowering the temperature. However, bacteria can overgrow urine samples at room temperature surprisingly quickly, especially in the summer, and many types of crystal are more likely to stay in crystalline form if the sample is kept cool. Therefore, on balance, it is probably better to store urine samples in the fridge if they cannot be dealt with immediately. Samples which are only required for chemical analysis (protein, phosphate, creatinine, etc.) may be frozen, but freezing will destroy the appearance of the sediment and the cytology.

Faeces

Again, samples may be refrigerated or frozen. Samples for trypsin estimation which cannot be dealt with the same day should always be frozen as this enzyme is fairly labile in faeces.

Other body fluids

No processing is required. These samples may be treated like plasma and kept refrigerated or frozen. However, do not freeze samples which are required for cytology.

Sending samples by post

This is the definitive Murphy's Law situation – anything that can go wrong most certainly will go wrong, if not the first time you make the mistake, at least eventually. Adequate packaging is essential – think about sorting offices, and guard's vans on trains.

Post Office packaging guidelines state that pathological specimens should be packed as follows:

(1) Placed in a securely sealed watertight container not exceeding 50 ml (this is the primary sample pot – note that this prohibits faecal samples, for example, being sent in plastic bags or examination gloves).

(2) Wrapped in enough absorbent material (e.g. cellulose wadding or cotton wool) to absorb all possible leakage in the event of damage.

(3) Sealed in a leak-proof plastic bag (when sending more than one specimen, separate containers with additional absorbent padding).

(4) Placed in either a clip-down container, cylindrical light metal container, strong cardboard box with full-depth lid, or a two-piece polystyrene box with empty spaces filled with absorbent material and the two halves firmly fixed together with adhesive tape.

(5) Padded bag as outer cover clearly labelled in bold capitals '**PATHO-**

LOGICAL SPECIMENS – FRAGILE WITH CARE' and sender's name and address so that Royal Mail can contact them in the event of damage or leakage.

For advice on sending larger specimens and non-standard packaging, customers should contact their Customer Service Centre on 0345 740740.

Certain particularly low-risk samples (microscope slides, *dried* blood samples, specimens fixed in formalin) merely require packaging that is 'robust and fit for the purpose'. Microscope slides should be placed in cardboard or plastic slide mailers (cardboard may have advantages, as plastics can do strange things to air-dried cells), and as formalin itself is hazardous it is preferable to fix histology specimens in the practice and pour off the formalin before posting – if this is impractical, then formalin-containing pots should be *extremely* well wrapped and padded.

Specially manufactured packaging systems which meet UN standard 650 are available to fulfil the requirements, and some laboratories supply these to their clients. However, use of the official standard system is not compulsory, and many laboratories simply supply the outer padded bags, leaving the practices to deal with the inner packaging. Whichever system is in use, it is important to take *great* care to observe the guidelines. In 1998–99 an attempt was made to impose an altogether more stringent packaging standard (UN standard 602) on the profession. This packaging is intended to contain dangerous pathogens (such as HIV) in the event of an explosive decompression at high altitude. It is many-layered, very expensive, very heavy, and the outer boxes have minimum dimensions too great to allow them to be posted in an ordinary pillar-box – they would have to be taken to a post office for despatch. Fortunately this was not implemented at the time, as the consequences for veterinary pathology would have been grave. However, the threat has not necessarily gone away, and it could take just one veterinary surgeon wrapping a sample carelessly to bring the whole thing back down on everyone's heads.

Be careful also to avoid over-wrapping samples. Yards of cellulose tape and dozens of staples are not necessary, and not appreciated by the person unwrapping the thing. It is quite possible for samples themselves to be damaged or spilled when trying to undo over-enthusiastic wrapping. Aim for a package which is both safe in transit and safe and easy to unwrap. Make sure that the correct request form(s) are included in the package, and that these are *outside* the outer plastic bag part of the wrapping so that a leaking sample will not render the form illegible. If you do not have a postage-paid pre-addressed container for the laboratory you are using, make sure that everything necessary (including the laboratory's full address and post code) is clearly written on the label, and that the package is weighed to ensure that the correct first class postage is affixed. Never, ever send laboratory specimens second class.

It is important to consider the time of posting relative to the perishability of the sample. Samples collected too late to catch the last post are better stored in the fridge overnight than allowed to lie in the pillar-box – especially in hot weather. However, the restoration of the Sunday postal collection has been a real boon for practices, and samples which catch that collection have a good chance of being in the laboratory on Monday morning. Bear in mind, however, that Sunday collections are limited and usually confined to main collection points (such as boxes located at post offices). It is advisable to post a notice of last collection times, including time *and place* of Saturday and Sunday collections, in the practice side-room near to where sample wrapping is being carried out. High temperatures are the main enemy of good sample preservation, and summer is the period when most trouble is encountered; however, in very cold weather samples may actually freeze overnight. This will completely wreck whole blood (and cytology), but will not harm anything else – another good reason for separating your biochemistry samples before posting.

First class mail is a good service, and the vast majority of samples posted this way will arrive the following morning. However, for particularly vital samples it is worth utilizing Royal Mail Special Delivery. This requires samples to be taken to a post office before a certain time (usually 4.30–4.45 p.m.), and the payment of a fee of a few pounds in addition to the normal postage, but guarantees next day delivery. Some practices use this service routinely – if a number of samples are being sent in one package it is quite economical, as of course the extra fee applies to the entire package.

Choosing and using an external laboratory

'Veterinary pathology can be practised only by individuals with the appropriate clinical and pathological experience, i.e. veterinary-qualified pathologists. Observance of this principle is in the best interests of animals, because it affects the quality of veterinary practice. Veterinary surgeons who do not follow this principle run additional risks of litigation, since they would be held liable in respect of diagnoses made by non-veterinary-qualified pathologists. These principles have recently been quoted in articles dealing with wider aspects of veterinary pathology and have also been affirmed by the Royal College of Pathologists. The RCVS emphasises to members the importance that it attaches to this principle and its opposition to the practice of veterinary pathology by non veterinary surgeons. The issue is not solely a legal one; it is primarily one in which individual veterinary surgeons should seek the highest possible standards in the best interests of their patients and the public.'

RCVS News, June 1994.

'Diagnostic veterinary pathology is covered by the definition of veterinary surgery and is legally undertaken only by veterinary qualified pathologists. The generation of objective numerical clinical pathology data (for example blood biochemistry and haematology) is acceptable only if it excludes diagnostic interpretation. Surgical and post mortem pathology is inherently diagnostic and is fully within the legal definition of veterinary surgery.'

RCVS Guide to Professional Conduct, 2000.

The message here is perfectly clear. A veterinary surgeon should not be using a non-veterinary laboratory, and this includes laboratories which advertise a 'veterinary' service but have no veterinary surgeon on the staff, and human laboratories, either NHS or private. NHS laboratories are explicitly forbidden by the Department of Health from soliciting veterinary work. Although it is not technically in breach of the Veterinary Surgeons Act for a veterinary surgeon to use a non-veterinary laboratory simply as a number-producer, this is a pretty pointless exercise. No matter what benefit might be gained in terms of speed of availability of results (assuming such a laboratory is very near at hand), it simply isn't worth it. A large component of the service offered by the professional veterinary pathology laboratory is the interpretive and diagnostic advice from the clinical pathologist, and in fact the laboratory is actually the practice's most accessible and frequently used second opinion referral service. It is unrealistic for a general practitioner to expect to be able to make the fullest use of clinical pathology data without specialist advice, and just as you wouldn't dream of referring a case (or sending X-rays or ECG data) to an unqualified person, you should not be telephoning a technician for diagnostic advice which he is, in any case, legally not allowed to give you.

Since the RCVS first began to take a firm line on this matter in 1994 there has been a marked and extremely welcome improvement in the quality of veterinary diagnostic laboratories. Most of the really dubious concerns are no longer in business, and almost all laboratories offering a service to the veterinary profession are now under the direction of a veterinary clinical pathologist. Even the practice in some lay-operated laboratories of referring results to a neighbouring general practitioner for comment has pretty much died out, and it is now normal practice for veterinary pathology to be a full-time speciality covering not just interpretation of results but professional direction of the laboratory as a whole. Thus, when selecting and using a laboratory, it is important to realize that you are dealing with a professional colleague, often a senior and specialist colleague, from whom you are seeking advice. A good relationship based on mutual respect and the exchange of clinical information is enormously advantageous to the practitioner.

There is no question as to whether or not to use an external laboratory. No practice can possibly undertake everything from bacteriology to histopathology to endocrinology, and even where some limited haematology or biochemistry analyses may be available in-house, there are enormous benefits in referring all routine non-emergency investigations. This point is discussed further in Chapter 18, but may be summarized as follows:

(1) Analyses carried out by a professional laboratory are nearly always substantially cheaper than the same analyses carried out using point-of-care analysers.

(2) Reliability of results is inevitably more certain when they come from a professional laboratory which operates strict quality assurance procedures.

(3)   Responsibility, should anything nevertheless go wrong, rests with the laboratory, not the practice.

(4)   The interpretive advice from the clinical pathologist adds a second opinion to case management which can be invaluable.

In addition, the restoration of Sunday postal collection has reduced the weekend mail 'black hole' quite considerably, and the almost universal acquisition of fax machines now allows hard-copy paper reports to be transmitted almost instantaneously. Thus the response time from the professional laboratory is generally better than it was some years ago.

It is of course possible, indeed quite likely, that use will be made of more than one laboratory. A mixed practice may send farm samples in one direction and small animal samples in another. Some laboratories offer particularly specialized services such as endocrinology which may be especially appropriate in certain circumstances. Nevertheless, the bulk of the routine work will tend to go to one place, and even where that laboratory may be referring certain tests on to another in its turn, there is much to be said for having all the laboratory work looked at as a whole by one pathologist rather than sending a little bit here and a little bit there. Consider also that certain privileges such as discount levels or the provision of free couriers may be conditional on a certain volume of work coming to one laboratory, and you may miss out on these all round if you spread your favours too thinly (or try to do too much in-house).

Accreditation of veterinary pathology laboratories is something which has been talked about for decades, but at the time of writing, although the talking is still going on, there is still no scheme in operation. As already said, standards in laboratories have improved very considerably in recent years and there is a good range of reputable establishments to choose from; nevertheless, it is still a case of *caveat emptor*, and the responsibility rests with the veterinary surgeon to choose wisely.

Types of external laboratory

There are a number of different types of external laboratory to choose from, and it is important to weigh up the advantages and disadvantages of each when deciding which to use.

(1)   Veterinary Investigation Centres. Farm work is the *raison d'être* of the VI Centres, and they provide a comprehensive, efficient and high quality service in this area. Although prices have risen in recent years due to a reduction in levels of subsidy, they still represent remarkably good value for the quality of service provided. Considering also the associated advisory service and the depth of local and national epizootiological information available it is difficult to see why a farm practice should choose to do other than make use of this service. It is a sad fact that the number of VI Centres has declined as 'rationalization' exercises necessitated by funding cuts have led to closures. Nevertheless, the backbone

of the service is still there, and it is in the interests of those who rely on its continuation to support it. On the other hand, although the VI Centres will accept samples from any species, companion animal, especially small animal, work is a very different field, and it would be surprising if a service so specialized in one direction should be able to perform equally well in the other. In particular, the areas under discussion, haematology and biochemistry, are generally less sophisticated in VI Centres than in other types of laboratory as it is an undoubted fact that so far as farm work is concerned, microbiology, serology and post-mortem work are much more important. The biochemistry which is done usually concentrates on those tests of particular relevance to farm work. Under these circumstances the VI Centre is not usually the first choice of laboratory for a small animal practice.

(2) Private veterinary laboratories usually specialize primarily in companion animal work, thus complementing the VI Centres. These laboratories are privately run, receive no state subsidy, and operate on a purely commercial basis. This is the area in which the quality of the service is most variable. Laboratories may be wholly-owned veterinary partnerships, or may be owned by a larger corporation. However, the important point is not who owns a laboratory but that it should be under the day-to-day scientific direction of a veterinary clinical pathologist with experience not just in interpreting results but in analytical biochemistry and haematology.

(3) Laboratories attached to large practices, which accept samples from other practices, are really a sub-species of the private laboratory and the points raised under point (2) above are equally applicable to this type of service.

(4) University veterinary schools. All six UK veterinary schools run their own diagnostic laboratories and most will also accept samples from practitioners. There can be no denying the quality of the results generated by these laboratories, which are usually also engaged in research work requiring a high degree of quality control, but there are some drawbacks so far as the private practitioner is concerned. These laboratories are primarily engaged in dealing with clinical samples from the patients on site and so are often not geared up to optimum turnover of outside samples. For example, assay runs are usually not timed to ensure that results catch the post, and very few of these labs work on Saturdays. In addition, when staff have teaching, research and administrative commitments, it can be much more difficult to contact someone to discuss a case. Extra perks such as 'free' postage and packaging materials, provided by most private laboratories, are not usually available. In spite of these factors this can be a useful option, particularly for practices situated close enough to allow hand delivery of samples.

Choosing a laboratory

First, resist the temptation simply to go for the cheapest. In laboratory work, as with everything else, price cuts are usually achieved by cutting corners. Cheaper, less reliable reagents may be used, and quality control and result checking may be omitted. It can, in fact, be quite difficult to compare prices, as laboratories which seem more expensive at first glance may have discount schemes for heavy users or reduced prices for follow-up tests which even out the difference. In addition, quoted prices for individual biochemistry tests are very seldom actually paid by anyone, and it is the prices within the commonly used profiles which are the important thing. Some laboratories will make an extra charge for clinical interpretation, while with others this is seen as an integral part of the normal service. Bear in mind, however, that laboratory work is (within reason) not desperately price-sensitive, and it makes much better clinical sense to choose on quality of service.

If you are fortunate to be close enough to a laboratory which provides a courier service then, all else being reasonably equal, it makes a great deal of sense to take advantage of this. Even without this service, being close enough to be able to send an owner or a courier of your own to deliver an emergency sample is a big advantage. However, beyond this distance location is of little concern. Postal services cover the entire country, and a sample from the north of Scotland has as good a chance of arriving the next day at a lab in the south of England as one from the next county. The only thing to be careful about is that certain postal routes seem to be particularly troublesome, and if you find that a particular lab is in a 'black hole' from your own location it may be that another (perhaps more distant) will be more suitable.

Virtually all laboratories will provide postage-paid packaging of one sort or another. Some will also provide other 'free' items such as sample tubes or even items of office equipment. However, once again you tend to get what you pay for, there is very seldom such a thing as a free lunch, and this sort of peripheral ought not to be allowed to sway a judgement which should be made on quality.

The quality of private laboratories has improved a great deal over the past 10 years or so, and it is rare to encounter the major solecisms which point to ignorance of up-to-date practice. Nevertheless, it is still worth nothing some points of which to beware.

(1) Incorrect or outdated terminology such as albumen for albumin, BUN for urea or SGOT/SGPT for AST/ALT.
(2) Non-SI units, e.g. g/100 ml (or g/dl) where you would expect mmol/l.
(3) Lack of provision of calculated values such as MCV/MCHC and absolute differential white cell counts.
(4) Improbable or impossible results being reported without comment. For example, MCV and MCHC results which are quite impossible for the species indicate serious inaccuracies within a haematology system, dog basophils are *very* seldom seen, and a potassium concentration of over 10 mmol/l is unlikely to be compatible with life.

(5)   Improbable significant figures, e.g. the reporting of a second decimal place in urea or glucose measurements. No assay is that precise, and reporting such figures reveals a fundamental misunderstanding.

(6)   Improbable reference values – for example, something like 0.00–12.00 mmol/l for dog urea, when you know that about 3–8 mmol/l would be far more reasonable. Improbable significant figures in reference values is another point – it is quite ridiculous to give the upper limit for glucose (say) as 5.83, implying that 5.84 is somehow 'abnormal', when the measurement itself cannot be that precise.

(7)   Reporting of tests alphabetically. Related tests should be grouped together, and although groupings may vary between laboratories, the choice should be reasonable.

Any laboratory that perpetrates these types of solecism is best avoided.

Attitude to spoiled samples is important. It is very tempting to praise a laboratory which gives you results every time, and to damn and blast one which returns forms as unable to test due to clotting (of haematology samples), haemolysis or lipaemia. However, a moment's thought demonstrates the fallacy there. It is certainly not to the advantage of a laboratory to refuse to analyse a sample, as they will lose the fee by doing this, but a reputable establishment will not report (potentially misleading) results from an unsuitable sample. Rather than criticizing this practice, it should be viewed as evidence of professionalism. Labs do *not* haemolyse samples or cause previously liquid samples to clot, and if you are experiencing this sort of problem you should be re-examining your sample processing procedures rather than shooting the messenger.

Design of test profiles should be intelligent and helpful. Many laboratories have adopted the approach outlined earlier in this book whereby the most useful tests to cover all the relevant differential diagnoses implied by particular presenting signs are grouped together. Well-designed profiles simplify test requesting, facilitate organization of the laboratory workload, facilitate interpretation, and discourage the parsimonious habit of requesting only one or two tests on a sample (which is often counterproductive as so little information is generated). It is impossible to lay down rigid rules about what should or should not be included, but if tests you would normally find yourself requesting as a group in a free-choice system are included in a profile, this is a good start. Beware the laboratory which insists you have analyses done which aren't appropriate for most patients, or which groups exclusively large-animal tests in the same profile as exclusively small-animal tests. Very long lists of tests are bad news, even if they seem like a bargain. The chance of relevant abnormalities being swamped in a huge amount of extraneous detail is quite high.

However, the most important asset of any laboratory is its people. Look for postgraduate qualifications among the veterinary staff, with scientific or academic qualifications (e.g. PhD, MSc, MRCPath, etc.) being more relevant than purely clinical certificates or diplomas, as it is important that a pathologist has expertise on the technical and analytical side as well as in interpreting the results. Technical staff with degrees or appropriate diplomas are also found in practically all high-quality laboratories.

If possible, try to arrange a visit to a laboratory you intend to use. Most laboratories are happy to welcome clients or potential clients, and it is always easier to assess a situation at first-hand. It is also easier to strike up a relationship with colleagues you have actually met.

Perhaps the most important thing of all is the relationship between the practice and the clinical pathologists. Are the comments and interpretations on the report forms constructive and appropriate? Is it possible to talk to the person concerned to discuss the case further – or to discuss a case even before the samples are sent in? Are such conversations useful and constructive, and do you have confidence that the person you are talking to really is an expert in the subject? Some laboratories operate a premium-rate telephone line service for interpretation and advice, while others offer this as part of the service without further charge. Only you can decide whether you are getting your money's worth from the former service.

Using an external laboratory

Once you are using the laboratory, try to keep up a two-way communication. Make a habit of supplying good clinical histories, and if further information is requested, supply that too. Respond positively to suggestions for improving sample collection or processing procedures. If you need further help, telephone, or send a fax or an email. If you are unsure of the most appropriate tests to request on a particular patient, ask, preferably before you collect the sample – this is much more constructive than guessing, and having to back-track later. Regular, routine communication is the best way to maximize the usefulness of any laboratory service, and to head off potential misunderstandings and disagreements before they arise. Bear in mind also that the clinical pathologist will welcome feedback, and if the final outcome of a case in which the laboratory has been particularly involved comes from another source (such as exploratory surgery), then an update will always be appreciated.

Finally, if you have any reason to suspect a laboratory error, contact the laboratory about it as soon as possible. No reputable laboratory will ever object to a reasonable request to check something, and it is always better to be safe than sorry. However, after a week or so, deteriorating samples and discarded samples may mean that it is impossible to be absolutely certain what (if anything) has happened. Not only that, if an error may have caused two patients' results to be transposed, it is vital that someone is alerted as soon as possible so that the other party to the mistake, who may have accepted the erroneous results without suspicion, can be advised of the situation.

Side-room Testing in the Veterinary Practice

Purpose and scope

The first and most important thing to understand is that a 'practice lab' and a professional pathology laboratory are two very different things, with different objectives. The professional laboratory offers a comprehensive in-depth analytical service aimed at allowing as full a work-up as may be necessary for each case, with particular attention being paid to accuracy and reliability. It is virtually impossible to duplicate this sort of service within a practice. Many procedures are simply beyond the scope of the practice side-room, many of the side-room methods which are available offer accuracy only of the 'approximate emergency guesstimate' standard, and attempts to offer even a partial 'routine' service within the practice inevitably generate overall costs which are substantially greater than the prices charged by the professional laboratories for an equivalent service.

Nevertheless, the practicalities of sample transport mean that in a genuine emergency some results may be required more quickly than they can be obtained from the professional laboratory, and in this situation approximate answers can certainly be better than none at all. In addition, simple monitoring of patients on treatment (such as diabetic monitoring) and some simple tests which are better performed on fresh samples (such as urinalysis) are well within the scope of the practice side-room. Thus the side-room should be seen as a complementary facility, specializing in the art of 'point-of-care testing', that is quick, simple and highly relevant tests which, though often somewhat approximate, can give invaluable information to help in decision-making *before* the results of the full laboratory investigations are available, or occasionally to help decide if there is, in fact, a need to proceed to a full laboratory work-up of a case. Such a facility requires little capital equipment, little in the way of expensive reagents, and the skills required are easily within the reach of the busy general practitioner and veterinary nurse. It is also highly cost-effective.

The other main function of the side-room is sample preparation and despatch, as described in the previous chapter. In fact the two functions fit well together – if one is in the habit of making blood films to send with haematology requests, it becomes quite a simple matter to take a quick look at a film in passing, and once plasma has been separated to send away for biochemistry it is easy to divert a few microlitres in the direction of the refractometer or the Merckognost strips in appropriate circumstances.

Haematology

This is an area where side-room tests can be extremely informative, yielding a comparable amount of information to a full haematology report, though sometimes in a qualitative rather than a quantitative sense. The two main procedures are PCV measurement by microhaematocrit and examination of a blood film.

PCV

The microhaematocrit measurement is accurate, it is employed by many professional laboratories and is arguably superior to machine-generated haematocrit results derived arithmetically from RBC count and MCV measurements. In addition to measuring the PCV, it is useful to record the colour of the plasma (icteric, lipaemic, haemolysed), and to note if the buffy coat (the layer of white cells between the plasma and red cell layers) is unusually thick.

Blood film examination

This is the central pillar of haematological investigation, whether in the practice side-room or the professional laboratory, and yields an enormous amount of information. Making a blood smear is *not* difficult, the skill is easily acquired with a little practice, and once acquired will not be lost. Rapid haemocytological stains are available which are very easy to use, simply requiring the slide to be dipped in three solutions in succession. Thus haemocytology is well within the scope of any practice with a microscope. Anyone who encourages you to believe that this is difficult or cumbersome and suggests an alternative 'easier' way of doing it, probably has something to sell you!

Information which can be gained from blood film examination includes the following:

(1)   Red cell morphology, including assessment of degree of regeneration present, degree of hypochromasia, and any abnormal forms such as spherocytes or leptocytes.

(2)   Qualitative assessment of platelet numbers, and any morphological abnormalities such as macro-platelets.

(3)   Approximate qualitative assessment of white cell numbers (it is useful to compare this guess with the thickness of the buffy coat).

(4)   Percentage differential white cell count, though the absence of a quanti-

tative total white cell count makes any attempt to express results as absolute numbers fraught with difficulty.

(5)   Presence of diagnostically significant or abnormal cells, such as juvenile/ band neutrophils, toxic neutrophils, reactive lymphocytes, atypical or leukaemic lymphocytes, or even mast cells in a systemic mastocytosis.

(6)   Presence of blood parasites.

White cell counting

The real deficiency in this system is the total white cell count. With practice, it is certainly possible to make an intelligent guess which may be sufficient for emergency use. However, it is helpful to have the capability of performing a haemocytometer white cell count, even if this is only used occasionally. (Staff competence can be checked and maintained by performing the count from time to time on a sample being submitted to the professional laboratory.)

Other haematology methods

Bleeding time, clotting time and clot retraction are all tests which have to be performed in the presence of the patient, and all are easily within the capability of the practice side-room. Cross-matching of blood for transfusion is not difficult, but it is labour-intensive and time-consuming. The card-presentation blood typing kits for dogs and cats are intended for practice side-room use and may eliminate the need for performing cross-matching.

Thus it is possible to obtain a good approximation to almost all the information on a haematology report, in the side-room, quickly and easily, without any capital equipment apart from the microhaematocrit centrifuge and the microscope, and without the need for expensive reagents.

Plasma biochemistry tests

This discipline is not as well served by side-room tests as haematology; nevertheless, about half a dozen methods are available, and those tend to be the analytes which are of most immediate relevance in the near-patient situation. The methods were, of course, originally developed for human use, but all give useful results on animal samples, at least as an interim measure.

The main item of capital equipment required is the centrifuge, as very few tests can be performed on whole blood. However, this is in any case an essential item of practice equipment. Many practices employ one dual-purpose centrifuge which will perform a microhaematocrit and separate plasma or serum for biochemistry. Although these can only handle small-volume tubes (about 1.5 ml), they are generally perfectly adequate for the purpose – two tubes can be used for patients with particularly high PCVs.

Total protein

This is performed by refractometry, and it is important when purchasing a refractometer to ensure that it has a total protein scale engraved as well as the scales for specific gravity and refractive index. No consumables are required. Total plasma protein agrees well with refractive index in a clear sample, but note that lipaemia and/or haemolysis will lead to erroneously high results. Peritoneal and pleural fluid protein can also be estimated on the refractometer, although very low-protein fluids (below about 5 g/l) may also be checked on the protein patch of a urine dipstick. Most refractometer protein scales are given in grams per 100 ml, so it is necessary to multiply the reading by ten to derive a result in grams per litre.

Urea

A side-room screening test based on a chromatographic reaction is available (Merckognost, Merck). This is more labour-intensive than the simple colour-comparison strips, but it is designed for side-room use by nurses, and results correlate quite well with standard laboratory methods. The test requires no laboratory instrumentation.

A very quick colour-comparison urea test using whole blood is also available (Azostix, Bayer; formerly manufactured by Ames), but the colour-comparison chart has only four patches, graded 2–5 mmol/l, 5–9 mmol/l, 10–14 mmol/l and 18–28 mmol/l; in fact, the maximum colour block should simply be graded as >18 mmol/l. Thus it provides no more than a quick indication of whether the urea is normal or elevated, with little differentiation between the merely raised and the very high. A useful strategy is to use the Azostix as a screen (they can be used during a consultation if necessary, as the test takes only 1 minute), and then use the Merckognost test to obtain a more accurate result on separated plasma whenever the Azostix indicates that an abnormality is present.

Although an exact 'urea meter' analogue of the glucose meters described below does not exist, urea results from reflectance meters (dry-reagent analysers) are respectably accurate on non-human blood. Two or three such instruments are on the market and are well worth considering as an alternative to messing around with paper strips. The machines which are capable of analysing whole blood are especially attractive in this context. It makes sense to choose the simplest instrument available – many of the other dry-reagent methods do not perform particularly well on non-human blood (see p. 321), and the temptation to extend the use of reflectance meters to analytes such as protein or enzymes is best avoided.

Glucose

The widespread use of home blood testing by human diabetics has led to an explosion in availability of pocket glucose meters, some of which are extremely cheap. These meters use fresh whole blood (though they will also read fluoride plasma), and results on non-human samples are satisfactory. The main application is, of course, in monitoring diabetic patients on treatment, and also in monitoring patients on fluid therapy (particularly where a dextrose-containing fluid is being given). Some caution should be exercised in using glucose meters for primary diagnosis – an immediate result is of course very valuable, but this should normally be regarded as an interim figure to be checked by the professional laboratory in due course. Naturally there will be cases where there is little or no doubt about the result, especially the patient who is grossly diabetic on first presentation, but odd things do happen sometimes, and in particular all apparent hypoglycaemias must be checked professionally. The phenomenon of 'glucose meter non-hypoglycaemia' (spurious diagnosis of hypoglycaemia caused by an under-reading glucose meter), well recognized in human medicine, is even more common in veterinary practice!

Blood glucose strips may also be read by eye against a colour comparison chart on the bottle. This can give extra information in very marked hyperglycaemias, as the meters usually read only to about 25 mmol/l, while the colour blocks go up to about 44 mmol/l.

Ketones

While urine is the preferred sample for checking for ketosis, in the absence of a urine sample a drop of *plasma* (not blood!) may be applied to the ketone patch of a urine dipstick for a qualitative result.

Cholesterol

Strip tests for cholesterol are available on the human market for use in clinics screening for coronary artery disease risk factors, but this is not a test of great relevance to the veterinary side-room situation, where cholesterol is not an emergency requirement.

Triglycerides

Hypertriglycerideaemia causes lipaemia, the milky/cloudy suspension which appears in some blood samples. This is readily appreciated by eye. Note that if the milky suspension rises to the top when the sample is left standing overnight, the cause is chylomicrons in the plasma, while lipaemia which does not separate on standing is due to free triglycerides. Practical diagnostic use is mainly confined to the horse, where hyperlipidaemia is a serious clinical concern, but it can also be helpful when performing a fat absorption test (see p. 133).

Bilirubin

Bilirubin is yellow, and easily appreciated as icterus in a plasma sample. With a little practice it is quite easy to grade the gross appearance as slightly/moderately/markedly icteric, and draw appropriate interim conclusions. Subtle changes in the shade of yellow may also give useful information; for example, haemolytic jaundice is often a light primrose shade, while liver disease can have a more orange appearance. Bilirubinometers which give a numerical result are available, but these are produced for use in paediatric intensive care, and are quite unnecessary in the veterinary practice side-room.

Note, however, that equine plasma always appears icteric to a greater or lesser extent, as the normal plasma bilirubin concentration is much higher than in other species, and that bovine plasma is also yellow in appearance (due to the presence of β-carotene) which makes icterus difficult to appreciate in this species.

Electrolytes

The obvious deficiency in the above list is sodium and potassium. Electrolyte measurement is such an important part of emergency and critical care that serious consideration must be given to acquiring the means of measuring these constituents.

The most accurate of the methods available for point-of-care use is the ion specific electrode (ISE). A range of such machines is available, many intended for near-patient use in human operating theatres or intensive care units and thus designed for use by appropriately trained nursing staff. However, these instruments are in a different class from the glucose meter or the refractometer, and staff who will be operating them need to be trained to a fairly high technical standard. Obsessive attention to calibration and quality control is also essential.

Electrolyte estimations are also available in conjunction with some reflectance meter systems, using dry-reagent or potentiometry methods; however, these are less well characterized than ISE technology for animal use and should be regarded merely as a very approximate guide.

Electrolyte analysers, whether ISE or other methodology, which accept samples as whole blood are particularly attractive for emergency or critical care use. However, it is very easy for haemolysis to go unrecognized in such a sample, and the resulting artefactual results (especially erroneously high potassium concentrations) to be interpreted clinically. Great care must be exercised to avoid this problem.

Critical-care meters

Reflectance-meter-type analysers have been developed for near-patient critical care testing in human medicine. Intended more for the accident and emergency department than the intensive care unit, and using whole blood as a sample, they may prove to be suitable for the veterinary practice. A range of tests is available in a variety of combinations, including urea, glucose, electrolytes, blood gases and haemoglobin. However, although they are marketed to veterinary practices, there are no method comparison data available to demonstrate accuracy on non-human blood. The methodology is also significantly more expensive than other side-room tests.

Urinalysis

Urine analysis is seldom an emergency requirement; nevertheless, the techniques involved are very simple and there is great advantage in examining a fresh sample. pH tends to increase with the age of the sample, crystals can redissolve, contaminant bacteria can overgrow the specimen, and the incidence of spurious colour changes on strip tests increases in old samples.

Specific gravity

The preferred method is refractometry, using the same instrument as for total plasma protein. The test is very quick, only a couple of drops of sample are required, and there are no consumables. The urinometer method (a graduated float) is also accurate, but comparatively messy and awkward to read, and requires a fairly large volume of sample to float the instrument. If you have urine dipstix which include a specific gravity reagent patch, *never use these under any circumstances* – the method is only valid for human urine and gives completely misleading results in animal samples. Obliterate the SG part of the colour comparison chart or scrape the patches off the strips if you have to!

Chemical strips

Several manufacturers, principally Bayer (formerly Ames) and Roche (strips formerly made by Boehringer), make a range of single or multiple urine test strips designed for various applications in human medicine. Unfortunately no one makes anything specifically for the veterinary market, but it is not difficult to make an appropriate selection. Perhaps the most useful multiple test combination is the 'Nephur-6-Test' (Roche). This includes:

pH (five blocks reading from pH 5 to pH 9)
Glucose (five blocks reading from zero to 55 mmol/l)
Leucocytes (four blocks reading from zero to about 0.5×10^9 WBCs per litre)
Nitrite (negative/positive reading)
Protein (four blocks reading from zero to 5 g/l)
Blood/haemoglobin (five blocks reading from zero to about 0.25×10^9 RBCs per litre, with some indication as to whether erythrocytes or free haemoglobin are present).

Many people also prefer the Roche strips because of the membrane over the reagent patches which aids colour matching, and because the timing of the various readings and the layout of the colour-comparison chart is simpler than with other manufacturers. In addition, they do not include the potentially misleading specific gravity patch.

The other useful combination for veterinary use is the 'Keto-Diabur-Test' (Roche). This consists of:

Glucose (eight blocks reading from zero to 280 mmol/l, more quantitative than the general strips)
Ketones (four blocks, reading negative to +++).

This is mainly required for the ketone block, which can be used with milk or plasma if a urine sample is unavailable.

Other analytes are available, but these can be associated with some problems:

Specific gravity. See above, this method is *invalid* in non-human urine.
Bilirubin. This can be helpful, but can also be misleading – some bilirubin can be found in normal canine urine, and false positive results are common in stale samples. In addition, strips with bilirubin always seem to include urobilinogen, which is not wanted.
Urobilinogen. Once again, this analyte is only of use in human medicine, and should not be included in a veterinary investigation. However, a strange colour change on the urobilinogen patch often signals that the strips have passed their expiry date!

Sediment examination

This is carried out by direct (unstained) microscopy of a drop of urine sediment, usually prepared by centrifuging the urine sample at 1500 rpm for about 2–3 minutes and pouring off the supernatant. Structures which can be recognized include erythrocytes, leucocytes, epithelial cells, various sorts of crystal, various sorts of casts, and even bacteria. Sediment examination is more reliable than the chemical strip in picking up leucocytes (the strip does produce both false positives and false negatives occasionally), and visualizing erythrocytes under the microscope is a much better way of distinguishing between blood and haemoglobin than trying to decide if the pattern on the reagent patch is uniform or stippled.

Professional laboratories also offer this investigation, and there is certainly something to be said for having the experienced technician examine your samples. In addition, some practices find it difficult to prepare the sample, as the high-speed microhaematocrit centrifuges often used as general side-room workhorses are not particularly suitable for this purpose. Nevertheless, the advantages of examining a fresh sample are considerable, and it is helpful to have the capability of performing the examination in the side-room. (Unfortunately it is not possible to make the preparation in-house and send it to the lab for examination, as the wet preparation will dry out and become unrecognizable in transit).

Pleural and peritoneal fluids

Many of the estimations which are useful in identifying these fluids can usefully be carried out in the side-room, often by minor adaptations of methods in use for blood or urine analysis.

Physical description. This should *always* be recorded by the person collecting the sample.
Protein. In a *clear* sample, a refractometer protein reading will give a reasonable approximation. Very-low-protein samples (recognizable by the fact that they froth little or not at all on shaking) may be cross-checked using the protein patch of a urine dipstick.
Cytology. A stained smear of the fluid can be examined in the same way as a blood film, and an actual count may be estimated using a haemocytometer if required.
Chyle. The rough 'chyle test' described on p. 178 can be performed in the side-room with appropriate safety precautions.
Urea. Beware of assuming that an ascitic fluid is urine simply from a 'high' reading on an Azostix strip or even the Merckognost – urine will have a urea concentration *substantially* greater than the concurrent plasma urea concentration. It may be necessary to dilute the sample to be certain.
Bilirubin. Once again, beware of assuming that an ascitic fluid is bile simply because it looks very yellow – jaundiced patients will have jaundiced body fluids, and neat bile appears almost black.

Again, all these tests, to a higher standard of accuracy and using more sophisticated methodology, are offered by the professional laboratories. If there is no great urgency there is much to be said for simply sending the sample off and letting them get on with it. Nevertheless, the methods described here are simple and can be very helpful even if only as an interim guide.

Cerebro-spinal fluid

Many of the methods listed above for peritoneal and pleural fluids are also applicable to CSF – protein using a urine dipstick, cytology of a stained smear, a white cell count can be performed by putting a drop of the fluid neat on a haemocytometer slide, and glucose can be estimated using a blood glucose meter. It is good practice when collecting a CSF sample to have a quick look at it in the side-room before sending it off to the laboratory, as examination of a fresh sample may reveal information which can be obscured by the time the sample has reached the laboratory.

Faeces

In a word, don't bother. Samples are messy and unpleasant to handle, and tests such as faecal trypsin or undigested food elements are not especially helpful in emergency situations. In addition, the most useful and commonly requested test on faeces (at least in small animal practice) is bacteriology, which is not a side-room test by any stretch of the imagination. Even parasitology, which is not particularly difficult, is hardly ever an emergency requirement. The sensible approach is simply to pack the samples securely and let the laboratory worry about the smell and the mess.

Virus serology

As this book went to press, an independent study revealed that (contrary to the assumptions in Chapter 13) current side-room FeLV kits miss one in 3 to one in 12 infected cats. FIV performance is a little better, but several kits still miss around one in 10 antibody-positive cats. The rationale for their use therefore seems very questionable. The side-room FIP tests should be avoided – again, this is not an emergency requirement, and this is a test which should definitely be left to the professionals.

Summary

A respectable range of emergency biochemistry estimations, some quantitative, some semiquantitative and some qualitative, is available to the veterinary surgeon without any great investment in capital equipment and without any need for special analytical expertise. As far as costing is concerned, the principles outlined on p. 312 also apply to the side-room emergency facility. However, capital investment is small, reagent costs are small, and most tests are quick to perform. Thus it is relatively simple to make such a facility pay for itself without greatly increasing the cost to the client.

Appendix I: Useful side-room methods

Haematology methods

Packed cell volume

The standard microhaematocrit is the method of choice for all veterinary laboratories. Several different systems are available for sealing the end of the capillary tube:

(1)   Heat sealing in a bunsen flame is the method of choice if mains gas is available.

(2)   Proprietary clay sealers (Cristaseal, Crit-o-seal, etc.) are the next best

thing, but the seal is not so reliable and the occasional tube will 'spin out' no matter how careful you are. They are no quicker than method (1), and so safer, as it is just as easy to break a tube in your fingers while twisting it into the clay pad as it is to burn your fingers when touching a newly heat-sealed tube.

(3) Machines are available which self-seal the tubes by pressing them against a rubber pad, but this method is very prone to leaks, especially as the rubber pad ages. In addition, results have to be read with the tubes still in the machine, against a printed scale. This is unreliable, especially if tube filling is not uniform.

(4) A miniature battery-operated version of method (3) has been marketed, but it is very fiddly to use, hard on batteries, and has poor precision and accuracy due to the short capillary tubes. Not recommended unless freedom from an electricity supply is essential.

Materials required

Sample of whole blood in anticoagulant (usually EDTA, but heparin will do)

Capillary tubes
Tissues
Bunsen burner and matches (or, if no gas supply, pad of clay sealer)
Microhaematocrit centrifuge
Microhaematocrit reader

Procedure

(1) Mix blood thoroughly by repeated inversion or rotary mixer.

(2) Remove cap and tilt sample so that a clear surface without bubbles can be seen. (Bubbles cause an air-lock in the capillary and make filling difficult.) Place end of capillary tube in blood and tilt sample tube further so that capillary can be held almost horizontally. Allow capillary tube to fill to two-thirds to three-quarters of its length with blood (the reader requires a column of blood 4–7 cm long).

(3) Wipe blood from outside of capillary tube.

(4) Hold capillary tube horizontally between thumb and first two fingers, with palm of hand facing upwards, and gently rotate it between the fingers. Gradually touch the very tip of the end with *no* blood in it to the edge of a hot bunsen flame, rotating it all the time. Only 1 mm of the capillary tube should touch the flame, and less than 5 seconds is required to seal it. If blood bubbles or turns brown, discard tube and start again. (It is important that the end of the capillary which is to be sealed is *completely* free of blood, so be careful not to let the blood run from one end to the other before sealing.)

(5) Hold capillary tube vertically, sealed end down. If blood column

immediately drops to the bottom, the seal is incomplete – discard tube and start again.

(6) Check that sealed end is both flat and symmetrical (see Fig. 17.1). Do *not* attempt to spin a misshapen tube. It is liable to break in the centrifuge and cause serious damage; if it survives it will give an inaccurate reading.

(7) Place tube in any groove in the centrifuge rotor, sealed end out. It is not necessary to balance tubes across the axis. If several tubes are being spun together make a note of the number of the groove each one is in.

(8) Screw inner lid down on rotor so that screw is finger tight. *Do not forget this step – you will regret it!*

(9) Close outer hinged lid. Make sure centrifuge is plugged in and mains switch is on. Turn timer to 6. Do something else for 6 minutes.

(10) Do *not* use the brake button to stop the centrifuge – it can damage the motor. Allow it to stop naturally.

(11) Remove the capillary tube from the centrifuge and check the colour of the plasma (haemolysed? icteric? lipaemic?) and the thickness of the buffy coat. Make a note of your observations.

(12) Place the capillary tube in the groove on the cursor of the micro-haematocrit reader. Adjust it vertically so that the bottom of the red cell layer is level with the bottom ('0') *line* (not the edge of the black area). Move cursor horizontally until the top of the plasma layer is level with the top ('100') *line* (not the edge of the black area). Adjust white reading line (knob on left) so that it passes through the buffy coat (the buffy coat/red cell junction if buffy coat is very thick). Read off result on scale at right-hand side (Fig. 17.2).

(13) Write down the result. The reader expresses it as a percentage, but the modern trend is to use a decimal fraction. Either will do.

(14) Clean up any spilled blood (cold water is best). Discard all used capillary tubes to glass bucket, and all tissues and used matches to yellow plastic bag. Make sure cap is replaced on sample tube and it is either discarded in the yellow plastic bag (glass bucket for Vacutainers) or placed in the fridge if not required again immediately. Put everything else back where you found it.

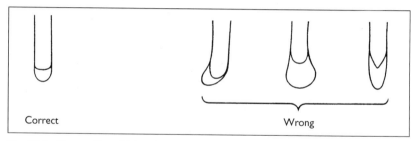

Correct   Wrong

Fig. 17.1   Heat sealing of PCV tubes.

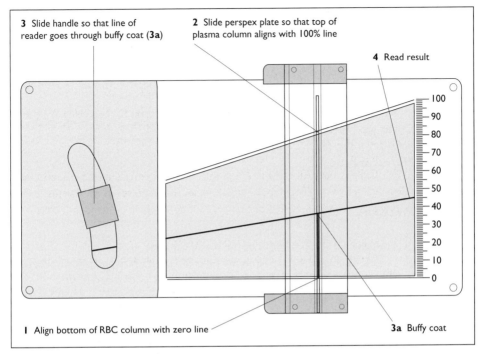

3 Slide handle so that line of reader goes through buffy coat (**3a**)

2 Slide perspex plate so that top of plasma column aligns with 100% line

4 Read result

— 100
— 90
— 80
— 70
— 60
— 50
— 40
— 30
— 20
— 10
— 0

1 Align bottom of RBC column with zero line

3a Buffy coat

Fig. 17.2   Microhaematocrit reader.

Note: A full 6 minutes is required to pack non-human erythrocytes properly; be sure to spin for the full period.

White cell counting

Although a rough guess at a total white cell count may be made from the appearance of the blood film and the thickness of the buffy coat, it is useful to have the capability to carry out a chamber count if required.

Haemocytometer kits are still often sold complete with two bulb pipettes to perform the red and white cell dilutions. These are very difficult to use accurately, and a nightmare to clean. It is much better to substitute a more accurate dilution procedure, though that does mean acquiring some sort of pipette capable of dispensing 0.95 ml (either a graduated glass pipette or a variable automatic pipette – see Chapter 18, Appendix III, for operation of automatic pipettes) into individual test-tubes (preferably tubes with caps; plastic centrifuge tubes will do), and either some 50 µl disposable capillary pipettes or a 50 µl automatic pipette.

Materials required

Sample of whole blood in EDTA
50 µl disposable capillary pipettes (green band)

Rubber mouthpiece for pipette

Tissues

Plastic tube containing 0.95 ml of Turck's fluid (capped). (It will save time if a batch of these is prepared in advance every week or so, but note that Turck's fluid is very susceptible to fading if exposed to light and so should always be stored in the dark)

Improved Neubauer haemocytometer slide (mirrored backed ones are best)

Cover slips at least 22 × 22 mm in size

Capillary tubes (i.e. PCV tubes)

Microscope

Procedure

(1) Make a 1 in 20 dilution of the blood sample.
   (a) Remove the cap from the tube of Turck's fluid and place it where it won't get knocked over. If no tubes with Turck's fluid already measured out are available you will have to dispense 0.95 ml from the stock bottle into a clean tube using a glass pipette.
   (b) Fit the disposable pipette (the end with the green band) into the plastic mouthpiece holder.
   (c) Mix blood thoroughly by repeated inversion or rotary mixer.
   (d) Remove cap from sample and place end of capillary pipette in blood. Put the other end of the mouthpiece in your mouth and by gentle suction draw the blood into the pipette until it is just above the black graduation line. Do not allow the blood to disappear up the pipette and into the rubber tube.
   (e) Remove the pipette from the sample and wipe all the blood from the outside. Then gently blot the end of the pipette until the end of the column of blood is *exactly* on the black line.
   (f) Place end of pipette in the tube of Turck's fluid (under the surface) and gently blow the 50 µl of blood into the solution. Then wash out the pipette with the solution by gently sucking fluid into the pipette and expelling it four or five times. Again take care that the solution does not get sucked into the rubber tube.
   (g) Remove the pipette from the tube, cap the tube and mix it thoroughly. Leave it to stand for 10 minutes to allow the red cells to be completely destroyed and the white cells to take up the stain. During this time, proceed with (h) and step (2).
   (h) Make sure cap is replaced on blood sample. Discard used capillary pipette to glass bucket and wash and dry rubber mouthpiece.
(2) Fit coverslip to haemocytometer slide to form a chamber of precise depth.
   (a) Make sure haemocytometer slide is clean.
   (b) Run your thumbs along the glass of the side sections, next to the

grooves (where you want the Newton's rings to appear). This makes it slightly greasy and helps the cover slip to stick.

(c) Remove a coverslip from the box without touching the centre and place it so that it half overlaps the area of the grid on the haemocytometer slide.

(d) Holding the slide firmly in both hands, use both thumbs to slide the coverslip towards a central position, pressing down firmly all the time. When you feel the resistance of the glass increase, Newton's rings are probably present. If the cover slip cracks, discard it and start again with a new one. *Take great care during this procedure not to scratch the mirrored surface of the slide!*

(e) Angle the slide up to the light to check for the presence of Newton's rings somewhere on each side of the cover slip (see Fig. 17.3). They look like fine rainbow stripes and they demonstrate that the two layers of glass are properly stuck together. Only when they are present is the chamber of the haemocytometer the correct depth. It is not essential for the cover slip to be straight, so long as the grid is completely covered and Newton's rings visible on both sides.

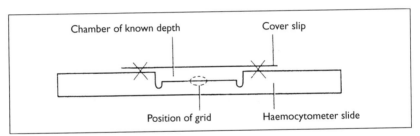

Fig. 17.3   Cross-section of haemocytometer slide and cover slip. × = position of Newton's rings.

(3) Fill the haemocytometer chamber with the diluted blood sample.

(a) After the 10-minute staining period is up, mix the blood sample dilution gently; then remove the cap and half-fill a plain capillary tube (PCV tube) with the solution. Touch the end of the capillary tube to the edge of the chamber you have formed over the grid with the cover slip, and allow the chamber to fill by capillary action. Do *not* fill the grooves on either side of the chamber.

(b) Leave the slide on the bench for a minute or two to allow the white cells to settle on the grid.

(4) Count the white cells.

(a) Switch on the microscope and move the condenser lens as *low* as possible.

(b) Place the slide on the microscope stage so that the grid is as central as possible. Select the lowest-power lens and move the stage up as high as it will go. Gradually bring the grid into focus. The first thing which comes into focus is usually the *bottom* of the slide, which shows up as scratches. Go past this and the next thing you see is the stained white cells (small dots) and the grid, if you are using a mirrored slide. On unmirrored slides the grid is much less easy to see and may not be visible until the next highest power.

(5)   Orientate yourself with the grid – at this power the whole grid pattern is in view. Then concentrate on the top left hand white cell counting square (large square made up of 16 smaller guide squares, marked 'W' on Fig. 17.4) and move it to the centre of the field. Move to the next highest power lens and refocus *carefully* – if the lens touches the cover slip it will come unstuck from the slide, you will lose the Newton's rings, the haemocytometer chamber will no longer be the correct depth, and you will have to go back to the start of step (2)!

(6)   *Either* adjust the slide so that the 'W' square is central and count all the white cells in it (using the guide squares to help). In normal animals expect about 30–50 cells. *Or* concentrate on the top left hand guide

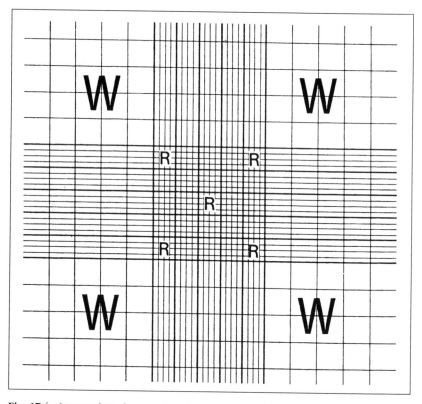

Fig. 17.4   Improved Neubauer ruling. R = squares used for red blood cell counts; W = squares used for white blood cell counts. On the actual slide, the *thick* lines are *triple* lines, and lines extend well beyond the boundaries of the grid.

square and move it to the centre of the field. Move to the highest power (*not* oil-immersion) and refocus *very very carefully*. Move each of the 16 guide squares into the field in turn and count the cells in each one. In normal animals expect about 2–4 cells per guide square. Add up the cells in all 16 guide squares. (It is a matter of personal preference which lens power to use to count the cells. The higher power makes it easier to distinguish cells from dirt specks.)

(7)   Move the slide so that the top right hand 'W' square is in the field and repeat step (6) for that square. Then repeat again for the bottom two 'W' squares.

(8)   Check that the variation between the numbers of cells in the four squares is no more than 10%. If it is greater than 10% the count is invalid due to irregular cell distribution (caused by poor technique or dirty glassware) and must be repeated. If the variation is acceptable add up the results for the four squares.

(9)   Divide this total by 20. Suffix your result with '$\times 10^9/l$'. This is the total white cell count of the sample (the factors take account of the dilution used, the size of the grid squares, the depth of the chamber and the number of cells counted); write it down. (See p. 296 regarding modification of this result which may be necessary if a significant number of nucleated red cells are present.)

(10)   Clean up any spilled blood (cold water is best). Clean the haemocytometer slide with distilled water (*never* rub the mirrored surface with tissues), dry, and return it with the rubber mouthpiece to the box. Turn off light on microscope and make sure the stage and lenses are left clean. Discard all used capillary tubes and coverslips to glass bucket, and all other disposables (used tube of Turck's fluid, tissues, etc.) to yellow plastic bag. Make sure blood sample is either discarded to the yellow plastic bag (glass bucket for Vacutainers) or placed in the fridge if not required again immediately. Put everything else back where you found it.

Haemocytometry can also be used for counting red cells (not recommended!) and platelets. The platelet method is exactly as above except that the diluting fluid is Rees–Ecker solution and the dilution used is 1:200, as for red cell counting (20 µl blood + 4 ml Rees–Ecker solution). The filled chamber should be left for 20 minutes to allow the platelets to settle – they appear as tiny refractile dots among the red cells. Count all the platelets in the 25 central (triple-lined) squares on the grid (see Fig. 17.4), and multiply this number by 2 to give a platelet count of $n \times 10^9/l$.

Preparation of blood films

The skill of making a good blood film is easily acquired with a little practice, and is well worth the effort. Some alternative methods based on vital staining have been marketed, either using pre-stained slides or mixing liquid blood and stain, then placing a drop of blood on the slide and covering with a coverslip. However, visualization of cell morphology is never as good as with a properly spread film, and the staining characteristics of the cells are often quite unlike the appearance of the standard Romanowsky-type stains seen in all textbooks and atlases. They are not recommended.

Mechanical slide spreaders which were used in large laboratories and produced very high quality, uniform films, seem to have fallen out of use, perhaps due to safety concerns regarding potentially infective human blood.

Materials required

It is suggested that slides are stored in a jar of alcohol or methylated spirits, and polished dry immediately before use. This degreases the glass and improves spreading quality.

Fresh blood sample in EDTA. Alternatively, blood without anticoagulant may be used *immediately* after collection, and some authorities recommend this for FeLV testing by IFA. However, in that case blood must be collected and spread within seconds.
Microscope slides cleaned in alcohol
Cloth for polishing slides (clean tea towel or a length of gauze folded several times)
Plain capillary tubes (i.e. PCV tubes)
Spreader – another slide with an unchipped, ground-glass edge. It is best kept in a beaker with some damp cotton wool in the bottom which makes it easy to clean between samples. Using a slide with the corner broken off allows the film to be made with two edges. Alternatively an unbroken slide can be used, offset to the degreased slide by 3–5 mm, which means that the film will have only one edge.

Procedure

(1)   Remove a slide from the jar of alcohol (use forceps to protect hands) and wipe roughly dry.
(2)   *Polish* one side of this slide. Hold the slide in the left hand, preferably using one end of the polishing cloth. Wrap a fold of the free length of the polishing cloth round the forefinger of the right hand and polish one side of the slide. Rub briskly and firmly, alternating this with breathing on the surface of the slide (as if you were polishing your glasses). Half a minute spent doing this thoroughly is well worth it in terms of the quality of the resulting film. Lay the slide on a clean area of bench, polished side up.
(3)   Apply drop of blood to slide.
    (a)   Make sure the edge of the spreader is clean, remove it from its beaker and wipe it dry. Lay it ready to hand.
    (b)   Mix blood sample thoroughly by repeated inversion or rotary mixer. Remove cap.

    (c)   Choose a capillary tube with an evenly cut end and half-fill it with blood.

    (d)   Holding the capillary tube perpendicular to the slide, place a fairly small spot of blood near to one end of the slide as shown in Fig. 17.5a. You may have to experiment a little at first with the size of the drop of blood – anaemic samples tend to need a larger drop than usual.

(4)   Spread the blood film.

    (a)   Place the edge of the spreader on the slide nearer to the centre than the drop of blood and at an angle of about 20° to the slide (see Fig. 17.5a and b). Draw the spreader back towards the drop of blood until it touches it, then encourage the blood to form an even line along the edge of the spreader by varying the angle of the spreader to the slide *without* moving the edge of the spreader.

    (b)   Push the spreader along the slide in one smooth movement, not too quickly, making sure that the edge of the spreader always remains in firm, even contact with the slide.

    (c)   *Immediately* pick up the slide by one end (don't touch the blood film!) and fan it about in the air to dry it. Instant drying is most important in preserving cell morphology, especially that of red cells.

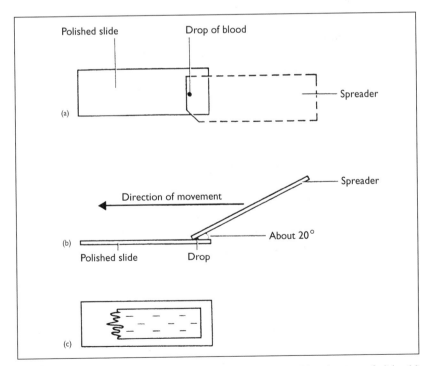

Fig. 17.5 Spreading of blood films: (a) top view of slide; (b) side view of slide; (c) appearance of finished blood film (top view).

If all has gone according to plan, the blood film should extend at least half way along the slide with a 'tail' which ends before the end of the slide (see Fig. 17.5c and Plate 1). The film should be fairly even with no gaps or holes in it, and should be thin enough to dry completely in about 5 seconds (fanning around). Experiment with the following three variables to achieve a good result:

(i)   Size of drop of blood. The larger the drop of blood the thicker the film and vice versa. Too much blood will produce a film which doesn't dry quickly enough and the tail may not fit on the slide.

(ii) Angle of spreader. Usually a fairly acute angle works best.

(iii) Speed of movement of spreader. Fast movement will leave the blood behind, slow movement will carry it along – aim for a compromise to get the tail in the right place.

The finished air-dried film may either be packed in a slide mailer to be sent to the laboratory or stained for further examination in the practice.

Staining of blood films

Many practices favour proprietary Romanowsky-type rapid haematological stains such as Diff-Quik or Rapi-Diff (Diff-Quik appears to be the favourite). For these stains, the manufacturer's instructions should be followed. However, they are not especially suitable for occasional use, as more will be spoiled or will fade unused than will be used. Leishman's stain is slightly more laborious, but it stores well, gives a good result, and (in contrast to the rapid stains) stained slides can be stored for years without deteriorating. It is also reputed to give better staining of mast cell granules.

Materials required

Well-made air-dried blood film
Staining rack – an enamel or plastic dish with a slide rack (two glass rods connected at either end by U-shaped lengths of rubber tubing) placed over it will save staining the sink.
Bottle of Leishman's stain
Buffered distilled water pH 6.8
Tissues and blotting paper
Microscope and immersion oil

Procedure

(1)   Place slide on staining rack over enamel dish, blood side *up*.

(2)   Pour on enough concentrated Leishman's stain so that slide is completely covered. Leave like this for 2 minutes.

(3) Add about twice as much buffered distilled water (pH 6.8) as you did stain. (Judge this approximately by eye – some will spill over into the dish anyway.) Leave this for *at least* 10 minutes. Staining is best if left for 20 minutes and even longer will not do any harm.

(4) Wash off the stain with plenty of distilled water. Immediately wipe the *back* of the slide firmly with a damp tissue to clean the stain from there. (Be very careful not to wipe the wrong side or you will have to start all over again!)

(5) Leave the slide to dry. Air drying is best, but careful blotting can be used if you are in a hurry. Never put immersion oil on a wet slide.

(6) Examine film under microscope. A low-power scan is useful, but cell morphology can only be seen properly with oil immersion. Note red cell size, shape, staining density and any abnormal staining (e.g. polychromasia). Note platelet numbers and size (remember that platelets may appear clumped if slide was not prepared from a very fresh sample). Note white cell morphology and state of preservation, and proceed with differential WBC count.

Differential white cell count

Materials required

Total white blood cell count of sample must be known
Well-made blood film stained with Leishman's or other Romanowsky-type stain
Immersion oil
Microscope
Some way of recording numbers of different cell types seen – purpose-made counter or pencil and paper
Good knowledge of the morphology of the different types of white cell

Procedure

(1) Perform low-power scan of slide to assess white cell distribution. If this is seriously uneven/clumped it is better to make another blood film.

(2) Apply a drop of immersion oil to slide and view under oil immersion. Adjust condenser up for optimum illumination. There are two systems of scanning the slide to ensure statistically valid counts.

    (a) *Battlement method:* Find the edge of the smear and start at the end nearest the tail. Scan three fields along the edge, moving away from the tail, then two fields into the smear, then two along, then two back out to the edge, then two along ... and so on as shown in Fig. 17.6.

    (b) *Straight line method:* Move the objective lens in a straight line parallel

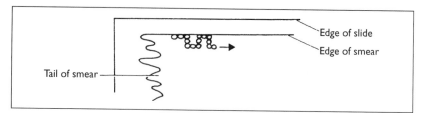

Fig. 17.6   Battlement method for performing a differential white cell count.

with the edge of the film and about 5 mm in towards the centre. Start near the tail and move away from it.

(3) Identify each white cell encountered and record. Normally keep going until 200 cells have been identified and counted, but for many purposes counting only 100 cells will be sufficient. If necessary, move to the opposite edge of the blood film to find enough cells. In severely leucopenic samples it may not be possible to find even 100 cells; in this case a result may still be reported but it is essential to record the number of cells actually counted. Unrecognizable degenerated cells ('smudge' or 'basket' cells) should not be included towards the total, but a check should be kept on the numbers encountered as if this is too high it can invalidate the count. Usually a sign of an old, mishandled or badly collected sample.

Nucleated red cells. The 'total white cell count' is really a total nucleated cell count, including any normoblasts present, and so it is important to include these cells in the differential count as if they were a category of white cell. Then, at step (5) below, allowance can be made for their effect on the total count.

(4) Express result for each cell as a percentage of the total (including any normoblasts).

(5) Using the total white blood cell count, calculate the *absolute* number of each cell type in circulation (as $n \times 10^9/l$) (see p. 50). Where significant numbers of normoblasts have been seen, the absolute number of normoblasts calculated at this point should be subtracted from the total 'white' cell count before it is finally reported.

(6) Clean oil from lens and put microscope away tidily. Either discard used slide to glass bucket or mark with patient identity and store in a safe place. Do not leave glass lying about on benches.

Clotting investigations

Clotting time

Note that simple observation of blood collected into a tube is a very poor guide to clotting time, as the time will vary with the size and type of tube, and repeated agitation of the tube will delay clotting. The following method gives a more standardized result. Note that the procedure cannot be undertaken by the person collecting the sample or holding the patient – an extra pair of hands is essential.

Materials required

The patient
Plain syringe and needle to collect blood sample (less than 1 ml will be sufficient)
Plain 5 ml glass tube
Stopwatch timer
Long glass capillary tube – these are normally drawn out in a bunsen flame from a section of glass tube immediately before use
Small piece of clay or plasticine to seal the end
Water bath or vacuum flask of water at 37°C
Cotton wool or tissues

Procedure

(1)   As soon as the needle enters the vein and blood is seen to enter the syringe, start the stopwatch.

(2)   Hold out the 5 ml tube so that 1 ml or so of blood can be transferred to it as soon as the needle has been removed from the syringe – the sampling procedure must be carried out as quickly as possible.

(3)   Fill the capillary tube with blood and seal one end with clay. If using a vacuum flask, ensure that the column of blood is no longer than the depth of the flask, but leave about 5 cm empty of blood at the sealed end to hold the tube with.

(4)   Place capillary tube in water bath or vacuum flask. Steps 1–4 should be accomplished within about 15 seconds.

(5)   Exactly 2 minutes from step (1) (10 minutes for horses), remove the capillary tube from the water bath, wipe dry the end away from the clay, and break off about 1 cm of tube. Inspect the broken ends as you draw them apart for any sign of a strand of clot running between the ends (Fig. 17.7b). Return the tube to the water bath as quickly as possible.

(6)   Repeat step (5) every 15 seconds (30 seconds for horses) until evidence of clot formation is seen. At this point, stop the stopwatch. The time shown is the clotting time.

Clot retraction

Note that this measurement requires fresh blood and therefore must be begun in the presence of the patient. A PCV result is also required to allow the result to be interpreted, and it will therefore be necessary to collect an EDTA sample at the same time.

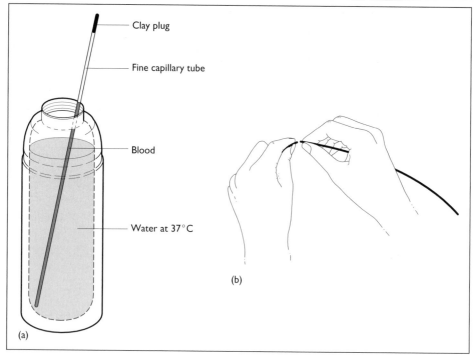

Clay plug

Fine capillary tube

Blood

Water at 37°C

(b)

(a)

Fig. 17.7 Performing a whole blood clotting time.

Materials required

At least 5 ml blood collected straight into a plain syringe
10 ml size glass boiling tube with graduation markings
Cork to fit this tube with a spiral coil of wire affixed at one end to the lower
surface of the cork so that the other end does not quite touch the bottom of
the tube when the cork is in place
Water bath at 37°C, with test tube rack

Procedure

(1) Immediately the sample has been collected, fill the glass tube exactly to
the 5 ml mark with blood.
(2) Fit the cork to the tube so that the coil of wire is suspended free in the
middle of the blood.
(3) Wait until the blood has clotted (usually about 5–10 minutes), then place
the tube in the water bath and incubate for 1 hour.
(4) One hour later, remove the tube from the water bath, and remove the
cork so that the blood clot is withdrawn adherent to the coil of wire. If
the clot does not come away cleanly but fragments or is friable, then clot
retraction is abnormal in any case.

(5)   Measure the volume of serum left in the tube by reading from the graduation marks.

(6)   Express the volume of serum as a percentage of the original volume of blood, e.g. 1.8 ml of serum remaining from 5 ml of blood would give a result of 36%.

Note that the expected volume of serum will vary with the PCV, and should normally be at least 90% of the plasma volume which would be present in the sample.

Bleeding time

Strictly speaking, this is not a laboratory technique at all, but a clinical measurement.

Materials required

The patient
Surgical clippers
Surgical spirit and swab
Petroleum jelly (Vaseline)
Method of producing a very precise skin wound – special double-bladed template lancets are available, but these do not work well in dogs and a no. 11 scalpel blade is probably better for this species
Circle of filter paper, about 10 cm diameter
Stopwatch timer

Procedure

(1)   Ensure that patient is adequately restrained. Local anaesthesia must not be used.

(2)   Clip the hair from the area of skin to be used and a reasonable surrounding radius. The usual sites are the inside of the pinna of the ear for dogs and the lip for horses.

(3)   Thoroughly clean the clipped area with spirit and allow it to dry (take care to avoid making the skin hyperaemic at this stage).

(4)   Cover the clipped area with a *very* thin layer of petroleum jelly.

(5)   Perform the skin incision. The standard bleeding templates are fairly satisfactory in the horse, but for dogs it is best to use a no. 11 scalpel blade to make a cut 1 cm long by 2 mm deep – mark the scalpel blade before cutting to ensure accurate depth. As the cut is made, start the stopwatch.

(6)   Fifteen seconds after cutting, and every 15 seconds thereafter, touch the edge of the filter paper circle to the *blood* (not the skin) so that it is absorbed into the paper – turn the circle by at least 1 cm each time so that a fresh area of paper is used.

(7)   As soon as no more blood can be absorbed on to the paper, stop the

stopwatch. This is the bleeding time, and it is normally under 5 minutes in most species.

Cross-matching blood for transfusion

(Note also that card-presentation blood typing kits are available for dogs and cats, intended for point-of-care use.)

Materials required

A sample of clotted blood in a glass tube, and a sample of blood in heparin from both the patient and the prospective donor(s). Each sample should be 5 ml if possible (though for cats you will simply have to manage with a lot less).
Materials to separate plasma and serum (see p. 302), including pasteur pipettes, as beads or jelly must not be put in the heparin samples
Isotonic saline (500 ml i/v infusion bag will be more than adequate, leaving some over for the next time)
Test tubes
Microscope slides
Microscope

Procedure

(1)   Set the clotted blood samples aside (preferably in a water bath at 37°C) to allow the clots to form and retract.
(2)   Centrifuge the heparinized samples as if for harvesting plasma (see p. 303), but when the separation is completed discard the plasma and retain the red cells.
(3)   Remove one drop (no more than about 0.25 ml) of concentrated red cells from the middle of each of the red cell packs (both donor and recipient), using separate pipettes.
(4)   Place each drop in a test tube containing 3 ml isotonic saline, mix and centrifuge.
(5)   Discard as much of the supernatant saline as possible from each tube, resuspend the cells in a fresh 3 ml aliquot of saline, mix and centrifuge again.
(6)   Repeat step (5) twice more.
(7)   Discard the last supernatant and resuspend the now washed red cells in a further 3 ml saline.
(8)   Harvest the serum from the clotted samples – these may be centrifuged along with the final washing of the red cells to save time.
(9)   Set up four test tubes as follows:
      (a)   Two drops recipient serum + two drops donor cell suspension.
      (b)   Two drops donor serum + two drops recipient cell suspension.

(c) Two drops recipient serum + two drops recipient cell suspension (control).

(d) Two drops donor serum + two drops donor cell suspension (control).

Allow all tubes to stand at room temperature for 30 minutes.

(10) Centrifuge all four tubes for 1 minute at 100 rpm.

(11) Examine the supernatant for significant haemolysis. Slight haemolysis is unimportant in canine blood, but any more than this in tubes (a) or (b), especially where (a) and/or (b) is haemolysed while (c) and (d) are not, indicates incompatibility.

(12) Check the tubes for agglutination. Agitate the tubes by gentle tapping to detect gross agglutination, and if this is not detected transfer a small drop from each tube to a slide and examine under the microscope at low power. Tubes (c) and (d) ought not to agglutinate. Any agglutination in either (a) or (b) indicates incompatibility.

Biochemistry methods

Tips for dipstix methods

These are 'dry reagent' chemistries which involve no sample processing and which produce a colour change visible to the eye which can be read by comparison with a colour chart printed on the bottle. The areas covered are urinalysis and a limited number of blood analytes (glucose and urea), and both Roche and Bayer produce a range of products.

Since these methods are intended for lay use they are all accompanied by comprehensive instructions and descriptions. It is important to take the time to read these properly before using the product, and an up-to-date copy of the package insert should be kept for reference, preferably in a display folder with all the other lab method sheets. There are a few general points to remember:

(1) Store strips at room temperature away from high humidity, in their original container, retaining the desiccator (either in the bottle or incorporated in the cap).

(2) Only remove the strip you are going to use from the bottle – do not return unused strips which may be contaminated. (*The author was only joking on p. 281 about scraping off the S.G. patch!*)

(3) Replace cap firmly immediately after removing the strip.

(4) Do not touch the reagent pad or let it touch other objects.

(5) Always follow manufacturer's instructions carefully and in full.

(6) Throw out all strips past their expiry date. With some strips the expiry date depends on when the bottle was first opened. It is therefore *essential* that this date be calculated and written clearly on the bottle when any new bottle is begun.

(7) Never transfer strips from one bottle to another. Not only can this cause

serious mix-ups with expiry dates, but in some cases the pigments used on the label colour charts are specially mixed for each new batch of strips and so results are not valid when read against the label of the wrong bottle.

These last two points mean that it is best to have only one current bottle of each type of strip in use at any one time, kept in a central place such as the practice lab or the dispensary. This ensures efficient use and avoids the need to throw out large numbers of time-expired strips. It is wise not to keep large stocks of these strips, again because of the expiry date problem, and so it is essential to keep a close eye on usage to ensure that you don't actually run out.

Plasma and serum separation

The precise method will naturally vary according to the make and model of centrifuge used. Note that any centrifuge of which it is physically possible to open the lid while the rotor is turning is DANGEROUS, illegal, and should never be used. The following instructions are generally applicable to most types of bucket or angled head centrifuge, but dual purpose microhaematocrit centrifuges mostly operate on a different principle, with special tubes being clipped to the rotor and a much shorter spin time being required (because of the higher speed). The manufacturer's instructions should be consulted regarding these models.

Materials required

Blood sample (with anticoagulant for plasma, without for serum)
Applicator sticks (for clotted samples)
Centrifuge
Centrifuge tubes (unless blood collection tubes will fit in centrifuge)
Water-filled centrifuge tube or blood collection tube to balance centrifuge
Support to place under tube in centrifuge well (where 5 ml tubes or smaller are being spun in wells designed for 10 ml tubes). Custom-made supports can be obtained, but improvisation is cheaper – another old 5 ml tube minus its cap, or a short length of thick plastic tubing
Test tube rack
Balance to check that centrifuge is evenly loaded across the rotor (not absolutely essential)
Pasteur pipettes and teat (plastic all-in-one pipettes are very convenient and safe for disposal) and/or beads or jelly (Serasieve) to separate cell and plasma layers
Plastic tubes (and caps) to store separated plasma or serum
Labels or indelible marker

Procedure

(1) (a) Samples in anticoagulant may be centrifuged immediately after collection.

    (b) Blood for serum harvesting must be left for at least 2 hours at room temperature (or preferably 37°C) to allow it to clot properly. After this time, open the tube and slide an applicator stick around the inner circumference to ensure the clot is free from the sides of the tube. The clot may be removed at this stage – this is optional.

(2) If your centrifuge will not take the blood collecting tubes you are using, transfer the blood sample to a suitable centrifuge tube.

(3) (Not essential but useful.) Add sufficient Serasieve or plastic beads to form a layer at least 0.5 cm thick above the red cell layer when spun. (These products have a specific gravity intermediate between cells and plasma and greatly aid separation.)

(4) Make sure the centrifuge is switched on both at the mains and the switch on the machine – otherwise the lid will not unlock.

(5) Place the blood tube(s) in centrifuge wells and ensure that the centrifuge is balanced across the rotor. If a tube is suspended in a well by its cap, the screw threads will give during centrifugation and the tube may break, and so it is necessary to place a suitable support under short tubes in long centrifuge wells (make sure the cap will still clear the rotor when the bucket has swung to a horizontal position). Approximate balancing by eye (i.e. matching items across the rotor, using water to match blood where necessary) is all that is necessary to stop the centrifuge leaping off the bench, but minor imbalances cause long-term stress to the rotor, so if you can bear the thought of balancing the tubes and buckets accurately on a balance you will prolong the life of the machine.

(6) Close the lid of the centrifuge, make sure both the 'speed' and 'timer' knobs are set to zero, then turn *first* the timer to 10 minutes, *then* the speed to 3000 rpm. Normally operate with the brake *on* (it only cuts in when decelerating). Do something else for 10 minutes.

(7) The lid should unlock automatically once the rotor has stopped. Remove the sample from the centrifuge, taking great care not to agitate it if no Serasieve or beads have been used, and place in test tube rack. Carefully transfer the supernatant (plasma or serum) into a plain plastic tube. If Serasieve has been used it is possible simply to pour off the supernatant. If beads have been used, pouring is just possible with care, but it is easier to use a pasteur pipette. If neither has been used take *great care* not to agitate the cell layers while pipetting – it is essential that no red cells get into the plasma or serum. Cap the tube. Close the lid of the centrifuge and switch it off.

(8) Make sure all necessary patient details are transferred to the plasma/serum tube, using either a label or an indelible marker.

(9) Return all balance tubes, supports, etc. to their places, discard all glass

(including glass sample tubes) to the glass bin and all other rubbish to the yellow plastic bag.

Refractometry

This method is used both for urine specific gravity and as a rapid point-of-care estimation of total plasma protein. A small, hand-held refractometer is employed (see Fig. 17.8). The instrument has an eyepiece with a variable focus at one end and a plate for sample application at the other. The method involves simply placing a couple of drops of sample on the glass plate, closing the lid firmly over the plate, and reading the result by holding the instrument up to the light and viewing through the eyepiece. The most suitable instruments have three scales visible (see Fig. 17.8c), one for refractive index which is not used, one for specific gravity of urine, and one for total plasma protein (usually in grams per 100 ml, so results must be multiplied by 10 to report as grams per litre). Always ensure that the correct scale is used for the measurement which is being made. The reading is taken at the boundary between the lower (bright) field and the upper (dull) field, twisting the eyepiece to achieve a sharp focus.

Once the reading has been taken, the instrument is simply wiped clean of sample with a tissue and returned to its case. Other than tissues and disposable pipettes, there are no consumables.

Urine sediment examination

Materials required

About 10–20 ml *fresh* urine
Centrifuge tube with pointed end (plastic universal bottles are also suitable)
Centrifuge
Pasteur pipettes
Microscope slides
Coverslips
Microscope

Procedure

(1)   Centrifuge sample at 1500 rpm for 2–3 minutes so that sediment is concentrated into a pellet in the pointed end of the centrifuge tube.
(2)   Pour off as much of the supernatant as possible without disturbing the sediment.
(3)   Resuspend the sediment in the last few drops of supernatant by tapping the tube sharply.
(4)   Place a drop of concentrated sediment on a clean microscope slide and cover with a coverslip, taking care to avoid trapping air bubbles under the coverslip.

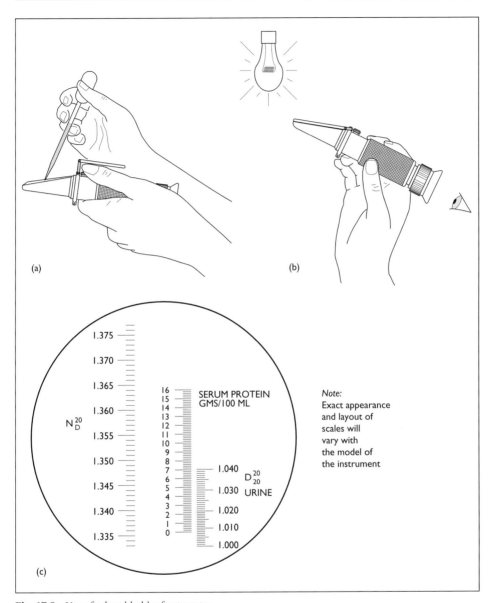

Fig. 17.8 Use of a hand-held refractometer.

(5) Examine the sediment under the microscope at low and medium power. Many different things can be identified:

   (a) Cells – red blood cells, white blood cells (usually neutrophils), epithelial cells, sperm.

   (b) Crystals – calcium carbonate ('cartwheels', normal in horse urine), calcium oxalate, calcium phosphate, magnesium ammonium phosphate, uric acid, leucine, tyrosine, cystine.

(c) Renal tubular casts – protein and mucopolysaccharide.
(d) Microorganisms – bacteria, fungi, yeasts, protozoa, parasite ova (it is useful to do a Gram stain on a dried smear of concentrated sediment to identify bacteria, etc., more closely).

18 The 'Practice Laboratory'

The side-room philosophy is one of complementing the professional laboratory, concentrating on quick and simple tests relevant to emergency and critical care, and referring all routine, non-emergency investigation. The philosophy behind what is usually described as the 'practice laboratory' is different. Although it is still, realistically, a 'near-patient' or 'point-of-care' testing situation, the aim becomes one of doing as much of the practice's laboratory work as possible in-house, and minimizing the use of the referral laboratory. This, of course, means acquiring specialized instrumentation to do biochemistry and perhaps also haematology analysis.

How desirable is a practice laboratory?

Superficially a practice lab can seem an attractive concept, and one readily reinforced by advertisements and sales representatives from companies eager to close a contract on analytical equipment. There is also, at least among some sections of the profession, a philosophy which regards the in-practice laboratory as progressive and praiseworthy in its own right, though this is not necessarily an attitude which is particularly well thought-out. Against this background it is useful to examine the rationale behind the concept somewhat more critically.

Speed of results

This is the most commonly cited reason for setting up a 'practice lab'. It is certainly true that results – or at least numbers – can be available substantially more quickly this way compared with the turn-round time of a professional laboratory. However, how great is the time saving really, and how much impact does it have on patient care?

Emergency care

This is often quoted as a major argument in favour of the in-house laboratory.

However, one has to consider what proportion of sample requests in a practice actually relate to genuine emergency situations, as opposed to more or less routine non-emergency case work-up? The answer is, of course, only a very small minority. Then, in what proportion of these genuine emergencies is immediate availability of extensive laboratory data likely to result in a significant modification to treatment? Again, most emergency cases are treated empirically based on history-taking and clinical examination, and there is often little immediate benefit in having comprehensive laboratory data to hand. Finally, accepting that there are indeed situations where laboratory investigations can be helpful in an emergency, is the information available from dedicated in-practice analysers significantly better than that from the simple side-room approach? The fact is that the tests most helpful in emergencies are, in general, those which the practice side-room should be able to deal with anyway – PCV, total protein, glucose, urea, that sort of thing. Electrolytes are, of course, a major advantage also, and this consideration is discussed in Chapter 17. There is a very good argument for investing in a dedicated instrument to measure sodium and potassium, but little rationale for requiring the bulk of routine tests to be on hand for emergency admissions.

Routine investigations

These make up the bulk of a practice's laboratory work. Most animals are out-patients, with samples being collected at one appointment and results available in time for the follow-up appointment. Even where an in-house laboratory exists, this doesn't change a great deal – the practicalities of sample separation and analysis mean that it is not feasible to have results available during the initial consultation, and it is seldom worthwhile to ask clients to wait in the waiting room until the analysis has been completed. In the chronic cases which make up the majority of a practice's patients, the difference between waiting an hour or so for in-house results, or anything from about 6 hours (with courier collection) to 3 days (with weekend post) for a professional report becomes much more one of client relations than real clinical benefit.

Another aspect which is less often appreciated is the matter of follow-up investigations. It often happens that a 'routine' profile will be requested one day, then shortly afterwards, either as a direct follow-on from these results or because of clinical developments, further tests are required which may not be within the scope of the practice laboratory. When the initial testing has been done by the professional laboratory this is very straightforward – the follow-up results can be emerging from the fax machine within half an hour of a telephone call. However, if the initial testing was done in-house, the question of sample transport to the laboratory still has to be tackled.

What really matters in the non-emergency case is, of course, not the speed of availability of the initial results, but the time taken to reach a diagnosis. While this may be slightly reduced by a 'practice lab' in the very straightforward cases (indeed, those cases which could probably be entirely dealt with by the simple side-room facility), experience demonstrates that in the more complex cases attempts to 'be your own pathologist' can actually slow down the investigation quite considerably. Several factors contribute to this, but the main issue is usually one of interpretation of results. Clinical pathology is a speciality like any other, and with the best will in the world the general practitioner with a limited in-house facility and a relatively small case throughput cannot hope to have experience equivalent to that of someone who scrutinizes scores of 'unusual' cases from many different practices every day. Sometimes doubts arise as to the reliability of the in-house results, and expensive tests are repeated and repeated. Sometimes hours are spent poring over textbooks, then more textbooks which contradict the first lot. Sometimes an irrelevant or spurious abnormality is latched on to, and days spent pursuing red herrings down blind alleys. Finally, samples may be sent to the professional laboratory, but even then a reluctance to repeat the initial basic tests can result in numerous unnecessary requests for specialized investigations which may not, in fact, be warranted.

In contrast, when the case work-up is carried out through the referral laboratory in the first instance, the second opinion input from the clinical pathologist frequently smooths a relatively direct path to the answer, and often elicits advice on treatment or prognosis based on seeing comparable cases on a daily or weekly basis. The superficially attractive 'fast track' of in-house analysis actually cuts a practice off from its most accessible second opinion. By their very nature, veterinary practices often have relatively little regular opportunity for case discussion and exchange of ideas with colleagues outside the practice, certainly compared with medical practices which are part of a much larger network of policy committees and consultants' reports. Daily contact with a referral laboratory can be very valuable in this situation, allowing dissemination of clinical experience and advice, and facilitating rational approaches to case investigation. This aspect of the professional laboratory service frequently more than compensates for the time taken to transport the samples to the lab, and has to be taken into account when comparing total contribution to patient care.

Monitoring patients on treatment

Critical care monitoring is of course important, but the situation is similar to that discussed above regarding emergency cases – the tests which are of most immediate value are those already covered by the side-room facility (assuming provision has been made for electrolyte analysis). In fact, too ready availability of routine tests (for both the critical-care patient and the recovering animal) can be counterproductive, as it often leads to over-investigation – tests (especially enzymes) which should only be repeated every week or two at the most may be run daily, just because the facility is there, and the inevitable minor fluctuations trigger quite unnecessary revisions of treatment or prognosis. This is a very good example of a situation where how fast you might *like* the results and how fast you may *need* them can be two very different things.

One situation where patient monitoring using in-house facilities is entirely appropriate is, of course, the stabilization of the diabetic patient, but once again this is adequately provided for by simple side-room techniques, and extensive analytical instrumentation is unnecessary.

Pre-anaesthetic screening

This subject is one which is frequently raised by those marketing laboratory equipment to veterinary practices, and regrettably the justification often appears to be more financial than clinical. As discussed in Chapter 15, the decision to request blood sample analysis before a general anaesthetic should be based on perceived risk, because of a known clinical reason for concern. If it is not standard practice in human medicine to run a 'blood profile' routinely before elective surgery in a young healthy individual, why should it be any different in veterinary medicine?

If a pre-anaesthetic screen is indeed decided on, for sound clinical reasons, the question of timing is crucial. The dream of those favouring in-house analysis appears to be to admit the patient on the morning of the scheduled surgery, already fasted and with the owners assuming that the operation is going to be done that day, to collect the pre-anaesthetic sample soon after admission, to do the analysis as quickly as possible, and deliver the results to the anaesthetist virtually as he is hovering over the patient with a loaded syringe. However, this is not the ideal approach. The reason for choosing to carry out a pre-anaes-thetic screen is precisely so that surgery can be reconsidered and perhaps postponed if something untoward is revealed. To this end, it is far preferable to have the results to hand at least 24 hours before the scheduled time of surgery, in time to halt the process if necessary *before* the owners begin to fast the animal (and perhaps withhold water overnight, which may not be the best advice if a renal problem might exist), and to avoid having the owner depart happily for work confidently assuming that his dog's dental surgery will go ahead as planned. The time to collect the pre-anaesthetic sample is during the initial consultation when the need for surgery is discovered, and even using ordinary postal services the results will then be available from the professional laboratory in time to allow proper consideration of their implications. Even if the opportunity to collect the sample is missed during the initial consultation, it is much better to arrange a nurse's appointment for blood sampling a couple of days before surgery than to rely on a last-minute in-house analysis on the day itself.

Client expectations

This aspect seems to be an increasing concern, possibly fuelled by some of the veterinary 'fly-on-the-wall' television programmes. Clients who may be quite used to the need to wait days or even weeks for results of blood tests from their GPs, suddenly expect a veterinary practice to be able to produce these almost instantly. There is no doubt that having a 'practice lab' scores easy points when advertising or promoting a practice to the public. Nevertheless, what may impress the client and what is in the best interests of the client's animals are not necessarily the same thing. If a practice has taken a considered decision to optimize side-room emergency testing but to refer all routine non-emergency investigations to the professional laboratory, it should be possible to justify this decision rationally to all but the most short-sighted clients. One suggested approach is to ask the client, if it were his own health which was on the line, which would he prefer – that his blood sample was analysed by the practice nurse on a small side-room machine, or that his sample was analysed by the specialist technicians in the hospital laboratory and a report sent out signed by the consultant clinical biochemist or haematologist? If you are confident that your approach represents best practice as you understand it, you should be able to explain this confidently and positively to your client and avoid sounding apologetic or half-hearted.

Legal liabilities

The question is sometimes asked, is it not opening a practice to the risk of legal action not to have a full in-house laboratory facility, when other practices may boast of the advantages of such a facility? In fact, the true position is quite the reverse. It is inconceivable that a practice which has taken care to ensure that emergency requirements are adequately provided for should be open to any sort of criticism for choosing to refer routine laboratory work to a professional laboratory, or for not having instant availability of the less urgent analytes (such as enzymes) for the emergency case. On the contrary, it is the practice which has chosen to run its own clinical pathology laboratory that is at greatest risk of litigation. When the analysis is done by the professional laboratory, then it is that laboratory which carries the can for inaccuracies, errors and mistakes. Quality assurance in the laboratory is a complex and painstaking exercise, and the lengths to which professional laboratories go to avoid errors are not often appreciated by the client. Even so, accidents do happen. When a veterinary practice is carrying out its own routine analysis, using staff with no specialist technical training (and sometimes instrumentation which was never intended by its developers to offer more than a 'side-room' standard of accuracy), the opportunity for something to go wrong must be even greater. However, the practitioner is choosing to take on this entire responsibility himself, including responsibility for proving (in a court of law if necessary) that results reported are correct. This is one reason why in-office analysis is seldom employed in the human field, even in private medicine. The risks to the general practitioner of taking entire responsibility for accuracy of laboratory results are perceived as being simply too great.

Financial considerations

However compelling the clinical arguments in favour of maximizing use of the referral laboratory, there often seems to be an underlying conviction that analyses carried out in-house must automatically generate more profit for the practice than analyses referred elsewhere. However, this is another assumption which fails to stand up to close scrutiny.

It is certainly true that availability of in-house analysis frequently increases a practice's *turnover*. There are several reasons for this. Firstly, more tests tend to be carried out per patient when laboratory facilities exist within the practice. However, whether these genuinely represent investigations essential to patient care is very questionable. The 'profiles' promoted by those marketing in-house analysers frequently include tests whose justification appears very slender – amylase done as a routine where no clinical suspicion of pancreatitis exists (or even worse, on cats, where the test is of no benefit in any case) is one example, bilirubin included even where the sample is quite obviously not at all yellow is another. Investigations are, on average, repeated more frequently by practices with their own laboratories, often more frequently than would appear to be clinically necessary: sometimes this is just 'because the facility is there', sometimes because the clinician is unsure about the interpretation and hopes that a repeat might yield a more clear-cut picture. Sometimes tests which might otherwise have been dispensed with are performed in-house, such as pre-anaesthetic screens on young, clinically healthy animals, or 'senior health checks' on clinically well dogs and cats – often no more than 7 or 8 years of age! Secondly, the price charged per test tends to be higher compared to the referral laboratory, simply because the tests cost so much more to run. These factors combine to produce an often impressive turnover attributable to the practice laboratory. However, it is not turnover as such which is important, but whether increased turnover leads to increased profit, in other words, are the total costs of the exercise more than covered by the income generated?

Calculating the true cost of in-house analysis is very much like calculating the total cost-per-mile of running a car. It is easy to see that petrol might cost, say, 10 p per mile. However, any taxi firm which calculated fares on that basis alone would soon be out of business! Items which should be considered in any realistic calculation of laboratory costs include:

Purchase or rental cost of instrument(s)
Maintenance costs, both contractual and occasional
Reagents used for paying tests
Reagents used for non-paying tests (calibration and quality control (QC) samples, out-of-range repeats, etc.)
Other consumables for both paying and non-paying tests
Calibration and QC material
LABOUR COSTS, both lay and professional
Cost of capital tied up in equipment

Cost of capital tied up in reagents and other stock
Pro-rata share of practice overheads (heat, light, power, rent, rates, etc.)

The most frequently overlooked significant cost item is labour. Running a laboratory is a time-consuming exercise, even with modern, user-friendly instrumentation. Not only do the required analyses need to be carried out, but calibration, quality assessment, trouble-shooting, staff training, cleaning and maintenance, stocktaking and ordering and so on, all take time. This is mostly nurse time, but not entirely – the veterinary surgeon always needs to be familiar with what is going on, to help where necessary, and to be involved in the training of lay staff. In addition, some allowance for professional time spent interpreting the results must be made. It is pointless to declare, as some do, that as the nurses are 'already there', then their time need not be taken into account. Unless your nurses work on a voluntary unpaid basis, their wages, etc., are a pro-rata part of the cost of every task they undertake, and must be included.

It is important to apply proper accountancy methods to this sort of costing. Various spreadsheets have been produced to enable the calculations to be made, and the final figures often surprise practitioners very much. Up to £5 or £6 *per test* is not unusual with some biochemistry systems, and this is, of course, the cost to the practice before any profit margin is included. Failure to appreciate the real cost of your analyses may easily lead you to charge your clients less than it is costing you to carry out the work.

Comparisons with the professional laboratory also have to be realistic. Prices listed by most labs for individual tests are usually comparatively high, but these prices are seldom actually paid by anyone. The price to look at is the price of the test *within the commonly used profiles*, and this tends to be less than about £2 per routine biochemistry analyte – quite substantially less in some laboratories. This also represents the *maximum* you will be charged – most laboratories offer prompt settlement discounts to regular clients, and many offer cut-price retests for follow-up repeat investigations. Effect on cash flow is also important. A professional laboratory will carry out the tests first, send an account after the end of the month, and allow (typically) 3 or 4 weeks for settlement. Thus the client's money (including your mark-up and the VAT) can be in your bank account well in advance of the work having to be paid for. This is much better for cash flow than having paid-for reagent packs sitting on a shelf waiting for the tests to be required. In addition, bear in mind that these bald price-per-test comparisons omit what is perhaps the most valuable service offered by the professional laboratory – the second opinion advice from the clinical pathologist.

The profit from laboratory work, as with everything else, of course depends not on who does the work, but on the difference between the costs incurred and the price charged. The substantially lower costs incurred by 'outsourcing' to the professional laboratory mean that the desired profit level can be more easily and reliably achieved by that route, and at a lower cost to the client. It is of course true that economies of scale are involved here, but attempts to achieve similar economies in the practice lab by churning out more and more 'routine screens' are largely missing the point. Small instruments designed to be used by nursing staff achieve this objective by packaging reagents in one-shot, single-sample units in such a way as to minimize operator manipulation. This results in irreducible reagent costs many times those of professional laboratories – you are paying for the convenience of point-of-care testing, and the system is not amenable to being scaled up. Simpler small instruments which use bulk reagents may offer the possibility of reduced reagent costs, but at the price of much more operator manipulation, hence increased labour costs and much greater opportunity for error. It is not until you come to the large 'number-cruncher' biochemistry analysers employed by the professional laboratories, where tiny volumes of bulk-packaged reagents are manipulated by complex instrumentation, that real economies of scale start to emerge – and this is at the level of hundreds of samples per day, and the machines are the provenance of the trained technician, not nursing staff.

The 'possession object'

In spite of all the arguments in favour of maximizing the use of the professional laboratory and confining side-room analysis to the genuinely useful tests in the genuine emergency, it is remarkable how many practitioners nevertheless embrace the 'be-your-own-pathologist' philosophy enthusiastically. Part of this may stem from a feeling that a practice which owns a comparatively sophisticated-seeming instrument *must* in some way be superior to a practice which does not, and that diagnostic results produced from such a machine are in some intangible way more valuable and thus more worthy of being charged for than results produced from relatively simple instruments such as the refractometer or the microscope. However, the comparison of total protein methods is a good example of how misleading this impression can be. Figure 18.1 shows the performance of three different methods compared with reference results. (The comparisons are presented as scatterplots, which are reasonably self-explanatory, but see p. 329 for a fuller explanation of the correlation statistics.) Figure 18.1(a) is a routine wet chemistry method; points are clustered close to the 1:1 line of coincidence and there are no outliers, which is the sort of performance that any practice aiming to replace the professional laboratory ought to be achieving. Fig. 18.1(b) is a hand-held refractometer; scatter is much wider than in (a), and there are a few outliers. This level of performance is fine as a quick guide in an emergency, which is exactly how the refractometer is used, but no one would dream of advocating it as a routine laboratory procedure. Figure 18.1(c) is a side-room reflectance meter; the scatter is substantially worse than the refractometer's, and there are a couple of extremely wide outliers. Even though the reflectance meter is a much more complex machine than the refractometer and costs considerably more to operate, it is giving poorer results.

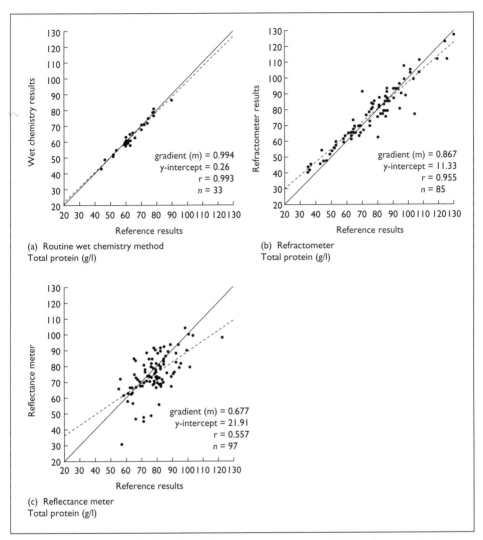

Fig. 18.1 Total protein results from three different instruments compared with reference methods.

The value of a result lies in its being right, in the right place, and at the right time – snazzy-looking instruments are not necessarily better than simple techniques, and having a result sooner than it is really required does not enhance its value – especially if it is less reliably accurate.

Accuracy of results

Although this is arguably the most important consideration of all, it is often sadly neglected by practitioners. 'Side-room' standards of accuracy are all very well in the genuine side-room situation, where a rough *interim* guide is what you want and what you know you are getting. Any important discrepancies will be revealed when the referral laboratory investigation proceeds in due course. However, if an in-practice facility is intended to *replace* professional analysis rather than to complement it, far more stringent standards must apply. A 'ball-park' figure is no longer acceptable. Maximum information extraction from the laboratory report relies on the ability to recognize fine detail, to appreciate the significance of small variations from normal, and to recognize crucial patterns inherent in the figures. To this end, a high degree of accuracy is required, a goal which professional laboratories spend a great deal of time and money achieving with various quality assessment and quality control schemes. If a practice laboratory is to replace this facility, standards of accuracy and reliability must be equally high.

This is not as easy as it sounds. Investigations which generate a pictorial result, such as radiography or microscopic examination, have their own in-built 'garbage detector' – the human eye. A badly focused X-ray plate or a micro-scope slide obscured by stain debris are easily appreciated as poor quality, and unlikely to give rise to a confidently asserted, but wrong, diagnosis. However, instruments which generate a list of numbers are much less easy to catch out. The confidence a clinical pathologist has in his own laboratory's results is based on a great deal that the client never sees – known control sera analysed fre-quently, with patient results never being issued unless these controls are satisfactory; participation in blind quality assessment schemes run by and for human hospital laboratories, with any unsatisfactory performance triggering a major investigation and troubleshooting exercise; and regular re-analysis of patient samples where the experienced eye has spotted an inconsistency, incongruity or possible error. The idea that 'the machine gave me that result, and so it must be right' never comes into it.

It is a very big decision to choose to take over this responsibility within the practice. Although the technicalities of the other main area of diagnostic investigation, radiography, are covered in the veterinary undergraduate course, virtually no instruction is given in laboratory techniques or laboratory man-agement – certainly not beyond the basic side-room procedures. It is only too easy to allow this ignorance of the subject, and the superficial credibility of the printed list of numerical results, to lull you into a false sense of security. Per-haps the day will come when anyone can pick up Dr McCoy's tricorder, point it at a patient, and be handed a 'full diagnostic readout', but it is not here yet and will probably not be along any time soon.

It is common to find that practitioners who are considering the purchase of a major item of analytical equipment have never even thought of asking the salesperson to show them an evaluation of the machine for the target species, against standard reference methods. This would be unheard-of in human medicine, where the sales representatives know they have to be thoroughly familiar with every technicality of the machine they are demonstrating, and expect to have to prove its performance to a sceptical and well-informed purchaser. The veterinary attitude often seems to be, 'I thought they wouldn't be allowed to market it unless it was accurate'. Not so. Although pharmaceutical sales are highly regulated through the Veterinary Medicines Directorate, and every product must have its product licence and its approved data sheet, so far as analytical equipment is concerned it is *caveat emptor*. It is entirely up to the purchaser to assure himself that an instrument meets his requirements – even the usual Advertising Standards legislation does not apply to items marketed to the professions, on the grounds that we are intelligent enough to be able to look after ourselves! This doesn't mean that everybody is out to rip you off, but it does mean that you can't afford to take *anything* on trust.

With a few specific exceptions such as the FeLV and FIV kits, virtually every single laboratory method sold to or employed by veterinary practices was originally developed for human use. This also applies to the simple side-room tests – most of these have never been formally evaluated for veterinary use and the manufacturers do not actively promote the products to veterinary surgeons. However, extensive practical experience and numerous small informal evaluations mean that, in general, one has a pretty good idea of what works and what doesn't. If we are lucky, performance is just about as good as it is on human samples – the diabetic glucose meters are a good example of this. On the other hand, some methods simply have to be avoided – the specific gravity patch on the urine dipstix is probably the prime example.

When it comes to larger items of equipment the situation becomes more complicated. Again the parent instrument has inevitably been developed for the human market, but then comes the 'vetification'. It can be very difficult to tell just how much alteration has really occurred between the parent machine and the veterinary model – it may be little more than painting it a different colour and adding 'VET' somewhere in the name, or there may have been quite extensive further development. In general, however, one finds that modifications tend to be confined to the internal computer software, and perhaps to the sample handling facility. The actual analysis itself is seldom if ever modified, as the viability of the whole exercise inevitably depends on the reagent packs supplied to the veterinary market coming off the same production line as those for the (much larger) human market. In many cases veterinary sales are handled by a secondary franchise-holder with no facilities for research into or implementation of significant changes to the methodology, while the primary manufacturer is focused on servicing the human market and has little interest in the veterinary field other than as an additional market for the existing product. Therefore, just because an instrument is capable of printing out the species of the patient or the practice logo on the report form doesn't mean that the methods employed have been modified or even validated for non-human samples.

As a general rule, instruments which employ the same basic analytical methods as those in routine use in professional veterinary laboratories tend to be reasonably promising, while those which employ novel methods can be more problematical. It is particularly in this latter category that it is vital to insist on seeing a thorough method comparison study, preferably from an independent source, using veterinary samples, including at least some from any species for which the instrument is to be used. Never accept remarks such as, 'Oh, I'm sure it works fine on wallabies' at face value.

Haematology methods

Particle (impedance) counters

The original cell counters which superseded manual chamber counting under the microscope were particle counters operating on the Coulter principle. The early models didn't particularly care what species the blood sample came from – one simply set the parameters to suit the appropriate cell size, and everything was fine. Later refinements designed to streamline analysis of human samples inevitably upset this to some extent, and attempts to provide multi-species operation on the more sophisticated models by means of bolt-on 'vet-packs' were often not entirely satisfactory, as they generally relied on arithmetical fudge-factors with inbuilt assumptions which were not necessarily applicable to every patient. More modern multi-species instruments generally perform quite well in experienced hands, but it remains the case that the basic machines with the fewest refinements are the best choice for veterinary laboratories and a spun PCV from a microhaematocrit is more reliable than a value calculated from a measured RBC count and MCV. The principles of particle counting are presented in Appendix I to this chapter (see p. 340).

Non-Coulter principles

More recently a new generation of human haematology analysers has been introduced, based on laser technology. Their introduction caused a great deal of trouble in the (human) quality assessment (QA) scheme. Until then, most QA distributions had been of horse or donkey blood, because of easy availability of relatively large volumes, and for safety reasons (animal blood does not transmit hepatitis C or HIV). The Coulter machines coped with these just fine. However, the non-Coulter machines, which perform beautifully on human blood, turned in quite silly numbers on the non-human samples. The eventual outcome was that the use of equine blood was discontinued, and all haematology QA distributions are now of human blood. Even if modifications are made to non-Coulter instruments their performance is never comparable to Coulter-principle machines on non-human blood, and they are best avoided for veterinary use.

Automated differential counts

One of the major advances in automated haematology in the human field has been the automated differential counter. These instruments use various tricks to produce not just a total WBC count, but to generate individual counts for each WBC type. Once again the machines developed for human use are very impressive, and in some respects (especially accurate tallies of low-number cells such as basophils) offer advantages over manual (microscope-read) differentials. Their forte is in the large routine hospital laboratory, where a significant proportion of samples are unremarkable. On fresh, uniform and well-collected samples they are an invaluable tool for disposing of the routine requests and allowing the haematologists to concentrate on the important ones. Even so, many haematologists report that they still perform manual differential counts or blood film examination on 50% or more of the submissions they receive.

Unfortunately the techniques used to differentiate the cell types for instrument counting are to quite a large extent species specific, and adaptations of the methods for veterinary use have been relatively disappointing. In addition, collecting uniformly good-quality samples from animals is not nearly as easy as it is with human patients, and this also creates difficulties. However, the main point is that these methods are for the large laboratory and the experienced haematologist with a workload of hundreds of samples a day, and their purpose is to reduce the number of manual counts which have to be performed. They should never be seen as the lazy way out of acquiring skill in blood film examination for the small laboratory. The blood film is the absolute central pillar of haematological analysis, and no laboratory, however small, can possibly claim to be competent in haematology without competence in film examination.

Centrifugation instruments

Another type of non-Coulter instrumentation which has been widely promoted in the veterinary market is the centrifugation technique, where WBC measurements are made by spreading the stained buffy coat by means of a float. Unlike the laser counters, which are sophisticated instruments designed for professional use, the centrifuges were never intended as anything more than point-of-care 'aids'. They produce a microhaematocrit PCV result, a total white cell count, a platelet count, and some also provide a partial approximate differential count which has the serious disadvantage of being unable to distinguish between lymphocytes and monocytes.

The drawback to this methodology is that the quality of the information generated is, on average, poorer than that obtainable from the simple micro-haematocrit-PCV-and-look-at-a-blood-film approach. Although the PCV is performed by centrifugation, correlation with microhaematocrit results is not particularly good (see Fig. 18.2a). The white cell counts generated are probably better than the sort of guess that can be made by scanning a blood film, but again, correlation with impedance counter results is not very good (see Fig. 18.2b). The partial differential WBC counts reported by this type of machine can vary considerably from manual counts performed on the same samples; in particular, the method frequently appears to overestimate eosinophils, and the

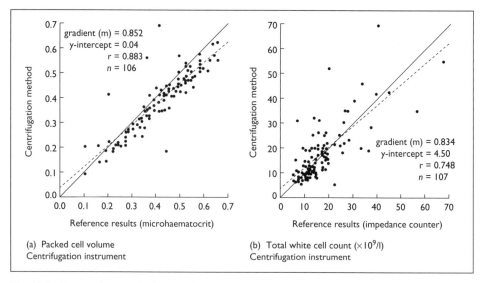

Fig. 18.2   Haematology results from a side-room instrument operating on the centrifugation principle compared with reference methods.

combined mononuclear cell counts (which do not differentiate between lymphocytes and monocytes) often bear little relation to the sum of these cell types taken from the manual count. The reported platelet counts also seem to vary considerably from the appearance of the blood film in many cases.

It must be borne in mind that these machines are not haematology analysers – their place really ought to be in Chapter 17, among the approximate side-room 'guesstimates'. If you are using one, it should be seen mainly as a means of obtaining a better estimate of the total WBC count than can be made from a blood film. If the PCV measurement is critical this should always be repeated by microhaematocrit, and a blood smear must always be used to estimate platelets and for the differential WBC count. These instruments are inappropriate as a replacement for the professional laboratory and their results should never be treated as more than an approximate interim guide.

Biochemistry methods

The principal consideration regarding biochemistry instruments is the distinction between traditional methods where the measurement is carried out by observing the change in optical density of a solution at a specified wavelength, now commonly referred to as 'wet chemistry' methods, and the more recently developed 'dry reagent' methods (or reflectance meters) which measure the change in *reflected* light from the surface of an opaque reagent patch. The principles of photometric analysis are presented in Appendix II at the end of this chapter (p. 343).

'Wet chemistry' methods

These methods are the general workhorse assays of the clinical biochemistry laboratory, and all that was available before about 1988. All published studies of biochemical reference values and changes with physiological or disease processes have used wet chemistry analysis, and it is regarded as the 'reference method'.

Fortunately most wet chemistry methods are not especially species-sensitive, and they have proved reliable in a wide variety of animals. This feature was formerly exploited by the external quality assurance schemes for human laboratories, and much use was made of equine and bovine plasma for both quality control and quality assessment. However, as with haematology, this has been superseded by the almost universal use of human material in spite of the higher risk of transmitting infectious diseases. Again this is a consequence of the introduction of more species-intolerant techniques, including dry-reagent methods.

In general, standard wet chemistry methods for most routine analytes perform well on non-human blood. However, there is a tendency when designing point-of-care analysers to incorporate all the parameters for each assay as factory-fixed settings with no opportunity for a lay operator to meddle. There is some justification for this attitude, but the problem is that it can prevent the small modifications to the assays necessary to optimize them for non-human samples which are standard practice in the professional veterinary laboratory. Thus even wet chemistry instruments need to be evaluated with care for veterinary use.

Two analytes of which to be particularly wary are albumin and alkaline phosphatase. Albumin (by the bromocresol green (BCG) method) seems to vary in performance between different manufacturers' versions of the same method, probably because of differences in the buffers used. Experience in veterinary laboratories is that a method which frequently reports dog and cat albumin results of greater than 40 g/l may be unreliable, and switching to another supplier may be advisable. Alkaline phosphatase is unusual in that two very different buffer systems are in regular use, and they give very different results. For veterinary use it is important to choose a method using diethanolamine (DEA) buffer, and methods using aminomethylpropanol (AMP) should be avoided. It does seem, however, that the AMP buffer is becoming more widely used in human medicine.

'Dry reagent' methods

The extension of reflectance photometry beyond the simple glucose meter began in the late 1980s. Early machines required a pre-dilution step, with diluted plasma then applied to the reagent strip. Performance of these machines was quite good, certainly adequate for point-of-care testing, but the pre-dilution step was disliked by operators and the instrument was discontinued when machines capable of handling neat plasma proved more popular in the human testing market.

Unfortunately, the elimination of the sample dilution introduced enormous problems when the methods were applied to non-human samples. The cause of the problem appears to be the 'plasma matrix effect', where the physical properties of the proteins in the sample interfere with the analysis. In wet chemistry methods the plasma is invariably diluted substantially as part of the analytical process, and problems with matrix effects are seldom a major issue. The application of undiluted plasma to a dry reagent layer is, however, a different matter. Methods which can be demonstrated to perform beautifully on human samples suddenly develop unacceptable scatter when non-human plasma is used. This effect is peculiar in that while any one sample will always give essentially the same result however often it is analysed, the relationship between this figure and the result from the reference method appears to be mostly a matter of chance. One sample may consistently read 30% above the correct value while another sample (from an animal of the same species) may read 20% below, which means that even correction by 'fudge factors' is impractical. The effect is worse with some analytes than with others, as demonstrated in Figs 18.3 and 18.4.

The routine wet chemistry urea method (Fig. 18.3) shows good clustering of the points along the line of coincidence, especially in the crucial lower part of the range where appreciation of the fine detail is important in recognizing pre-renal effects and in identifying below-normal results. This is an average performance rather than superstar status, but this level of accuracy is very important in a routine diagnostic method where a reliable urea result is essential for the pattern-recognition process. In contrast, the reflectance

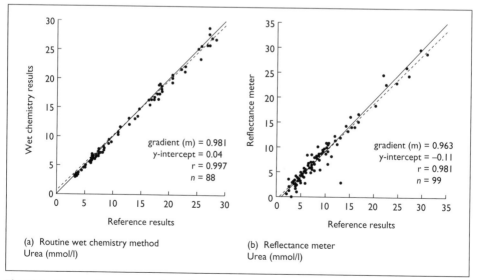

(a) Routine wet chemistry method
Urea (mmol/l)

gradient (m) = 0.981
y-intercept = 0.04
r = 0.997
n = 88

(b) Reflectance meter
Urea (mmol/l)

gradient (m) = 0.963
y-intercept = −0.11
r = 0.981
n = 99

Fig. 18.3 Comparative accuracy of wet chemistry and dry reagent methods for urea.

meter demonstrates a much wider scatter, and results close to the reference limits are not exact enough to allow appreciation of metabolic and circulatory effects. It is thus unsuitable for routine work-up of a non-emergency case. Nevertheless, the method is linear, with only one real outlier, and even that result would have been unlikely to have been seriously misleading in the short term. Considered as a 'point-of-care' emergency method, this reflectance meter method would be genuinely useful.

As with the urea method, the performance of the wet chemistry ALT assay

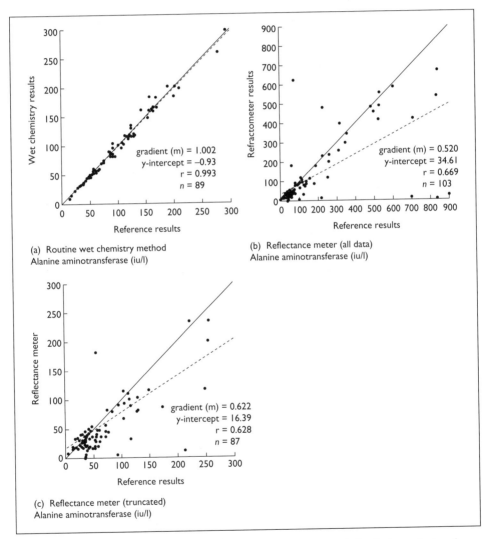

(a) Routine wet chemistry method
Alanine aminotransferase (iu/l)

(b) Reflectance meter (all data)
Alanine aminotransferase (iu/l)

(c) Reflectance meter (truncated)
Alanine aminotransferase (iu/l)

Fig. 18.4   Comparative accuracy of wet chemistry and dry reagent methods for alanine aminotransferase (ALT): (b) displays the points for all the samples checked on the reflectance meter, while (c) presents only those with results less than 300 iu/l, to allow more direct comparison with the wet chemistry results shown in (a).

(Fig. 18.4) is a reasonable average, and demonstrates the sort of accuracy which should be an achievable goal for any laboratory performing routine diagnostic investigations. Again points are clustered close to the line of coincidence, and those which are a little off only deviate from the target value by a relatively small percentage. There are no gross outliers. In contrast, the scatter seen with the reflectance meter is much more marked. However, unlike the reflectance meter urea method, there are also several serious outliers – at least six of the 103 samples tested gave results which could be considered dangerously misleading, involving both underestimation and overestimation. It is therefore questionable whether a method like this should be considered even as an emergency point-of-care assay.

Modification of dry reagent methods for non-human samples would require either pre-treatment of the samples (e.g. by dilution or deproteinization) or re-engineering of the reagent strips/slides, possibly for each species individually. This problem has not yet been seriously tackled, and reflectance meters should be recognized as having major limitations in the veterinary laboratory.

Choosing suitable instrumentation

If, after careful consideration, you do decide that having a routine clinical pathology lab in your practice is appropriate, choice of instrumentation is crucial. Always bear in mind that if the facility is intended to replace the referral laboratory rather than complement it, accuracy and reliability standards *must* be comparable to those of the professional laboratory. Thus methods chosen must be appropriate.

Haematology

Moving from a simple spin-a-PCV-and-look-at-a-blood-film system to a full haematology analysis does not, in fact, offer such a huge advantage as might be supposed. The main difference is, of course, having an accurate total WBC count, which then allows accurate calculation of the absolute differential WBC counts. Beyond that, the effect is marginal. Haemoglobin measurement is only useful in its own right to assess the size of the circulating erythron in patients whose haematology samples are too grossly haemolysed to allow a PCV tube to be read – which one hopes will not occur very often! Other than that, it simply permits calculation of the MCHC, but hypochromasia can be assessed at least as well by visual inspection of the red cells on the blood film. RBC counts also are virtually never interpreted as they stand, being simply used to calculate the MCV. Again, cell size can be assessed at least as well by inspection of the blood film. Some instruments also offer the possibility of a platelet count, but while having a numerical result is nice, again platelet numbers can be adequately estimated from the blood film.

Facilities to avoid include machine-generated PCV results and automatic differential WBC counts. In animal blood, the spun PCV is a more accurate measurement than a machine-generated figure (which is a calculation based on measuring the MCV and the RBC count, and difficulties can arise because the instruments were originally developed to cope with the larger human erythrocyte). In addition, having PCV and RBC/Hb measurements completely separate is an invaluable internal quality control – if the resulting MCV and MCHC values are credible for the species in question, and match the appearance of the blood film, it is extremely unlikely that any mistake has been made. In contrast, an all-in-one machine measurement is quite capable of generating a very credible, but wrong, set of results – due to poor sample mixing for example.

The only method to consider for differential WBC counting is blood film examination. The automated differential counts available by machine are simply not sufficiently reliable on non-human blood, especially if the sample quality might not be absolutely perfect. In particular, these methods should never be used as a lazy way of avoiding having to look at blood smears. As explained above, the *raison d'être* of automated differential counting is to reduce the number of blood film examinations which have to be made in the busy human laboratory, by screening out the obviously unremarkable samples. Not only does the methodology not transfer particularly well to non-human blood, this approach is simply not appropriate for the small veterinary practice facility, where looking at every blood film should be standard practice. It cannot be too often or too strongly stated, YOU CANNOT RUN A HAEMATOLOGY LABORATORY WITHOUT EXAMINING BLOOD FILMS, and the more you examine the better you will be at it.

As discussed on p. 318, haematology analysers for the veterinary laboratory should be Coulter-principle machines (particle counters, impedance counters), as laser technology is unsuitable for non-human samples. All that is required is a total WBC count, an RBC count and a haemoglobin concentration, and perhaps also a platelet count. Availability of further measurements is not only unnecessary, adding to the cost of the machine without adding to its usefulness, it is undesirable, because when a measurement (such as a calculated PCV or an automated differential WBC count) is available there is an almost irresistible temptation to use it, rather than carrying out the procedure by the more accurate manual method.

Although these machines have come a long way since the original basic particle counters and some effort has been expended to make them easier to use, it must never be forgotten that these are laboratory instruments. They need quite a lot of care and attention to keep them performing correctly – cleaning, calibrating and so on – and as a general rule the amount of user care and maintenance needed will turn out to be about two or three times that implied by the salesman when the machine is demonstrated. Staff who will be operating the machine require training to a fairly high standard, as running these instruments is a task really more appropriate for a laboratory technician than a nurse. Quality control and quality assessment must also be carried out *obsessively* – this is the only way to ensure confidence in the patient results.

Biochemistry

For the reasons explained above, wet chemistry methods are essential when moving beyond simple glucose and urea estimations. Reflectance meters, like centrifugation-type haematology machines, are only appropriate as an emergency approximation.

Suitability for lay use is essential when choosing an instrument. The machine itself should be clearly set out with the appropriate parts clearly labelled, and there should be no opportunity for ambiguous instructions to be mis-interpreted. Both written instructions and packaging of reagent units should be simple and unambiguous. The number of operator steps should be reduced to a minimum, and it is also important that, as far as is possible, operator steps should be non-critical (e.g. transferring 'some' sample into a receptacle where the exact volumes required are then pipetted by the machine is preferable to requiring a nurse to use an automatic pipette accurately). The machine's optical performance and the chemistries must be stable with little drift, so that recalibration need not be performed too frequently. In addition, calibration should be as simple as possible, as errors when calibrating can have disastrous consequences. Finally, reporting of results should be clear – if possible, choose a machine which provides a printout of results with the patient identity (as entered by the operator at the start of the analysis) included. This minimizes problems caused by misreading of digital readouts or mix-ups of results between patients. An instrument which scores well on these criteria will inevitably be more expensive than a simple machine which puts all the responsibility on the operator – in particular the minimizing of critical operator steps is usually achieved by the use of quite expensive single-shot reagent presentation.

The range of analytes available should be appropriate. Having the *right* tests is much more important than having a huge number of analytes available. For a routine laboratory, all the tests included in the relevant profiles discussed in Chapter 15 should be available, but availability of further, more esoteric tests (such as uric acid or triglycerides) should not be seen as a plus point for a machine which is not otherwise ideal. It is also important to check that the methods for albumin and alkaline phosphatase are appropriate for veterinary use (see p. 321). Look also at the points listed for external laboratories on p. 272 – some of these are also relevant to point-of-care analysers. Instruments should use SI units as standard, and report a *reasonable* number of significant figures (second decimal places on things like urea and glucose are just a non-sense, and reveal fundamental misunderstandings). Reference values, if given, should also be credible, and should again avoid ludicrous significant figures.

Flexibility is extremely important, and a feature on which some small side-room machines score badly. It is certainly highly desirable to be able to run a group of tests for one patient as a single operation – nothing is more frustrating than having to stand waiting for the urea test to finish so that you can start the creatinine. However, you should be the person to choose the appropriate group of tests or profile for each patient, not the salesperson. Reject any machine designed only to allow a single inflexible profile to be run for all patients, and any machine on which it appears you will be forced to run tests you do not want in order to get the results you do want – or to buy reagent packs you don't need along with those you do. It is also absolutely essential that single tests can be run if required. This is important for several reasons. You may find that a single result in a profile looks suspect, and want to repeat it – you should not find that you have to repeat the entire profile, which can be extremely expensive and time-consuming. Often one single analyte will be reported as 'out of range', meaning that the result is higher than the upper level of sensitivity of the assay. It is vitally important that you dilute the sample appropriately and re-run the test to get a true numerical reading, both for the sake of maximum pattern recognition information and to allow an accurate assessment of improvement at follow-up sampling, and this again requires that the test be run singly. Also, you may sometimes require only a single test as a check-up on a patient on treatment. Reagent packs for point-of-care analysers are expensive enough without being obliged to carry out more tests than required.

Assessing instrument performance

Once you are seriously interested in a haematology or biochemistry machine which seems suitable, it is necessary to satisfy yourself regarding performance. Remember, nobody is licensing these machines for veterinary sale or checking that they perform adequately; it is entirely up to you to ensure that what you sign up to will not endanger your patients.

It is necessary to understand something about the ways in which perfor-mance can be measured, and the meanings of the terms used to describe performance.

Precision is a measure of consistency or repeatability. To assess this, the same sample is analysed a number of times (typically 20), and the *coefficient of var-iation* (CV) is calculated

$$CV = \frac{SD}{\bar{x}} \times 100(\%)$$

where $\bar{x}$ is the mean result and SD the standard deviation. This should be done for every analyte, preferably at two levels, one high and one low. Two different types of precision are traditionally considered; the 'within-batch' variation and the 'between-batch' variation. The former is calculated by running all 20 repetitions together in a single batch, and the latter by including the test sample(s) in each of 20 different batches of tests. With the advent of random-access analysers (where the tests are performed as needed rather than in batches of a single analyte) the latter measurement becomes less clearly defined; however, it is common practice to substitute 'day-to-day' variation, running the test sample once every working day until the 20 repetitions are achieved.

Acceptable CVs do vary from analyte to analyte, and within-batch precision tends to be rather better than between-batch precision, but for most methods a CV of less than 5% is generally regarded as reasonable.

It is most important to understand, however, that precision has nothing at all to do with accuracy, that is whether the result is 'correct'. It is perfectly possible to have excellent precision, but still be miles away from the target value. This can be illustrated by considering a marksman aiming at a target, as shown in Fig. 18.5. In (a) the shots are clustered closely together (good precision), and they centre on the centre of the target (good accuracy). However, in (b), although the shots are still clustered together and thus the precision is just as good as in (a), they are well off-centre of the target (poor accuracy). In (c) the precision is poor, while in (d) poor precision is accompanied by marked bias. Strictly speaking, *bias* describes a situation where the direction and magnitude of the deviation from the target value are constant between samples – this is usually a problem of calibration. *Scatter*, which is much more serious, describes a situation where the deviation varies from one sample to another – one may be consistently 2 ft out at 10 o'clock while another may be just as consistently 3 ft out at 6 o'clock, and simply straightening the rifle barrel isn't going to fix this.

Accuracy is assessed by comparing numerical results with results for the same samples produced by a reference method – a method comparison study.

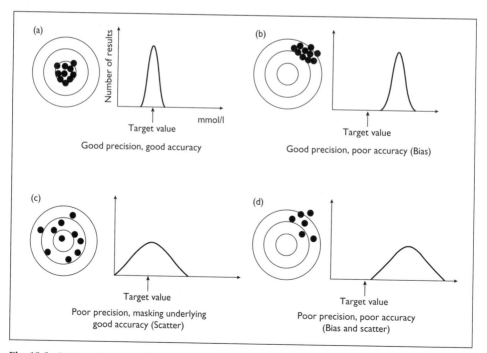

Fig. 18.5 Precision/accuracy. What is the difference? Examples assume a sample of known 'target' value has been assayed a large number of times.

Samples should, of course, come from the species which the machine will be used to analyse. Side-room instruments are generally evaluated against a large professional laboratory machine which is itself known to be performing well in all aspects of quality assurance. About 100 samples are analysed in parallel for each test, with a spread of concentrations covering the full physiological range (normal and abnormal) of the assay, and presented as a scatterplot with the reference method on the x-axis and the test instrument on the y-axis. Various examples of such scatterplots are shown in Figs 18.1–18.4. The solid line on each graph is the line of coincidence (or 1:1 line) which represents perfect agreement between the methods, while the broken line is the line of best fit of the points. Correlation statistics are also calculated – the *correlation coefficient* (*r*) describes the degree of scatter around the line of best fit, while the *gradient* (*m*) and the *y-intercept* of the line of best fit indicate bias (that is how far the line of best fit deviates from the line of coincidence, which has a gradient of 1.00 and an intercept of 0.00).

The correlation coefficient is, in fact, affected to some extent by the spread of values included, and a narrower range of values will give a lower result than a wide one for a similar degree of scatter. However, as a general rule one is looking for better than 0.99 for routine assays with a fairly wide spread of data points analysed, while methods where only a narrower spread of points is available (such as the total protein method shown in Fig. 18.1(a)) should still do better than 0.98. Ideally the line of best fit should be almost indistinguishable on the graph from the line of coincidence, with a gradient very close to 1.00 (0.95–1.05 at the worst), and a y-intercept close to zero (considering the units of the assay concerned).

Having said all that, however, a great deal can be appreciated simply by inspecting the scatterplots, without delving too deeply into the statistics. It is fairly clear that Figs 18.1(a), 18.3(a) and 18.4(a) represent decent performance which could be relied on for routine case work-up, while 18.1(b) and 18.3(b) would be practical for side-room emergency use but are not good enough for the routine laboratory. Figures 18.1(c), 18.2(a) 18.2(b) and 18.4(c) really shouldn't be allowed anywhere near anything describing itself as a laboratory.

Another point to consider is the practicality of the instrument for use by lay operators (that is nurses or vets as opposed to trained technicians). Precision and method comparison studies are often carried out entirely within the laboratory, with experienced technicians operating the test machine. Good performance in such a study is valuable in that it demonstrates that in the right hands the instrument is capable of producing the goods. Nevertheless, this performance may not be repeatable by the sort of person who will be required to operate the machine in real life. It is therefore advisable to ask in addition for equivalent results for a field study, where a trial machine has been placed in a veterinary practice for on-site evaluation. The centrifugation instrument and reflectance meter data in Figs 18.1–18.4 are from a field study.

This all involves a great deal of work, especially when a couple of dozen different haematology and biochemistry analytes may be involved. It is, of course, quite ridiculous to expect every prospective purchaser to carry out all these evaluations himself before purchase, not to mention a serious waste of resources. This work should all be done and tabulated before the instrument is put on the market, and the data should be available to be seen by potential purchasers. It is always more reassuring if the work has been carried out by someone other than the manufacturer, for example a university or research laboratory. It is disappointing, however, how seldom this information can actually be produced by those marketing laboratory instruments to the veterinary profession, which does rather raise the question as to whether the machines have been evaluated at all (rather than simply re-badged from human models), or if they have been, why is everyone so coy about the results? If a company cannot produce a respectable set of method evaluation data when requested, go no further with that instrument, no matter how many other practices may have succumbed. Go and talk to one of their competitors.

It is also, unfortunately, necessary to be very critical in your appraisal of any evaluations you might be shown. Some publications may *seem* to show that the machine is performing as required, but closer inspection can reveal that they in fact show no such thing. The things to look out for include:

The precision-only study. Precision is only a small part of the evaluation; the thing you are really interested in is the accuracy – the method comparison study. If accuracy is good, precision almost looks after itself. If you are shown an evaluation which only looks at repeatability (even if it is compared to the repeatability of a reference instrument) and offers no clue as to whether the result is actually *correct*, ask yourself what it is they are trying to hide.

The same-method comparison (which mainly concerns reflectance meters). The reference method for the comparison study *must* be the standard professional veterinary laboratory wet chemistry method. A study which shows that a veterinary reflectance meter gives exactly the same results as the human version of the same machine is of no value, because it completely begs the question of whether the results from animal samples compare well with the true reference method. If you are shown a study like this, consider carefully why the manufacturers chose this approach, rather than using a wet chemistry reference method.

Fudging the issue. Some published method comparisons can be rather coy about what it is they have actually demonstrated. Sometimes only selected scatterplots for the better analytes are displayed, with the poorer performance of the other analytes concealed in a table of correlation statistics (interpretation of scatterplots is fairly intuitive, but it takes a lot more effort to figure it out from the statistics alone). Sometimes scatterplots are drawn which aren't square, have different scales on the x and y axes, and do not display the line of coincidence (this is very naughty). Sometimes no scatterplots are shown at all. Sometimes methods are graded as 'satisfactory' on very lenient criteria, more suitable for the interim emergency situation rather than the routine laboratory. Scrutinise anything you are shown with great care!

Irrelevant data. A thick pile of paper can look very impressive – and very daunting – but if it all consists of studies on human samples, or studies on methods you are not interested in, or peripheral issues such as influence of haemolysis and lipaemia, it doesn't carry much weight.

In short, look for the scatterplots. A complete set of scatterplots (using wet chemistry reference methods) which look more or less like Figs 18.1(a), 18.3(a) and 18.4(a) is good news. If you are being shown something else, or if the salesperson doesn't appear to know what a method comparison study *is*, look elsewhere.

Finally, be very careful of instruments which incorporate any form of 'interpretation' of results. The development of an artificial intelligence program to interpret clinico-pathological data would be a very major undertaking, and it has never been seriously tackled in the veterinary field. The sort of 'guide' or 'suggestions' which might be tacked on to a point-of-care instrument is likely to be superficial at best, at worst actively misleading. The program may not even have been written by a veterinary surgeon. If you are shown a machine which generates suggested interpretations you yourself can easily see are spurious, consider very carefully whether the numerical data it produces, which are less easy to judge, can be relied on with any greater confidence.

Once you have found a manufacturer and an instrument you are happy with, you will of course want to try it out. It is important to keep your feet on the ground at this stage. Try using it yourself, and try teaching a nurse to use it. Is it really as user-friendly as you want it to be? Will you be tempted to skip essential maintenance or calibration routines because they are too onerous? Will you be chewing the crockery as its tubing blocks up for the fifth time in an hour? Are you finding a high proportion of 'out of range' results, and if so are you prepared to keep diluting the samples and repeating the analysis until you get a numerical result? (You wouldn't accept 'out of range' on a professional laboratory report, would you?) Is your nurse spending so long wrestling with the analyser that other duties are suffering?

You should also run at least a dozen samples, with a good spread of results, in parallel on the new instrument and through your usual clinical pathology laboratory. Bear in mind that even a very poor method with a lot of scatter will often have at least half its results relatively close to the line of coincidence – look again at Fig. 18.1(c). It is human nature to cheer the good shots and quietly forget about the less good ones. Therefore, plot your own scatterplots and inspect them dispassionately. Even a dozen points should give you an idea of whether or not you are reproducing the published performance capability of the instrument.

Only when you are really comfortable that you are doing the right thing should you go ahead with the purchase. Remember, while you can switch pathology laboratories any time you like, once you have invested in instrumentation of your own you will have to live with that choice for several years.

Setting up the laboratory

When setting up laboratory procedures, the concept of *quality assurance* should be a major consideration at all levels. This refers to the entire laboratory exercise being designed to ensure high-quality error-free results, and covers everything from sample reception through formal quality control and quality assessment, to laboratory safety and accurate record-keeping. Bear in mind also that the COSHH (control of substances hazardous for health) legislation applies to the laboratory in the same way as to the rest of the practice, and compliance should be ensured – it is convenient to deal with this when standard operating procedures (SOPs) are being written.

General necessities

Space.   Requirements should not be underestimated. It is not necessary to dedicate a whole room to the laboratory alone, but any activity which shares the room should be compatible with usual laboratory safety precautions. This rules out such things as the tea room or an office where secretarial staff are continually at work, but lab work can coexist happily with such things as a storage area (drug store or back files) or isolation kennels. The latter can be particularly useful as it enables a single person to carry out emergency tests out of hours while keeping an eye on the patient. The lab area should be comfortably warm and well lit, and not so far from the hub of practice activities that staff feel isolated while using it. Adequate electrical points (at least six) are essential, as is a gas point for a bunsen burner. The floor should be impervious, free from cracks, and easy to clean, e.g. well-fitted lino or lino tiles. Solidly fixed benching is necessary, 900 mm high and 600–750 mm, deep, with enough length to allow all the lab equipment to be arranged conveniently and permanently (it is very annoying to have to put the microscope in the cupboard whenever you want to use the centrifuge, or vice versa) and enough additional clear space to work on. Three metres of benching is probably the absolute minimum and even this is likely to be cramped. The bench surface should be impervious and easy to clean, e.g. Formica. Wood is not very satisfactory. There should be a sink with hot and cold water and space for a small fridge (with freezer compartment) – this may fit under the bench. At least one drawer unit and one double cupboard unit should also be fitted under the bench, positioned to allow clear knee space under the working area, the microscope and the analysers. A narrow shelf (about 150 mm wide and the same above the bench) is useful along the back of the bench for things like stain bottles, but it is often best to leave the wall behind the bench clear for the display of detailed operating instructions rather than to go in for lots of wall-mounted cupboards. Space should also be allowed for a desk and a filing cabinet (for things like instrument manuals and documentation, quality control data, and possibly patients' result forms).

Furniture.   Requirements have mostly been dealt with above. At least two comfortable lab stools or high chairs will also be needed, plus an ordinary chair for use at the desk. Several firms specialize in the supply of custom-built laboratory fittings, but it is possible to have quite satisfactory fittings installed more cheaply by a local joiner. A third possibility is to make use of a specialist supplier of fitted kitchen units. When deciding on the layout of the laboratory and the positioning of each item of equipment it is important to arrange equipment for each test and related tests close together and as conveniently to hand as possible, and to aim for a logical progression of the sample along the bench as it is processed. This prevents tiring and time-wasting criss-crossing around the room.

Staffing.   Staffing of the laboratory requires careful consideration. It is generally uneconomical to use veterinary staff for technical duties, and most of the routine testing will usually be the responsibility of the nursing staff. It is unfair to expect nurses to carry out lab tests in their coffee breaks, and staff duties should be organized to allow sufficient time for this work. It is probably best to arrange for a single person to have primary responsibility for the lab work during normal working hours – this is not to imply that this person does nothing else, but that he or she gives priority to dealing with lab requirements as they arise. If this duty is rotated, perhaps weekly, it ensures that all members of the lay staff acquire and retain the necessary expertise, which is invaluable for out-of-hours and sickness cover, and ensures that staff do not become stale and bored.

Training.   It is obviously essential to ensure that all staff to be involved in this duty receive adequate training. Unless the practice operates a system of having a nurse on call out of hours it will also be necessary to give all the veterinary staff basic training in performing those tests which are likely to be required in an emergency, in order to make full use of the facilities. Good quality training requires *time*, and sometimes money, and adequate provision should be made for this. Nearly all suppliers of laboratory analysers undertake to arrange staff training on their machine, and courses and evening classes in general laboratory work are available. However, it is dangerous to rely too heavily on outside training and there are a number of advantages to having staff trained 'on the job' by a member of the practice staff, usually the veterinary surgeon with primary responsibility for setting up and running the laboratory.

(1)   Training can be tailored to the practice's own particular methods, and can encompass the whole area of running the laboratory rather than just how to perform a number of tests.

(2)   Training can be accomplished with minimum time away from work or disruption to work routine.

(3)   Training can be regularly reinforced as necessary and immediate help given when problems are encountered.

(4)   If the person who is responsible for lab supervision also trains the staff then the supervisory duties become much easier and more realistic – otherwise it can become a case of the blind leading the partially sighted!

If this system is to be followed then it is obviously essential that the responsible veterinary surgeon must first become thoroughly familiar with all the equipment, the methods in use and the things which can go wrong. It is also a good idea to try to acquire some training in the art of training – there are very specific techniques which make training easier and more effective. Careful attention should be given to the production of written standard operating procedures (SOPs) for every task, in sufficient detail to allow someone unfamiliar with the task to carry it through if necessary. These instructions should be clearly typed and either displayed on the wall (if they will be referred to frequently) or bound in a loose-leaf or display folder. Ensure that they are kept up to date and amended wherever they prove to be unclear or inadequate. Clear and detailed SOPs take time to produce, but will save much more time in training, reminding and troubleshooting. They will also be invaluable to colleagues performing lab tests out of hours.

Paperwork.   Once the furniture is installed and the equipment purchased, some thought should be given to the logistics of ensuring that the system works as smoothly as possible. The absolute minimum paperwork for each sample is a basic request form, incorporating the following information:

Requesting veterinary surgeon
Unambiguous patient identification
Date and time of sampling
Nature of samples (e.g. 'EDTA and heparin blood')
Analyses required
Some means of recording that the tests have been carried out, by whom and at what time.

A supply of these should be kept in every consulting and operating room.

It is helpful to site an 'in tray' (plastic cat litter trays are very good) somewhere convenient, in which all samples together with their request forms are placed. A clear notice should be displayed beside the tray to indicate who is currently on lab duty so that that person can be tracked down if the sample is urgent. This system can also double as a gathering point for samples to be sent to external laboratories, together with their appropriate forms, so that the same person can deal with the packaging and despatch. He or she should be responsible for checking the tray regularly and dealing with samples as they arrive.

Modern analysers, even for the small laboratory, usually include the facility to print out individual patient reports, which may eliminate the need for the laboratory day-book and a comprehensive report form. However, some thought has to be given to tests performed away from the analysers, such as microhaematocrit PCVs, manual differential WBC counts, urine test strips and sediment examination. Provision may be made for these on the lower part of the request form, so that it doubles as a result form, or some thought may be given to adding handwritten results to the printouts produced by the analysers. If the results are to be entered into the patients' computer records then it may be practical to work directly on to the 'report' form, which is then filed in the laboratory, and so omit using a separate day-book to record results. However, some practices will find it necessary to use a day-book to record results as the samples are analysed, with results then transcribed on to a reporting form (which may still be part of the request form) which is returned to the patient's records.

Some thought should also be given to storage of results. If everything can be stored on computer and associated with the patient's record, so much the better. However, many systems only allow for a summary of laboratory data to be incorporated in the records, and in that case a clearly cross-referenced filing system is essential to enable the full report to be retrieved when required. Good laboratory practice demands that not only original results but original quality control data be preserved – when deciding on your record-keeping system, consider how you would respond if the accuracy or reliability of a result were ever challenged in court.

Running the laboratory

If close attention has been paid to the points raised above when the laboratory is set up then the minimum of attention should be necessary to keep it running satisfactorily. However, as with any system where staff operate on a rota system, it is essential to have one person in a permanent supervisory role to ensure that standards are maintained. This person should normally be the veterinary surgeon who set up the laboratory, but some of the more routine duties may be delegated to a senior nurse. It is important to set aside some time regularly every week to go into the laboratory and ensure that everything is satisfactory, and to budget for this time and effort when costing out the laboratory. The supervisor should be prepared to organize or deal with everything in the following areas.

Quality control

This is an extremely important concept and it is absolutely vital that an appropriate quality control (QC) system is operated in all laboratories carrying out diagnostic work. In larger laboratories quality control involves the analysis *every day* (sometimes more often, especially when out-of-hours emergency runs are performed) of two samples with known results – usually one in the normal and one in the pathological range. Limits of acceptability for these results are pre-set, using 'state of the art' criteria rather than clinical usefulness. If results for an assay fall outside these limits then the assay is recalibrated until the QC is satisfactory, and only then are patient results accepted. If this happens regularly then rigorous troubleshooting is instituted. Quality control results are also statistically analysed to provide a measure of the *precision* of the assay, which expresses the ability of the lab to get the same result repeatedly day after day (see Fig. 18.5). The statistic used is the coefficient of variation (CV). Target CVs vary between assays, but for most simple techniques a value of less than 5% is desirable.

In a practice lab with a fairly high throughput the same system should be adopted. Where throughput is lower, and the lab is perhaps not used every day, minimum frequency for QC is weekly. Again, one normal and one pathological sample should be run for each assay. It is useful to have the new duty nurse do this each Monday morning at the start of the duty rota – this enables her to refamiliarize herself with the procedures and gives a true 'between-batch' figure for precision. Results should be both recorded in a dedicated notebook (name of operator, date, lot number of QC serum and all results) and plotted on a graph as illustrated in Fig. 18.6. This is known as a Levey–Jennings plot. Better still, it is fairly easy to set up a computer spreadsheet for this, so that graphs are plotted and CVs calculated automatically as results are entered. The graph allows the general situation to be assessed very quickly by the supervisior, and it allows easy appreciation of certain warning signs – seven consecutive results either rising or falling, or seven consecutive results either above or below the previous mean value, spell trouble and should be investigated.

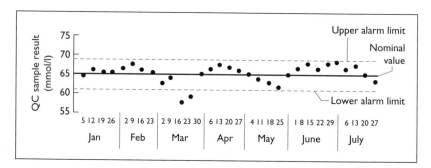

Fig. 18.6 Example QC results recorded graphically. Method is 'out of control' if (a) two consecutive 'outlier' values occur, e.g. in March, (b) seven consecutive falling (or rising) values occur, e.g. in April/May, or (c) seven consecutive results above (or below) the nominal value occur, e.g. in June/July. If possible, it is better to derive your own nominal values and alarm limits for each batch of QC serum, for your own methods. Assay the QC sample every day for 10 days; nominal value is the mean and the alarm limits the $\pm 3SD$ values. Mean should be within manufacturers' specified tolerances and CV should be reasonable for the method.

The most satisfactory way to approach this is to purchase freeze–dried lyophilized QC sera. These are available from a number of sources, including most suppliers of biochemistry analysers – in this case they will have specific target values listed for that particular analyser which makes it easier to establish your acceptable limits for each batch of serum. Specially preserved whole blood for haematology QC use is also available. It is best, to choose non-human-based products whenever possible, because when the label announces 'treat as patient sample' it really means 'treat as if potentially hepatitis B and HIV infective', which is not the same thing at all in a veterinary laboratory. Human-based products must always be handled with gloves. Be sure to follow manufacturer's recommendations regarding storage and reconstitution, or you may find deteriorating QC material masquerading as an analytical problem in your statistics. Haematology QC material must always be mixed *extremely* thoroughly to avoid cumulative errors caused by sequential removal of unrepresentative aliquots.

Quality assessment

In larger laboratories quality assessment involves the reception from an outside source of one or more samples every 2–4 weeks whose results are *unknown* to laboratory personnel. This is analysed as if it were a patient sample and the results reported to the scheme organizer. The lab's performance is then graded by the organizer in relation to all the other laboratories participating in the scheme. Pedantically speaking, quality assessment (QA) measures inter-laboratory (national) precision, but in practice the consensus mean is taken as being the 'correct' value and QA is thus considered to measure the *accuracy* of each method, which is in effect the ability to get as close as possible to the 'right answer' (see Fig. 18.5).

Again it is impracticable for a small practice laboratory to join one of the large, organized QA schemes, but the QA principle can be applied to the practice lab. There are two ways of going about this. A patient sample (haematology and/or biochemistry) may be split in two and the duplicate sent for analysis by a trustworthy external laboratory – be sure to optimize sample preservation and posting times to avoid penalizing your own lab for the effects of a deteriorated sample. Alternatively the supervisor may take a commercial QC sample of a different batch from that in routine use and with assigned values for the method in use given by the manufacturer, and submit this as if it were a patient sample.

The frequency of this exercise should be about once per month, but it is important to ensure that it is distributed evenly between all the operators on the rota. It is preferable, if possible, that operators should only know in general that this system will be run and should not be able to identify the actual samples. However, once all the results are available it is important to discuss them with the people involved – praise for work well done is always appreciated, and if something has gone wrong it will be necessary to investigate the problem.

Some instrument manufacturers operate their own QA schemes within their own user group. These can be useful, but take care that you are not simply joining a cheerleader club designed more to reassure than to test the system.

Statistical analysis of QA performance is complicated and it is probably best just to assess whether, clinically speaking, each result is acceptably close to the target. It is also vital to do more than shrug helplessly if results are *not* acceptable. Once identified, problems must be tackled and rectified, and a poorly performing assay must not be used for patient samples until this has been done and acceptable performance proved. It is important to include the costs of this exercise in the fixed costs when calculating the running costs of the laboratory.

Calibration

This does not apply to every system, but many instruments have standard curves which require recalibration from time to time, either at set intervals or when the QC results have been observed to be drifting. It is helpful if the supervising veterinary surgeon can carry out this task personally, as this ensures uniformity of technique and allows them to maintain familiarity with the machine. A full set of QC samples should always be run after calibration to check that everything has been done correctly, and the system is then ready for anyone simply to come along and run the samples. It is important to keep a record in the QC book of when the machine has been recalibrated.

Stocktaking

Nothing is more annoying than suddenly running out of some insignificant but vital consumable. It is therefore important to keep a list of all such items which are required in the laboratory, to check current stocks against this list weekly, and to ensure that anything which is running low is reordered in good time. This task may be incorporated into drug stocktaking procedures.

Technical matters

It is preferable to have one person who is responsible for the laboratory instrumentation, for matters such as organization of regular servicing, routine checking of instrument function, arranging any repairs which might be necessary and generally providing a liaison with the instrumentation and laboratory supply companies. Most companies prefer to deal regularly with the same person in a practice, particularly when that person is knowledgeable about laboratory matters, and this is the best way to maintain a good relationship with company representatives and ensure that you are kept abreast of new developments in the field.

Training

The need for adequate initial training has been discussed above, but it should always be remembered that training is a continuous process. Existing staff require regular reinforcement of their training, with particular attention being paid to the eradication of bad habits, and additional training will be required when new equipment is purchased or new methods are introduced. The training of new members of staff is extremely important, and sufficient time should be allocated to allow this to be done in a friendly, sympathetic and unhurried way before the new employee is left in a responsible position. Remember that poorly trained staff lack confidence, take far longer than necessary to carry out a task and are unreliable.

Troubleshooting

It is very helpful if staff know that there is one person on whom they can rely for help if they get into difficulties in the lab, or to whom they can show a doubtful-looking report for checking. Any problems which surface via the QC or QA schemes will also require investigation and correction.

Laboratory safety

A list of safety rules should be drawn up and displayed in the laboratory, and these should be strictly enforced. They should include:

(1) No eating, drinking, smoking or applying cosmetics in the room.
(2) Suitable protective clothing (e.g. lab coat) to be worn at all times, but it must be removed before meals or tea breaks.
(3) Strict attention must be paid to instructions for waste disposal.
(4) Extinguish bunsen burner when not in use.
(5) Wear gloves at all times when handling calibration or control samples of human origin.
(6) Wash hands before leaving the room.

Particular attention should also be paid to the safety of all electrical appliances (safe wiring, and correct fuses in plugs) and the gas supply. Centrifuges in which the lid can be opened while the motor is running are *strictly illegal*, and bucket-type centrifuges should be fitted with a lock which ensures that the lid cannot be released until the rotor has *stopped*. Most refrigerators are liable to explode if inflammable solvents are stored in them, and a notice forbidding this should be posted on the door. It is good practice to cover all working areas of the bench with a specially produced protective paper (Bench-Kote) and to replace this whenever it becomes soiled. In addition to the standard first aid kit, an eyewash bottle should be readily available. An efficient fire extinguisher should be close to hand in any room where a bunsen burner is operated.

Waste disposal

This has important safety implications. There are three categories of waste in a basic haematology/biochemistry laboratory and appropriate containers should be provided for each one. The correct place for all waste generated should be specified in the SOPs for each test. *Needles and blades* should be disposed of in the same way as in surgery, i.e. in a rigid, securely closed container. *Glass*, whether broken or not, must not be placed in a plastic sack, and a metal or plastic bin should be provided for this. It is also useful to provide a small bench-top glass bin on the haematology bench to facilitate quick disposal of the numerous capillary tubes, coverslips and slides used. *Everything else* may be placed in plastic sacks. It is usual to use yellow sack for contaminated material (to be incinerated) and a black sack for the ordinary rubbish. Again, it is useful to place a small box on the biochemistry bench for easy disposal of small items such as used pipette tips, which aids tidiness. Ensure that bench-top waste containers are emptied into the main receptacle at least daily.

It should be the clear responsibility of a named person to make sure that all waste bins and bags are properly emptied and disposed of, and not allowed to become over-full.

Cleaning and tidying

All staff should be trained to tidy up as they go and to replace everything in its proper place when the work is finished. General cleaning may be carried out by the duty nurse or by a cleaner, but whoever is responsible must be properly instructed in the correct procedures for cleaning lab instruments and the areas where particular care is required. The insides of centrifuges get particularly messy, and it is important to check benches and floors for overlooked cover slips, capillary tubes and microscope slides, which can accumulate in odd corners. Cleaning should not be neglected, as a dirty or untidy lab is a dangerous lab.

Appendix I: Principles of electronic resistance (impedance) particle counting ('Coulter principle')

This method has been applied to blood cell analysis since the 1950s and is well characterized for multi-species use. The instrument contains a transducer with an aperture of an exact size, and two electrodes, one inside and one outside the aperture. This assembly is immersed in an electrically conductive diluent which allows a DC current to flow between the electrodes (Fig. 18.7). Blood cells, which are non-conductive, are suspended in the diluent. When a cell passes through the aperture it decreases the flow of current, increasing the resistance between the electrodes. This causes a voltage change (the 'cell pulse') between the electrodes proportional to the volume of the cell (Ohm's law, $V = I \times R$, where V is the voltage, I is the current and R is the resistance). These small voltage changes have to be amplified, and electrical interference, artificial signals and the effects of temperature are eliminated in the electronic circuitry.

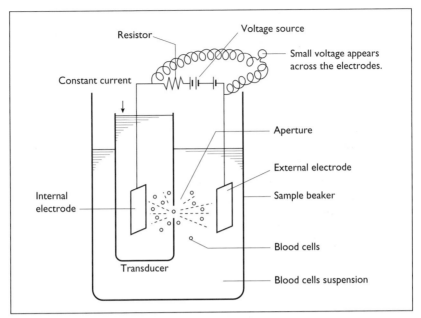

Fig. 18.7   Schematic representation of an electrical impedance particle counter.

A statistical 'coincidence correction' is also applied to allow for the effect of two cells passing through the aperture simultaneously, an incidence which obviously varies with the cell count.

An electronic 'threshold' or 'discriminator' is set to screen out very small pulses which might be noise or electrical interference, so that only objects the right size to be cells are counted. This is achieved by plotting cell counts at every different threshold level to obtain a cumulative cell size distribution curve (Fig. 18.8). The solid line is the cumulative pulse height (particle size) distribution curve, with the activity at the left-hand side of the graph (small particles) being 'noise'. The flat portion, or plateau, represents the boundary between the noise and the cell, and the optimum setting of the discriminator is around a third of the way along the plateau. The broken line is the ordinary cell size distribution curve which is derived from the cumulative plot.

Older Coulter counters were very flexible, with the operator being able to control the aperture, threshold and other parameters of the system, which enabled optimization of the instrument settings for particular species. More modern blood counters are usually comparatively rigid, being optimized for human cells, but it is still generally possible to adapt their operation for veterinary use. However, human red cells (at around 80–90 fl) are larger than the erythrocytes of any of the domestic mammals, and once one gets a long way from this size, problems can arise. Goat red cells are particularly small, but sheep can also be difficult to cope with in some systems. Smaller red cells obviously come closer to platelets in size, creating difficulties both in avoiding

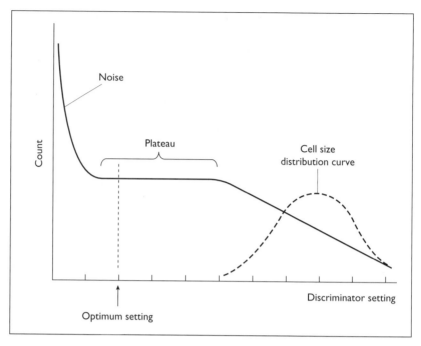

Fig. 18.8 Cell size distribution curves. The solid line is the cumulative curve, showing the relationship of the optimum discriminator setting to the plateau, and the broken line is the ordinary cell size distribution curve.

counting some platelets as red cells, and in adapting the method to count platelets in whole blood.

In red cell counting the cells are simply suspended in a dilution of isotonic fluid, counted at the appropriate discriminator setting, coincidence corrected, and the result multiplied by a factor to allow for the dilution ratio. As the size of the cell pulse is proportional to the volume of the cell it is also possible to derive MCV and PCV values in this way; however, it is arguably preferable to perform PCVs by the microhaematocrit method when dealing with non-human samples, especially in the practice side-room situation (see p. 284).

To count white cells by this method, it is first necessary to eliminate the red cells from the suspension. This is done by adding a lysing agent to the WBC dilution aliquot, which destroys the cell membranes and dissolves the cytoplasm, leaving only the (leucocyte) nuclei as countable particles. (This is why impedance counters cannot be used for white cell counting in birds and reptiles – the nuclei of the red cells also remain in suspension, completely overwhelming the number of white cell nuclei (see Plate 12). Camel blood can also be a problem because the erythrocyte membrane is very resistant to lysis.) After lysis, counting proceeds as for the red cell counting.

Exact procedures vary between machines, and some automate the entire process. However, the usual method is to make an initial 1:500 dilution of the sample, which will be used to count the white cells and measure the haemoglobin photometrically in the machine (all cell counters incorporate a basic photometer flow cell operating on the transmission/absorbance principle (see Appendix II below) for this purpose). Immediately an aliquot of that dilution is removed and further diluted to obtain a second 1:500 000 dilution for red cell counting. Automatic dilutors are available to simplify this procedure. The higher dilution is used unchanged, at the machine's RBC settings. The first dilution is further treated by the addition of a set volume of lysing agent. This both prepares the suspension of WBC nuclei for counting and releases the haemoglobin in the RBCs free into solution. A haemoglobin reagent (which contains cyanide, and must be handled with strict safety precautions) is included in the lysing agent. After waiting (usually 30 seconds) for complete lysis to occur and for the cyanmethaemoglobin reaction to go to completion, this dilution is passed through the machine at the WBC/Hb setting. The sample stream is split, part going through the transducer for white cell counting and part going through the photometer flow cell for haemoglobin measurement.

Total white cell counting on mammalian blood is virtually species-insensitive. However, refinements of the system to discriminate between different types of leucocyte (automated differential counts) most certainly are not. Although veterinary instruments with this facility are available, they have been developed by tinkering around with the human-cell instruments rather than being designed from the start for the target species. Veterinary haematology laboratories should always back up an automated differential count by scanning a blood film, and if there appears to be a discrepancy, a manual count should be performed. In the practice side-room situation it is wise, and much safer, to avoid automated differential counting entirely and make use of *all* the information available from the blood film (see p. 276).

Appendix II: Principles of ultraviolet/visible photometry

Ultraviolet/visible photometry is the main technique of concentration measurement in the biochemistry laboratory. Methods involve the production (or occasionally disappearance) of a chemical compound which has an absorption peak in the measurable UV/visible range and whose concentration is directly (or inversely) related to the concentration of the substance under investigation. The optically measurable compound may be formed directly with the substance under investigation (analyte), or may be the end-product of a linked series of reactions, in this case usually involving the use of specific enzymes.

For each of the common analytes there is usually a choice of methods involving different reaction sequences. In general the measurement of *substrates* (i.e. analytes which are not enzymes) is carried out by *end-point* methods, where the reaction is allowed to go to completion and the concentration of the final product measured, while *enzymes* are measured by *kinetic* methods, where several measurements of optical density are made while the reaction is proceeding in order to quantify the *rate* of the reaction, which is related to analyte concentration or activity. However, with the development of automatic reaction rate analysers many of the newer substrate methods are also kinetic, as this can reduce incubation periods and hence total analysis time quite considerably. One of the most useful reactions for kinetic methods is the $NAD^+ \rightleftharpoons NADH$ reaction which can be conveniently linked to a wide variety of reactions via the appropriate enzyme/substrate chains and which can be easily monitored at the UV wavelength of 340 nm (NADH absorbs at 340 nm, NAD^+ does not).

Transmission/absorbance photometry

This is the traditional measurement technique for the familiar 'wet chemistry' methods and depends on the well-known Beer–Lambert law:

$$A \text{ (or OD)}_\lambda = \varepsilon C \text{ (at a 1 cm path-length)},$$

which simply means that the absorbance (or optical density) of a substance at a given wavelength (λ) and in a cuvette 1 cm in diameter is equal to its concentration (C) times its extinction coefficient (ε), a constant which defines the substance's intrinsic ability to absorb that wavelength of light. The wavelength chosen for measurement is usually as close as possible to the peak extinction of the substance, to maximize sensitivity, while staying as far away as possible from the absorbance wavelengths of likely interfering substances such as haemoglobin and bilirubin. Where a grating spectrophotometer is used the exact wavelength can be set with as narrow a 'window' as required, but it is more usual in clinical biochemistry to use a (cheaper) filter photometer in which the wavelength is set by placing a coloured filter between the light source and the cuvette. With this system it is necessary to choose the filter supplied which is closest to the optimum wavelength for the method.

End-point methods

Based on this theory, it is easy to construct a 'standard curve' (which ought to be a straight line over the operating range) relating the original concentration of the analyte under investigation to the final absorbance of the reaction mixture at the chosen wavelength (see Fig. 18.9). While it is necessary to use a large number of standards to characterize a standard curve initially, especially to define its linear range, many established methods can be run quite satisfactorily using only two-point or even single-point (plus blank) calibration. It is not usual to read absorbances of over about 1.5 units as the logarithmic nature of the scale makes readings above this value imprecise. Even below this value, care should be taken to use only readings on the linear part of the standard

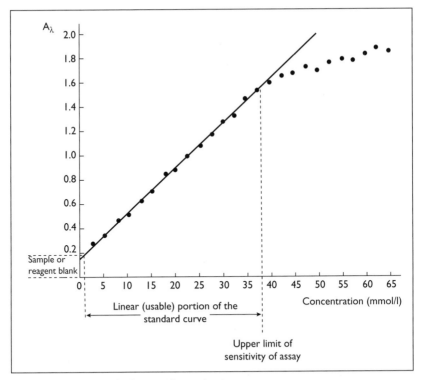

Fig. 18.9 Typical standard curve of an end-point assay.

curve, which often flattens out at some stage into an unusable plateau. This means that for the standard sample volume there is always an upper limit of sensitivity for any method, and when values over this limit are obtained it is essential to go back and repeat the assay with a diluted sample (or a smaller sample volume) to get a reading on the linear part of the standard curve, and then multiply up the result. Another point to watch concerns the blank, or zeroing. Many methods can be zeroed quite adequately using distilled water, as the reagent absorbance at the chosen wavelength is negligible, but where this is not the case a 'reagent blank' of reagents only with no sample must be prepared to define the level of they y-intercept of the standard curve (see Fig. 18.9). It is important to know which methods require this. So long as the measurement wavelength is sufficiently far away from those of possible interfering substances in the sample then this is all that is required, but certain methods (e.g. inorganic phosphate) use wavelengths so close to possible interference (e.g. from haemoglobin in a haemolysed sample) that a 'sample blank' containing all ingredients (reagents and sample) but in which no reaction is allowed to take place must be prepared from any highly coloured sample in order to achieve a genuine concentration reading. The requirement for a sample blank for every sample with some methods doubles the actual reagent costs and total running time for these assays.

Kinetic methods

These methods rely on the arrangement of the reaction chemistry so that the rate of a reaction which can be followed by the appearance (or disappearance) of a substance with an absorption peak in the measurable range (e.g. NADH) is proportional to the concentration (or activity in the case of enzymes) of the analyte under consideration. This means that the absorbance of the reaction mixture must be measured not once but several times for each individual sample. Manual kinetic measurements usually involve four or five readings over 2 or 3 minutes, while automatic analysers often take a large number of readings every second over perhaps 15 seconds to cut down analysis time. Whichever method is used, the aim is essentially to calculate the gradient of the ΔA (ΔOD) line and relate that to the concentration of a substrate analyte or the activity of an enzyme analyte (see Fig. 18.10). Note that the x-axis in this case is time, not concentration. The reaction shown is one of increasing absorbance, e.g. $NAD^+ \rightarrow NADH$, but a decreasing reaction (e.g. $NADH \rightarrow NAD^+$) is equally possible and useful. Again there are certain constraints which must be borne in mind. The reaction seldom sets off at its true rate the instant the

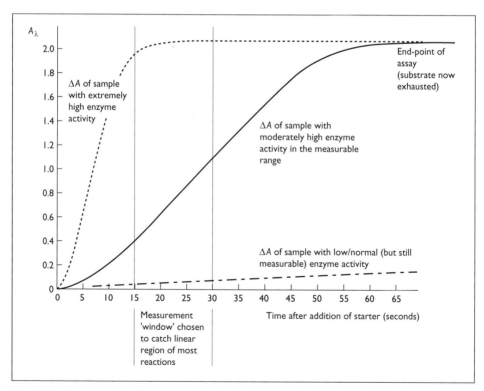

Fig. 18.10 Measurement of enzyme activities by the kinetic method. Note that during the measurement 'window' the ΔA of the extremely high activity sample which has reached substrate exhaustion is virtually the same as that of the low/normal sample. The giveaway is the much higher initial absorbance, and the reaction is also slightly non-linear.

reagents are mixed (the last thing to be added is termed the 'starter' as it starts the reaction) and the readings should not be begun until such time as even the slowest sample may be assumed to have reached its linear stage. On the other hand, the reaction cannot keep going indefinitely and there is a very real danger that in some samples the whole affair may be over and done with before measurements are begun. This is particularly likely where a very *high* activity of an enzyme analyte is present in a sample and is due to all the substrate supplied by the reagent solutions having been consumed – '*substrate exhaustion*'. The net effect is that by the time the readings are taken the ΔA value is, in fact, very small (see the dotted line on Fig. 18.10) and unless vigilance is exercised a very *low* enzyme result may be reported. The giveaway clue is that the first reading of the series, the '*initial absorbance*', is far higher than it ought to be (or lower in the case of a decreasing reaction) if this were simply a very slow reaction, and that the apparent enzyme activity is improbably low. Any sample where this effect is spotted must be diluted and re-run. Any automatic reaction rate analyser worth its salt should sense the initial absorbance of each reaction and 'flag' for checking any with evidence of substrate exhaustion, but this is a phenomenon which must be clearly understood with all reaction rate methods to avoid an extremely pathological enzyme activity being reported as normal.

Practical application in the laboratory

Modern point-of-care biochemistry analysers take care of all the measurements and calculations for each assay invisibly, so that it is no longer necessary for the operator to write down absorbance readings of standards, plot a standard curve, then read off the patient results from the graph – or worse still, follow a reaction rate with a pencil and a stopwatch. Instead, results are reported directly as mmol/l, or iu/l, or whatever. This is enormously labour- and time-saving, and when everything is going to plan it improves reliability by eliminating human error from the readings and the calculations. However, the resulting tendency to treat these analysers as a sort of 'black box' is not without its dangers.

Clear understanding of *how* a machine operates is absolutely essential when it comes to troubleshooting and problem-spotting. You need to have a firm grasp of the principles outlined above, and then understand how your own analyser actually puts these into operation. How many filters are there, and how are they changed? How is each test blanked? How many actual measurements does the machine make for each test? (End-point methods are often two-point, a sample or reagent blank, then a single absorbance measured at a fixed time after starting the test, when it is assumed that the reaction will have reached completion. Kinetic methods may also be two-point in small point-of-care analysers, but this makes some very heavy assumptions regarding the linearity of the reactions; see Fig. 18.10.) What are the upper and lower limits of sensitivity for each test? Does the machine have the capacity to spot substrate exhaustion in a kinetic method (again see Fig. 18.10)? Will the machine generate an error message with badly haemolysed or lipaemic samples, or will it simply print out a random result?

Just as you should not be taking X-rays without a clear understanding of the principles of radiography (no matter how easy your X-ray machine is to operate), you should not be undertaking laboratory analyses without the same understanding of the principles involved. This in turn leads to a good understanding of what can go wrong and how, and generates a healthy scepticism when faced with improbable results. Many point-of-care analysers are intentionally designed to be tamper-proof, on the grounds that non-technically-trained operators can do more harm than good if they are allowed to meddle. This is probably a wise precaution. Nevertheless, a good grasp of what is going on inside your 'black box' allows rational investigation of apparent problems, simplifies identification of correctable errors, and ensures that technical assistance is sought when necessary.

Reflectance photometry

This principle has been in use for quite a long time in the form of simple glucose meters designed to take the subjectivity out of dipstick reading, and in the 1980s several manufacturers extended its application to cover a range of biochemistry analytes. Initially the instruments were aimed primarily at the near-patient market, but larger instruments suitable for routine use (the Vitros series) have become quite widely used in large (human) hospital laboratories. As the name implies, these instruments measure *reflected* rather than transmitted light, sensing the colour change of a wet pad of originally solid-state reagents when sample is added. The actual measurement is performed by an *Ulbricht sphere* (Fig. 18.11). The mathematical principle of operation is not the Beer–Lambert law but the *Kubelka–Munk function*

$$f(R_\infty) = \frac{\varepsilon C}{S}$$

where S is the scattering coefficient.

The differing mathematics have some practical implications:

(1)   The useful K–M curve goes on longer, which potentially reduces the requirement for diluting the sample to keep the readings on the usable range (although the function is not, in fact, linear and must be linearized by mathematical transformation within the machine).

(2)   The slope of the K–M curve is shallower, which means that with identical precision in the measuring instruments the error in reflectance photometry is about twice that of transmission/absorbance photometry. This means that more precise instrumentation is needed to keep the inherent error of the methods down to acceptable levels.

(3)   The wavelengths of light involved in reflectance are quite different from those used in transmission/absorbance measurements, which has the

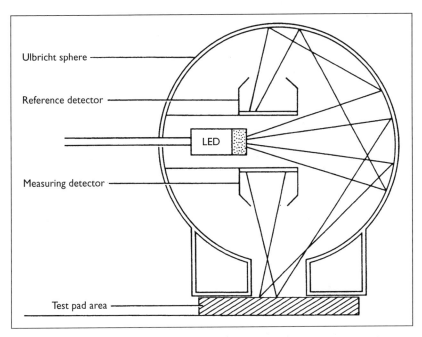

Fig. 18.11 Simplified scheme of the operation of the Ulbricht sphere used in reflectance photometers.

practical advantage of moving the measurement wavelengths well away from those of potential interfering substances such as haemoglobin in most cases.

Apart from these mathematical differences, the general principles of end-point and kinetic methods are fairly similar to those outlined for transmission/absorbance methods. Calibration, however, is generally a two-point process using genuine or simulated plasma-based calibrators, as the physical properties of the sample have some significant effects in the solid phase. This is the source of the problems with the 'plasma matrix effect' which creates difficulties with many dry reagent methods for non-human samples.

Even the early reflectance photometers were conceived from the start with the lay operator in mind, the aim being to allow them to be used on the ward by nursing staff. The concept of the 'black box' (blood in – numbers out with little or no opportunity for operator intervention or error, and no necessity for the operator to understand what they were doing) was much discussed. The much greater user-friendliness of these instruments compared with the relatively cumbersome nature of the wet chemistry analysers available at the time encouraged their adoption in veterinary practices in spite of the (not well publicized) problems with non-human plasma. However, a realization of their limitations has encouraged manufacturers to apply the same principles to the design of wet chemistry instruments for lay operation, and in veterinary terms dry reagent technology is best confined to glucose and urea measurement.

Appendix III: Use of automatic pipettes

Automatic pipettes are greatly to be preferred for clinical laboratory work for a number of reasons: they are much quicker and easier to use than glass pipettes; they are more accurate at small volumes; they do not involve any suction by mouth (which can be dangerous); and the disposable tips mean that glassware washing is eliminated. They are quite expensive, but if well cared for will last a lifetime.

Pipettes of this type may be obtained in either single pre-set volumes or (more expensive) variable volume designs. A variable pipette covering 200–1000 µl plus one or two smaller set-volume pipettes are probably the most economical. Models with automatic tip ejection are preferred as they avoid the need to handle contaminated tips. Make sure you buy good quality tips which fit your pipettes properly, and *always* throw away the used tip between samples or solutions (used tips may be washed, but this is usually uneconomically laborious).

In these pipettes the plunger has two 'stops', the first of which defines the measured volume while the second provides an added push to spit out the last drop from the tip. There are two possible ways of operating them.

Direct pipetting (see Fig. 18.12a)

(1) Fit a fresh tip to pipette.
(2) Depress plunger to first stop.
(3) Immerse end of tip in fluid to be pipetted.
(4) Release plunger gently, avoiding turbulence.
(5) Wipe excess fluid from outside of tip with a tissue (take care not to touch the end of the tip, or you will blot away some of the contents).
(6) Touch end of tip to the inside of the vessel you are pipetting into.
(7) Depress plunger gently to first stop then continue sharply until it is fully depressed to the second stop.
(8) Discard tip.

This is the method usually described in instruction booklets, but it often results in under-delivery of more viscous fluids such as equine plasma.

Reverse pipetting (see Fig. 18.12b)

(1) Fit a fresh tip to pipette.
(2) Depress plunger all the way to the second stop.
(3) Immerse end of tip in fluid to be pipetted.
(4) Release plunger gently, avoiding turbulence (if fluid travels far enough up the tip to touch the pipette itself, this method should not be used).
(5) Wipe excess fluid from outside of tip with a tissue, taking care not to touch the end.

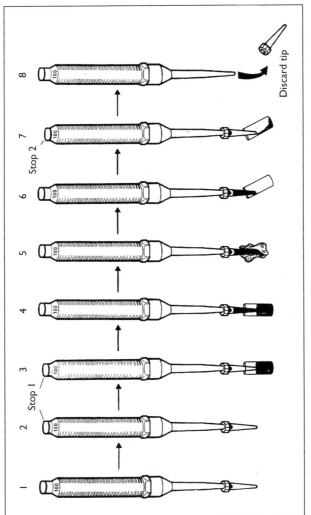

Fig. 18.12(a)   Stages of direct pipetting using a standard two-stop automatic pipette.

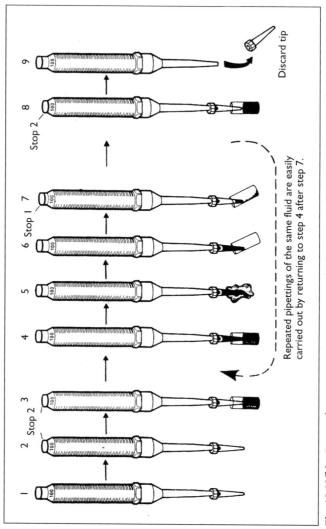

Fig. 18.12(b)   Stages of reverse pipetting using a standard two-stop automatic pipette.

(6)   Touch end of tip to the inside of the vessel you are pipetting into.

(7)   Depress plunger gently to the first stop.

(8)   Return pipette to original container of fluid and depress plunger fully to the second stop to replace excess.

(9)   Discard tip.

This method ensures full delivery of viscous samples and is inherently more precise than the direct method. It is also much easier on the fingers when repeat aliquots of the same fluid have to be pipetted (you simply go up and down to the first stop for each aliquot). However, it is not suitable where there is insufficient extra dead space in the tip to take the excess fluid.

Note that in neither of these methods is the tip rinsed out – the volumes set are *delivery* volumes.

Suggested Further Reading

Major reference works

Feldman, B. F., Zinkl, J. G. & Jain, N. C. (2000) *Schalm's Veterinary Haematology*, 5th edn. Lippincott, Williams and Wilkins, Philadelphia. ISBN 0683306928

Kaneko, J. J., Bruss, M. L. & Harvey, J. W. (1997) *Clinical Biochemistry of Domestic Animals*, 5th edn. Academic Press, New York. ISBN 0123963052

Other veterinary textbooks

Bellamy, J. E. C. & Olexson, D. W. (2000) *Quality Assurance Handbook for Veterinary Laboratories*. Iowa State University Press, Ames. ISBN 0813802768

Bush, B. M. (1991) *Interpretation of Laboratory Results for Small Animal Clinicians*. Blackwell Science, Oxford. ISBN 0632032596

Cowell, R. L. (1998) *Diagnostic Cytology of the Dog and Cat*, 2nd edn. Mosby, St Louis. ISBN 081510362X

Fudge, A. M. (2000) *Laboratory Medicine: Avian and Exotic Pets*. W. B. Saunders, Philadelphia. ISBN 0721676790

Harvey, J. W. (2001) *Atlas of Veterinary Haematology*. W. B. Saunders, Philadelphia. ISBN 0721663346

Jain, N. C. (1993) *Essentials of Veterinary Haematology*. Lea and Febiger, Philadelphia. ISBN 081211437X

Michell, A. R. (1988) *Renal Disease in Dogs and Cats: Comparative and Clinical Aspects*. Blackwell Science, Oxford. ISBN 0632018186

Schalm, O. W. (1980) *Manual of Feline and Canine Haematology*. Veterinary Practice Publishing Company, Santa Barbara. (This book, which contains an extremely good collection of colour plates, is sadly out of print, but library copies may be consulted.)

To avoid confusion, it is important to keep a table of conversion factors to SI units to hand when consulting US texts which use non-SI units.

Relevant books relating to human medicine

Hoffbrand, A. V. & Pettit, J. E. (1992) *Essential Haematology*, 3rd edn. Blackwell Science, Oxford. ISBN 0632019549

Mayne, P. D. (1994) *Clinical Chemistry in Diagnosis and Treatment*, 6th edn. Arnold, London. ISBN 0340576472

Piccoli, G., Varese, D. & Rotunno, M. (1984) *Atlas of Urinary Sediments: Diagnosis and Clinical Correlations in Nephrology*. Raven Press, New York. ISBN 0890005070

Smith, A. F., Beckett, G. J., Walker, S. W. & Rae, P. W. H. (1998) *Lecture Notes on Clinical Biochemistry*, 6th edn. Blackwell Science, Oxford. ISBN 0632048344

It is unwise to adopt procedures and recommendations from human medicine without checking on their applicability to veterinary species; nevertheless, it is advantageous to acquire some familiarity with the field. These human texts have the advantage over major veterinary reference works of being UK publications, thus using more familiar language and SI units. They are aimed at the medical undergraduate/house physician, and contain some very practical common sense.

Index